WITHDRAWN
University of
Illinois Library
at Urbana-Champaign

The Molecular Virology and Epidemiology of Influenza

The sixth of a series of occasional colloquia on aspects of infection which are of current concern to clinicians and scientists.

National Institute for Biological Standards and Control
21st–23rd September 1983

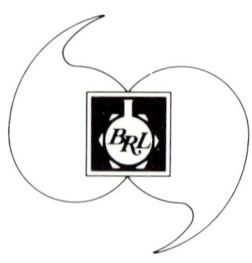

ACADEMIC PRESS INC. (LONDON) LTD.
24/28 Oval Road,
London NW1

United States Edition published by
ACADEMIC PRESS INC.
(Harcourt Brace Jovanovich, Inc.)
Orlando, Florida 32837

Copyright © 1984 by
ACADEMIC PRESS INC. (LONDON) LTD.

All Rights Reserved
No part of this book may be reproduced in any form by photostat, microfilm, or any other means, without permission from the publishers

British Library Cataloguing in Publication Data

The Molecular virology and epidemiology of influenza.
1. Influenza viruses
I. Stuart-Harris, Sir Charles H.
II. Potter, C.W.
616.2′030194   QR201.I6

ISBN 0-12-674740-7

Printed in Great Britain at the Alden Press, Oxford

The Molecular Virology and Epidemiology of Influenza

Editors

SIR CHARLES H. STUART-HARRIS

Emeritus Professor of Medicine
University of Sheffield

C. W. POTTER

Department of Virology
University of Sheffield Medical School
Sheffield

1984

ACADEMIC PRESS
(Harcourt Brace Jovanovich, Publishers)
London   Orlando   San Diego   San Francisco   New York
Toronto   Montreal   Sydney   Tokyo   São Paulo

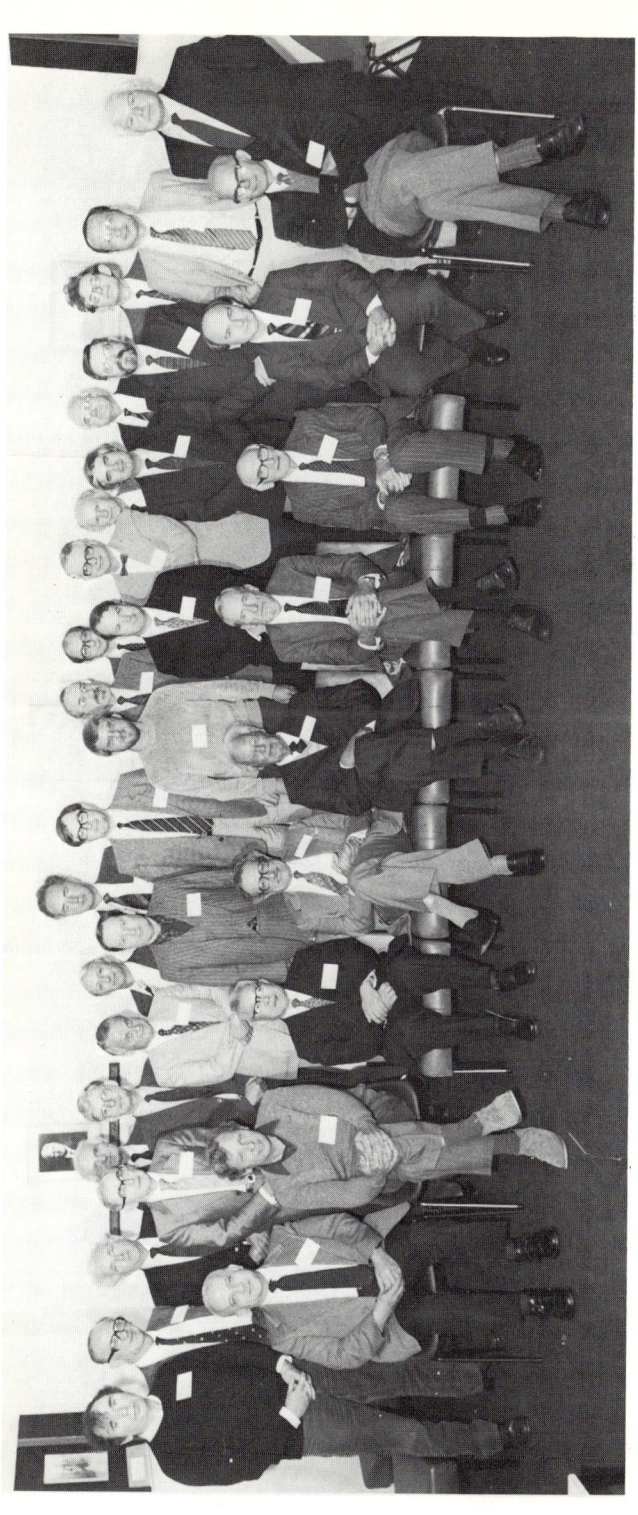

Back Row: H. Smith, A. Percival, H.P. Lambert, J.W.G. Smith, J.D. Williams, H.-D. Klenk, K.F. Shortridge, R.B. Couch, A.P. Kendal, R. M. Chanock, R.G. Webster, D.A.J. Tyrrell, G.G. Brownlee.

Middle Row: J.J. Skehel, F.W. O'Grady, C. Scholtissek, W.P. Glezen, G.W. Both, B.R. Murphy, B.W.J. Mahy, W. Fiers, P. Palese, G.C. Schild.

Sitting: H.F. Maassab, W.G. Laver, C.M. Chu, F. Assaad, Sir Christopher Andrewes, E.D. Kilbourne, Sir Charles Stuart-Harris, W.R. Dowdle, C.W. Potter.

Frontispiece: Participants

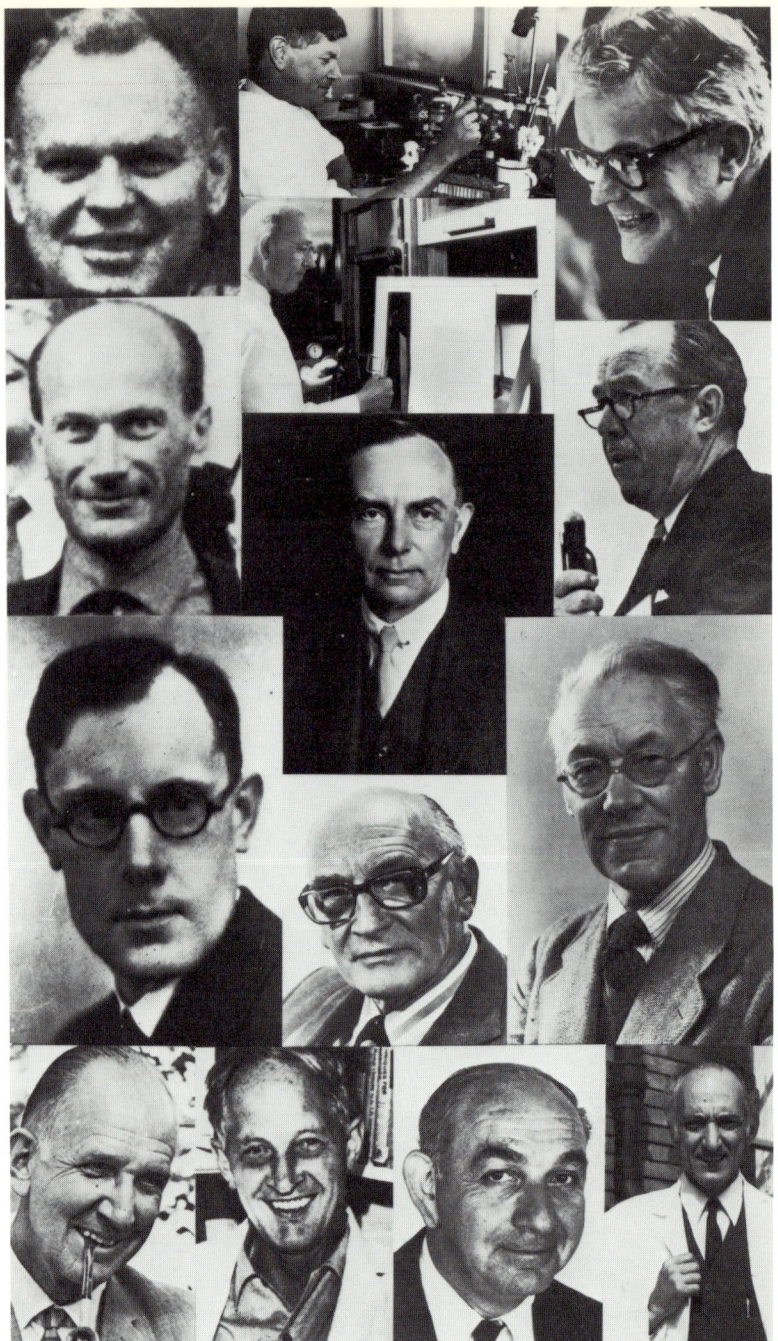

Pioneers

Top row: F.M. Davenport, F.M. Burnet (upper), A. Gottschalk (lower), G.K. Hirst.
Second row: S. Fazekasde St Groth, P.P. Laidlaw, T. Francis.
Third row: Wilson Smith, C.H. Stuart-Harris, C.H. Andrewes.
Bottom row: R.E. Shope, W. Schäfer, M.M. Kaplan, H.G. Pereira.

Preface

When the subject of this Sixth Beecham Colloquium on Aspects of Infection was first discussed, it was suggested that there were at least two ways in which influenza could be an appropriate topic in our series of studies. The first and most obvious was to seek a way of picking-up the thread of molecular virology in influenza work, or secondly, to deal more widely with the problem of influenza. Always at the back of our minds was the fact that 1983 would celebrate the jubilee of influenza research just 50 years after the paper by Smith, Andrewes and Laidlaw in the *Lancet* recording the success which crowned their efforts with the ferret.

Molecular virology is a difficult subject. Structure has always been a matter of opinion in the development of knowledge of the behaviour of viruses. Prior to the birth of new information, arising from the application of *E. coli* to the growth of haemagglutinin, the study of H1, H2 and H3 among the influenza virus A strains seemed to be irreproachable. Suddenly, however, there was an abundance of new material, freed from its host and available for all. Although we are still lacking vision in knowing what to do about it one obvious way was to see how H1 varied from H2—and this work brought about the analysis of the computer without which no one nowadays can move. Now that we can tackle the structure of large molecules by X-ray three-dimensional crystallography there is much new information on the location of antigens to be obtained—and this has been started. So the science of molecular virology in relation to influenza has seemed to flow on at a truly remarkable speed.

Meanwhile, the older method of realising that epidemics were occurring and then working to prevent them, had received a blow from a different direction. In 1977 there appeared the first return of the H1N1 virus—the A/USSR/77 virus. Quickly we all began to be aware of the new-old virus recirculating along the lines of its first appearance, or so it seemed until the handicap of an age-restriction was realized. Since then everything, epidemiologically speaking, has been different. The virus of the new generation is apparently milder than its precursor and influenza epidemics of this sort do not kill. Still the H3N2 viruses are about and breathlessly a watch is kept on the entire picture. So this new phenomenon, which may be merely what has been occurring before, of two viruses instead of one, is following along on entirely orthodox lines.

The mixture of these two major topics provided us with the opportunity of drawing the contributors to this volume together for a splendid new attack on a very old problem. It is fitting that the old building, in which the colloquium was held by kind invitation of the Director of the National Institute of Biological Standards and Control, Dr J. W. G. Smith, was once the home of the National Institute of Medical Research, where Smith, Andrewes and Laidlaw carried out their fundamental work.

March 1984
Sheffield

SIR CHARLES STUART-HARRIS

List of Participants

C. Andrewes, "Overchalke", Coombe Bissett, Wilts SP5 4LS, UK
F. Assaad, Division of Communicable Diseases, World Health Organization, 1211 Geneva-27, Switzerland
G. W. Both, Senior Research Scientist, CSIRO, Genetics Research Laboratories, P.O. Box 184, North Ryde, NSW 2113, Australia
Professor G. G. Brownlee, Sir William Dunn School of Pathology, South Parks Road, Oxford OX1 3RE, UK
R. M. Chanock, National Institute for Allergy and Infectious Diseases, Building 7, National Institutes of Health, Bethesda, Md. 20205, USA
C. M. Chu, Institute of Virology, Chinese Academy of Medical Sciences, 100 Yiug Xiug Jie, Xuan Wu Qu, Beijing, 100052, China
R. B. Couch, Department of Microbiology and Immunology, Baylor College of Medicine, Texas Medical Center, Houston, Texas 77030, USA
W. R. Dowdle, Director, Center for Infectious Diseases, Department of Health and Human Services, Atlanta, Georgia 30333, USA
W. Fiers, Laboratory for Molecular Biology, State University of Ghent, Ledeganckstraat 35, B-9000 Ghent, Belgium
W. P. Glezen, Department of Microbiology and Pediatrics, Baylor College of Medicine, Texas Medical Center, Houston, Texas 77030, USA
A. P. Kendal, Chief, Influenza Branch, Division of Viral Diseases, Center for Infectious Diseases, Department of Health and Human Services, Atlanta, Georgia 30333, USA
H.-D. Klenk, Institut für Virologie, der Justus-Liebig-Universitat Giessen, 6300 Giessen, Federal Republic of Germany
E. D. Kilbourne, Department of Microbiology, The Mount Sinai Medical Center, One Gustave L. Levy Place, New York, New York 10029, USA
H. P. Lambert, Consultant Physician, St. George's Hospital, Blackshaw Road, Tooting, London SW17 0QT, UK
W. G. Laver, Microbiology Department, The John Curtin School of Medical Research, P.O. Box 334, Canberra City, ACT 2601, Australia
H. F. Maassab, The University of Michigan, School of Public Health, Department of Epidemiology, 109 Observatory Street, Ann Arbor, Michigan 48109, USA
B. W. J. Mahy, Division of Virology, Laboratories Block, Addenbrooke's Hospital, Hills Road, Cambridge CB2 2QQ, UK

LIST OF PARTICIPANTS

B. R. Murphy, National Institute of Allergy and Infectious Diseases, Department of Health and Human Services, National Institutes of Health, Bethesda, Maryland 20205, USA

F. W. O'Grady, Department of Microbiology, University Hospital, Queen's Medical Centre, Clifton Boulevard, Nottingham NG7 2UH, UK

P. Palese, Department of Microbiology, The Mount Sinai Medical Center, One Gustave L. Levy Place, New York, New York 10029, USA

A. Percival, Department of Bacteriology and Virology, University of Manchester Medical School (Stopford Building), Oxford Road, Manchester M13 9PT, UK

C. W. Potter, University of Sheffield Medical School, Department of Virology, Beech Hill Road, Sheffield S10 2RX, UK

G. C. Schild, National Institute for Biological Standards and Control, Holly Hill, Hampstead, London NW3 6RB, UK

C. Scholtissek, Institut für Virologie, der Justus-Liebig, Universitat Giessen, 6300 Giessen, Federal Republic of Germany

K. F. Shortridge, Department of Microbiology, Pathology Building, Queen Mary Hospital Compound, Hong Kong

J. J. Skehel, World Influenza Centre, National Institute for Medical Research, Mill Hill, London NW7 1AA, UK

H. Smith, Department of Microbiology, South West Campus, The University of Birmingham, P.O. Box 363, Birmingham B15 2TT, UK

J. W. G. Smith, Director, National Institute for Biological Standards and Control, Holly Hill, Hampstead, London NW3 6RB, UK

C. H. Stuart-Harris, Department of Virology, University of Sheffield Medical School, Beech Hill Road, Sheffield S10 2RX, UK

D. A. J. Tyrrell, M.R.C. Common Cold Unit, Harvard Hospital, Coombe Road, Salisbury, Wilts SP2 8BW, UK

R. G. Webster, St. Jude Children's Research Hospital, 332 North Lauderdale, P.O. Box 318, Memphis, Tennessee 38101, USA

J. D. Williams, Department of Medical Microbiology, The London Hospital Medical College, Turner Street, London E1 2AD, UK

ORGANIZING COMMITTEE

Chairman—Sir Charles Stuart-Harris, CBE

Professor H. P. Lambert

Professor F. W. O'Grady

Professor A. Percival

Dr G. C. Schild

Professor J. D. Williams

Contents

Preface   vii

List of Participants   ix

Influenza A in Ferrets, Mice and Pigs   1
SIR CHRISTOPHER ANDREWES

Influenza—World Experience   5
F. ASSAAD, T. BEKTIMOROV and K. LJUNGARS ESTEVES

Epidemics and their Causative Viruses—Community Experience   17
W. P. GLEZEN, H. R. SIX, D. M. PERROTTA, M. DECKER and W. JOSEPH

Pandemics and Animal Influenza Viruses   39
R. G. WEBSTER, V. S. HINSHAW, C. W. NAEVE and W. J. BEAN

Studies on the Haemagglutinin 61

J. J. SKEHEL, R. S. DANIELS, A. R. DOUGLAS,
M. WANG, M. KNOSSOW, I. A. WILSON and
D. C. WILEY

Influenza Virus Neuraminidase: Structure and Variation 77

W. G. LAVER, P. M. COLMAN, C. W. WARD,
J. M. VARGHESE, G. M. AIR, R. G. WEBSTER,
V. S. HINSHAW, L. BROWN and D. JACKSON

Structure, Genetics and Role of Non-glycosylated Proteins 101

C. SCHOLTISSEK

Immunological Reactions and Resistance to Infection with
Influenza Virus 119

R. B. COUCH, J. A. KASEL, H. R. SIX, T. R. CATE and
J. M. ZAHRADNIK

Cellular Immune Responses to Influenza Antigens—A Brief
Review 153

G. C. SCHILD

Evidence for Host Cell Selection of Antigenic Variants of
Influenza A(H1N1) and B Virus 163

G. C. SCHILD, J. S. OXFORD and R. G. WEBSTER

Pathogenesis of Influenza Virus Infection in Ferrets, a
Model for Human Influenza 175

H. SMITH and C. SWEET

The Role of the Haemagglutinin as a Determinant for the
Pathogenicity of Avian Influenza Virus   195

HANS-DIETER KLENK, W. GARTEN, F. X. BOSCH
and R. ROTT

The Basis of Attenuation of Virulence of Influenza Virus for
Man   211

B. R. MURPHY, M. L. CLEMENTS, H. F. MAASSAB,
A. J. BUCKLER-WHITE, S-F TIAN, W. T. LONDON
and R. M. CHANOCK

Prospects for Stabilization of Attenuation   237

R. M. CHANOCK, B. R. MURPHY, C-J LAI,
L. J. MARKOFF and B-C LIN

Molecular Determination of the Epidemiology of
Influenza—A Reconciliation of Approaches   257

E. D. KILBOURNE

Outlook for the Control of Influenza   269

D. A. J. TYRRELL

Subject Index   303

Influenza A in Ferrets, Mice and Pigs

SIR CHRISTOPHER ANDREWES

When I cast my mind back 50 years, I think first of all of an episode in late January in a room, my laboratory, two floors up in this building, when Wilson Smith and I were working out a strategy for tackling the influenza problem. Whilst we were doing this, my temperature went up and I began to have the first symptoms of 'flu. So Wilson Smith washed out my throat and took the proceeds to put into a variety of experimental animals by a variety of routes and I went home to bed. As you know, it turned out that the ferrets were susceptible to the disease and, when I came back a few days later, the first ferret was sneezing.

But then we ran into trouble because our stock of normal ferrets had got infected with distemper and for some little while we did not know where we were with a mixture of 'flu and distemper in the animals. Fortunately, early in March at a time when the epidemic in the general population had stopped, Wilson Smith got the 'flu and there was good reason to believe that he had got it from a ferret. In fact, what we had done was very cleverly to clean the virus up by passing it through Wilson Smith who was not susceptible to distemper.

Things went happily ahead after that and, if we look a few weeks ahead, we see Wilson Smith, P. P. Laidlaw and myself meeting every morning at Mill Hill at what were then the Medical Research Council's farm laboratories. We would put on rubber coats and wellingtons and make clinical rounds on

"The Molecular Virology and Epidemiology of Influenza" (Eds Sir Charles Stuart-Harris and Professor C.W. Potter). Academic Press, London, New York and Orlando, 1984.

our ferret isolation hospital. We would wade through a shallow tray of Lysol and be swabbed down with Lysol and then go and see the first ferret. He would have his rectal temperature taken and we would make notes as to his general liveliness, nasal discharge and sneezing, and then we would be swabbed down again with more Lysol and go on to the next ferret. After we had completed our rounds we would go back to the laboratory, perhaps with one ferret to be killed to pass on to more animals or for other experiments.

On one such occasion, I had prepared some material for the experiment and there was some surplus so, in an optimistic spirit, I injected that into a number of mice. A few days later some of them had lung consolidation and thereafter we had a more convenient animal for further work.

I had for some time been friendly with Dick Shope. We had told him about our ferret results and he had found that swine 'flu also would go in ferrets, so I now passed on the glad tidings about the mice and he passed the news on to Dr Thomas Francis who was then working on human influenza at the Rockefeller Laboratories in New York. This caused considerable embarrassment because he had just found out independently that mice were susceptible and he was under pressure to publish his results quickly before we could publish ours. But, of course, Dr Francis was having none of that and the upshot was that, a few days later, we had a cable from New York urging us to publish our results quickly so as to clear the air, and this we did.

Dick Shope's contribution to knowledge about influenza was very considerable, quite apart from his discovery of the swine influenza virus. He had described, and repeatedly emphasized, how outbreaks of swine influenza could occur simultaneously in a number of farms some distance from each other and with no communication between one and another. He deduced that the virus had somehow been seeded in those herds and then was activated by some stimulus, probably meteorological. He further held the view, which was quite unorthodox at that time, that the same sort of thing might apply to influenza in man. Shope's belief that swine lung worm was the key to the mystery has not gained general acceptance, but even if we leave that on one side his contribution to our knowledge about influenza was considerable.

It is very easy to be an armchair virologist and think up experiments for other people to do, and it is generally a waste of time! So it is with considerable hesitation that I suggest the slogan "Back to the pig". We very badly want to know for certain that influenza can be latent in a population, we want to know how it manages to do this, where it is hiding and in what form. We cannot easily look in human beings for virus, or part of it, in every part of the respiratory tract from the nose to the deepest alveolus, but it could be done in a pig—and you need not waste the rest of the pig either! It would, of course, have to be a pig from a herd which was known to have periodical outbreaks of influenza and it would have to be done in between outbreaks. I find it hard to believe that all the modern techniques of biochemistry and of molecular biology will forever fail to detect the virus, or part of it, if it is there. If we can find out what it is doing and how, we shall be a great deal further on. We might find out more about what is the stimulus which converts a latent virus into an active disease-provoking one. We might find out whether or not this provocation, as Shope used to call it, converts the carrier into a diseased animal or whether, as Hope Simpson suggests for man, it makes the carrier, whilst still free from symptoms, into a profuse shedder of virus to infect his friends and relations.

Knowledge of all this might tell us more about how an outbreak of influenza starts. In my belief, the influenza virus does not have it all its own way. We know that for some years in the last century 'flu was apparently absent from the scene, and in this century during the last few years it has not been able to do very much, so the virus is vulnerable and that, I feel, is our chance.

Influenza—World Experience

F. ASSAAD, T. BEKTIMIROV and K. LJUNGARS-ESTEVES

Division of Communicable Diseases, World Health Organization, Geneva, Switzerland

INTRODUCTION

Influenza is a problem that has always aroused the interest of scientists and laymen alike because of its capricious behaviour and the failure so far to control the disease.

Of the three influenza viruses, A, B and C, only virus A has the potential to cause pandemics. It is associated with high morbidity and mortality, and occurs in man, animals and birds, and it is the virus that attracts most attention. Influenza B is associated every now and then with epidemics of high morbidity and mortality. Influenza C causes sporadic disease, is rarely recognized, and has attracted very little attention.

INFLUENZA A

Influenza A has a unique characteristic which makes it stand out: it has the

"The Molecular Virology and Epidemiology of Influenza" (Eds Sir Charles Stuart-Harris and Professor C.W. Potter). Academic Press, London, New York and Orlando, 1984.

ability to cause widespread outbreaks and epidemics and has no respect for frontiers, spreading from one country to another, affecting people of all ages.

The Human Disease

The severity of influenza varies considerably. Young, otherwise healthy, adults experience relatively mild symptoms after the first 24 hours of illness in bed, but seven to ten days may elapse before they are able to return to work. This means seven to ten days of manpower lost and in an influenza outbreak 30% or more of the labour force may be affected by the disease at the same time.

The principal characteristic of influenza in those with a previous history of chest or heart disease is the likelihood of pulmonary complications, and deaths from influenza are largely encountered in those with chronic disease. In the aged the degree of illness is increased and death may occur relatively suddenly with few warning signs. This damaging effect on the older members of the community, in particular those with pre-existing chronic disease, has led to the use of "excess" mortality in depicting influenza activity. The observed number of deaths during winter is compared to an expected mortality curve (constructed on a mathematical model). Excess mortality indicates an influenza outbreak and the degree of excess corresponds to the severity of the outbreak (Assaad *et al.*, 1973). No other disease causes such a dramatic increase in deaths in winter. This demonstrates one of the enigmas of influenza, i.e. the seasonal reappearance after having completely disappeared during the summer. Epidemics may disappear for one or more years but, after a short respite, they have always recurred.

THE HISTORICAL BACKGROUND

The early history of influenza cannot be established with any certainty. For at least the past 400 years epidemics of illnesses with shivering, cough, aching pains and sweating suggestive of influenza have been recorded in many countries. One can read of widespread illness in Queen Mary's court in the sixteenth century, of thousands falling ill in certain towns in the seventeenth century, and the well-documented epidemic of 1732 which was recorded in Paris in February, in Naples in March, spreading throughout Europe and to America, where it began in New England and spread southwards to the Caribbean, Mexico and Peru. Major outbreaks probably occurred in 1781–2, 1800–2, 1830–3, 1847–8 and 1857–8. In 1889 the first so-called Asiatic influenza pandemic was heralded in Bukhara in the USSR and swept all over the world with high morbidity and mortality. Eleven years later, in 1900, another epidemic became rife throughout Europe. By the time of the 1889–90 pandemic most doctors had accepted the germ theory and research workers tried very hard to find a bacterium as the cause. This they did, and called it Pfeiffer's influenza bacillus. In 1918, in the wake of the First World War, the great Spanish influenza pandemic came causing very high mortality and tremendous social and economic disruption. By 1918 it was known that some diseases were caused by microbes smaller than bacteria, the "filtrable viruses" (Beveridge, 1977). Nevertheless, it was Shope in 1931 who first isolated the influenza virus from swine before it had been demonstrated in man. This had to wait until Sir Christopher Andrewes and his team isolated the influenza virus in man in 1933. Since then, the amount of information that has been accumulated about the virus is considerable, but the behaviour of the virus remains bewildering and many gaps remain to be filled on the actual epidemiology of the disease.

The accounts of a Florentine family in the fourteenth and fifteenth centuries used the word "influence" to suggest an unusual conjunction of planets at times of epidemics of coughs, colds and fever. The word "influenza" was thus derived as a descriptive name for the epidemics due to "influences". Thomas Willis in 1658 said that the outbreaks occurred "as if sent by some blast of the stars" (Stuart-Harris and Schild, 1976). Science has since made huge strides forward but influenza still has a science fiction flavour about it. In 1978 Hoyle and Wickramasinghe wrote that the virus was formed in the galaxy and that it could be carried in meteoritic dust that would hit the earth as it crossed the debris of a new long-period comet.

In 1978 Hope-Simpson linked the appearance of new influenza virus subtypes with peaks in sunspot activity. More "celestial" hypotheses will undoubtedly be put forward until the detailed information on the virus which has been accumulated can explain its behaviour.

In a rather different sphere of endeavour, namely molecular virology, double-stranded DNA copies of the RNA gene coding for the haemagglutinin glycoproteins from human H2 and H3 pandemic strains of influenza virus have been cloned. DNA sequence analysis has provided the nucleotide sequence of an H2 and an H3 haemagglutinin. Comparison of the amino acid sequences of these haemagglutinins is revealing the extent of sequence changes in antigenic shifts and drifts (Gething *et al.*, 1980).

Pandemic Periodicity

In this last half of the century the decennial (actually 11-year) periodicity of pandemics has been striking: 1946, 1957 and 1968. Since 1968, i.e. over the last 15 years, the Hong Kong family of influenza A has been prevalent. Only two clear-cut pandemics occurred early in the century, in 1900 and 1918. "Serological archeology" can detect the footprints of earlier viruses by antibody studies in older people. Thus our backward reach is limited by the human lifespan and takes us only to the 1880s. The method is further limited because it identifies only antibody to those antigenic determinants of the surface antigens we use as our probes.

However, this approach has given us an intriguing glimpse of the past and suggests that H antigens of the Asian or 1957 virus circulated in 1889, and that the Hong Kong virus had its antecedent in 1900. However, to complicate the picture further, antibodies against A/equine/2 influenza virus H antigen (which is cross-related to the H3 of the Hong Kong virus), as well as antibodies to the Hong Kong virus, were demonstrable in the sera of older people exposed to the epidemic of 1900. It is interesting to note that the antibody to the neuraminidase antigen detected in these sera reacts with the equine and not the Hong Kong neuraminidase, indicating that the virus of the 1900 pandemic was certainly not identical to the present Hong Kong subtype. In 1929 a substantial increase in mortality probably marked the replacement of swine influenza with the H1N1 subtype. These observations have suggested a periodic recycling of influenza virus major antigens every 70 years or so (Kilbourne, 1977).

CIRCULATION OF THE INFLUENZA VIRUSES IN THE COMMUNITY

Since 1977, two novel events have marked the epidemiology of influenza and have shattered two previously-held concepts (Ennis, 1978).

In 1977 strains of the influenza A subtype H1N1, i.e. possessing the antigens of the viruses that caused epidemics in humans from 1946–57, returned after an absence of 20 years from man, and spread widely throughout the world.*

When an influenza A virus which bears haemagglutinin (H) and possibly also neuraminidase (N) surface antigens serologically distant from those of former human viruses, it has been commonly accepted that widespread epidemics or a pandemic would ensue. The effect of dual change is exemplified by events in 1957 when the Asian virus bearing H2N2 surface antigens not previously recognized among human influenza A viruses replaced the viruses of H1N1 antigen subtype. Following this was the

* The reappearance of the swine influenza virus in 1976 in a military camp in New Jersey, United States of America was short-lived. The virus failed to spread beyond the limits of the camp.

largest influenza pandemic recorded since the 1930s. The 1968 pandemic was caused by the Hong Kong virus in which a change was noted only in the H antigen, the neuraminidase remaining as it was during the Asian decade.

The arrival of the variant A/England/42/72, first isolated towards the end of the A/Hong Kong outbreak in 1972, caused sharp outbreaks which surprised everyone, as there was only a slight degree of drift of the H3 antigen from the prototype Hong Kong virus. Nevertheless, it was the cause of large epidemics in the 1972–3 season. As expected, the variant virus A/Victoria, which showed a large degree of antigenic variation in the H antigen, caused large outbreaks in the 1975–6 season.

The reappearance of influenza A(H1N1) strains in 1977 did not, however, result in the suppression of H3N2 viruses, except perhaps for a few months in some countries. Another concept of influenza epidemiology to be revised is that within a family of influenza A viruses the latest variant, once established, usually chases away all other members of the family.

Since 1979, there have been at least three members of the A/Hong Kong family circulating at one and the same time. In the 1979–80 season, A/Texas/1/77, A/Bangkok/1/79 and A/Bangkok/2/79 were detected. During the 1980–1 season, a variant which reacted equally well with sera prepared against A/Bangkok/1/79 and A/Texas/1/77 appeared and later became the more prevalent variant without completely replacing the other three. A/Belgium/2/81 was later chosen as a reference for this cross-reacting variant. These four variants were subsequently isolated all over the world and in 1982, a fifth variant, A/Philippines/2/82, further expanded the Hong Kong family. During the 1982–3 influenza season, A/Belgium/2/82-like strains remained the most common, and A/Philippines/2/82 accounted for about one-fifth of all isolates. The three older variants were still encountered, albeit infrequently (Table I).

Also in the H1N1 family there has been some overlap between the different variants circulating. The first one to become prevalent, A/USSR/90/77 is still being isolated, although for some time the second variant to appear, A/Brazil/11/78, seemed to take over completely for a few years. During the last season, 1982–3, the most common variant was A/England/333/80 but another variant, A/India/6263/80 was also isolated, and, as mentioned, A/USSR/90/77 in one or two countries (Table II).

INFLUENZA B

The first influenza B strains were isolated in 1940 during a moderate epidemic in New York. Influenza B virus seems to progress by causing localized outbreaks chiefly in school-children and sporadic cases in adults.

TABLE I
Variants of influenza A(H3N2) virus prevalent in the world, 1968–83

	1968	1969	1970	1971	1972	1973	1974	1975	1976	1977	1978	1979	1980	1981	1982	1983
A/Hong Kong/1/68	——	——	——	——												
A/England/42/72					——	——										
A/Port Chalmers/1/73						——	——									
A/Scotland/840/74							——	——								
A/Victoria/3/75								——	——							
A/Texas/1/77										——	——	——				
A/Bangkok/1/79												——	——	——		
A/Bangkok/2/79												——	——	——		
A/Belgium/2/81														——	——	
A/Philippines/2/82															——	——

TABLE II
Variants of influenza A(H1N1) virus prevalent in the world, 1977–83

	1977	1978	1979	1980	1981	1982	1983
A/USSR/90/77	———	———	———				
A/Brazil/11/78		———	———	———	———		
A/England/333/80				———	———	———	———
A/India/6263/80				———	———	———	———

But every now and then it causes not only a high morbidity but also high mortality. For example, during the epidemics in 1962 and 1966 the case-fatality rate was as high as in epidemics of similar size due to virus A.

Towards the end of the 1970s the influenza B variant, B/Hong Kong/5/72, was gradually supplanted by new variants, which in the 1978–9 season caused high morbidity and mortality in the upper age groups in a number of countries in Northern Europe. By 1979–80, one of these new variants, B/Singapore/222/79 had become firmly established. It hit the United States of America and Canada during this season and caused considerable illness among all ages and excess mortality among the aged. At this time there was virtually no influenza A in North America. Scotland, which escaped influenza B in 1979, felt the brunt of the epidemic in 1980. Since then, influenza B/Singapore/222/79 has caused widespread outbreaks in parts of Eastern Europe in 1980–1, in Japan, Australia and again in Scotland in 1981–2. It was the main influenza virus isolated in the German Democratic Republic during the season 1982–3 and it followed the wave of influenza A outbreaks in many other European countries.

It is hard to discern the influence of antigenic variations upon the prevalence of influenza B. The viruses isolated during some of the larger outbreaks possess haemagglutinins with distinct variation from the preceding ones and it would seem that influenza B virus variations are progressive with no apparent return of strains showing the antigenic grouping of former years. From an epidemiological standpoint influenza B outbreaks come and go at relatively longer periods of time than influenza A—in a four to six year span. Perhaps the relatively slow antigenic drift of the influenza B virus enables the population to adapt itself to the change. The relative lack of change in the neuraminidase may be a further stabilizing factor.

PREDICTION OF EPIDEMICS/PANDEMICS

There have been attempts, with varying success, to predict epidemics in a given community. The method used is based on the testing of sera from a wide age-range for HI antibody to known variants. The method could be used for short-term predictions of events but does not indicate their future magnitude. It has apparent limitations, not least because it depends on the availability of an antigenic variant before it starts an outbreak.

There has been some belief in one feature of influenza pandemics, i.e. the 11-year periodicity, and in one hypothesis, i.e. the recycling of the influenza A virus. Put together, one could theoretically predict the coming pandemic. In fact this conceptual framework was behind the scare which the swine influenza outbreak in New Jersey aroused: a 1918 pandemic revisiting. What has happened since has shaken the belief in forecasts. It would seem more profitable to keep a close watch on the influenza virus to detect the earliest changes that would sound the alarm. However, it is only through international collaboration that a surveillance system can work, which in turn brings to the fore the coordinating role of the World Health Organization.

WHO Programme

Since its Constitution in 1947, the World Health Organization has been collecting and disseminating information on current influenza A and B viruses and their extent of epidemic/pandemic spread. The WHO programme provides an early warning system for the emergency of new or altered antigenic sub-types, which is the basis for the formulation of the influenza vaccine.

Today, global surveillance of influenza is maintained through the efforts of a network of 108 National Influenza Centres in 76 countries throughout the world. Fifty-two centres are located in 44 developing countries and 56 in 32 industrially developed countries. These centres are designated by national health authorities and form part of the WHO programme by formal recognition by the Organization.

REFERENCES

Assaad, F., Cockburn, W. C. and Sundaresan, T. K. (1973). Use of excess mortality from respiratory diseases in the study of influenza. *Bull. WHO* **49**, 219–233.

Beveridge, W. I. B. (1977). "Influenza: the Last Great Plague. An unfinished Story of Discovery." Heineman, London.

Ennis, F. (1978). Influenza A viruses. Shaking out our shibboleths. *Nature* (Lond.) **274**, 309–310.

Gething, M. J., Bye, J., Skehel, J. and Waterfield, M. (1980). Cloning and DNA sequence of double-stranded copies of haemagglutinin genes from H2 and H3

strains elucidates antigenic shift and drift in human influenza virus. *Nature* (Lond.) **278**, 301–306.
Hope-Simpson, R. E. (1978). Sunspots and flu: a correlation. *Nature* (Lond.) **275**, 86.
Hoyle, F. and Wickramasinghe, C. (1978). "Diseases from Space." Dent, London.
Kilbourne, E. D. (1977). Influenza pandemics in perspective. *J. Am. Med. Assoc.* **237**, 1225–1228.
Stuart-Harris, C. H. and Schild, G. C. (1976). "Influenza. The Viruses and the Disease." Edward Arnold, London.

DISCUSSION

Brownlee I am not an epidemiologist but in Dr Assaad's slide of the recent H1N1 field strains it was shown that the A/USSR/77 was still being isolated in the 1982–3 session.

Assaad It has been isolated in very few countries.

Brownlee Is there a gap in the incidence of A/USSR/77 between 1977 and the present? I thought that the A/USSR was no longer being isolated but there is a continuous line from 1977 through to 1983.

Assaad It all depends on what you mean by a "stop". We have the southern hemisphere and the northern hemisphere. It may have stopped in one hemisphere but not in the other. What do you mean by "stopped"? Do you mean a month or two months? What do you mean exactly?

Brownlee I am really asking you what you mean.

Assaad We simply divide the world into two, as Skehel and Kendal know, as regards the influenza season. For instance, from 1 October to the end of March is one season for the northern hemisphere and this is the relaxed period for the southern hemisphere. If we do not find any isolates during any one season then we can call it a "stop", but not before then.

Brownlee I take it your definition is six months?

Assaad Yes.

Tyrrell May I raise a question on the present status of the work on monitoring animal influenza in relation to human diseases. Martin Kaplan worked on that for many years against many disappointments though now the whole situation has changed. I think it would be good if there could be continued efforts to keep the two areas of study in relation to each other.

Assaad Due to the lateness of the 'bus I had a discussion with Webster on this and he told me that I would be getting within a week or two a big paper on avian/swine—you cannot really call them swine/avian for it is very difficult to know which to put first—in Europe, which he has been carrying out with 15 laboratories and which would show the shifts or drifts in animals. These studies are continuing.

Tyrrell Is the WHO still interested?

Assaad Yes.

Schild You mentioned sub-types. We now know of 13 haemagglutinins and nine neuraminidases and the issue is whether there is a limitless number of sub-types or a finite number. In recent years although intensive surveillance of animal influenza has gone on, particularly in birds which have representatives of all known influenza A sub-types, the number of new sub-types seems to be dwindling; although I think effort is continuing to look for them. Perhaps the situation is not as bad as you might have suggested and there may be a limited number.

Assaad I hope so, but again, we were thinking we would close at 12 until Webster's laboratory brought up the gull business (Hinshaw *et al.*, 1983). So you have 13 haemagglutinins. I agree with you really that if they had been much more frequent we would have picked them up. Shortridge in Hong Kong has been doing this intensively. Dr Chu is here and he has also been doing this extensively. Certainly if there had been many more around we would have picked them up. I hope that is true anyway.

Shortridge With respect to the animal surveillances carried out in Hong Kong there are some haemagglutinin sub-types which we have not encountered. However, there is preliminary serological evidence of human exposure to such viruses.

Assaad Is that 13?

Shortridge They are haemagglutinin sub-types 8 and 13.

Assaad But within the 13?

Shortridge Yes, within that 13, so the possibility does exist that they are around but are not amongst the avian isolates recorded in the surveillance to date. It is all a matter of the level of surveillance, isolation technique and so forth. Indeed, serological evidence suggests human exposure to all 13 sub-types.

Couch Have all 13 sub-types infected humans?

Shortridge We have started a preliminary study of people in the Pearl River Delta and there is a certain amount of evidence that we do have antibodies to all 13 HA sub-types in the human population of the Delta, but not so much in the urban areas. One might infer, therefore, that there are still perhaps some other sub-types around that we have not as yet detected.

Kilbourne One might infer also that there is unsuspected cross-reactivity among haemagglutinin antigens.

Shortridge That cannot be entirely ruled out at this stage.

Kilbourne I would like to add that not only is there the matter of the finite antigens, but—and this really addresses the point you have anticipated—how many haemagglutinin antigens are capable of significantly affecting man, because there may be structural constraints in the haemagglutinin molecule.

Shortridge This is totally unknown territory and I think it will take a long time to unravel that one.

REFERENCE

Hinshaw, V. S., Air, G. M., Schild, G. C. and Newman, R. W. (1983). Characterization of a novel haemagglutinin subtype (H 13) of influenza A virus from gulls. *Bull. WHO* **61**, 677–679.

Epidemics and their Causative Viruses—Community Experience

W. PAUL GLEZEN,[a] H. R. SIX,[a] D. M. PERROTTA,[b] M. DECKER,[b] and S. JOSEPH[c]

[a]Influenza Research Center, Department of Microbiology and Immunology, Baylor College of Medicine, Houston, Texas, [b]School of Public Health, University of Texas Health Science, Houston, [c] McGregor Health Association/Prucare, Houston, Texas, USA

A special programme for surveillance of influenza epidemics and their consequences was initiated in Houston and Harris County, Texas, USA in December, 1974. Surveillance of influenza virus infections has been maintained by culturing specimens from patients presenting to sentinel primary care facilities (Glezen and Couch, 1978; Glezen et al., 1980) and by longitudinal observation of representative families with young children (Taber et al., 1981). The primary care facilities are strategically located throughout the county and serve patients in all socioeconomic and ethnic groups. The physicians are asked to culture all patients presenting with acute respiratory illnesses throughout the year. Complete pediatric care is provided for children in the Houston Family Study. The family members are cultured at the time of each respiratory illness and paired serum

"The Molecular Virology and Epidemiology of Influenza" (Eds Sir Charles Stuart-Harris and Professor C.W. Potter). Academic Press, London, New York and Orlando, 1984.

specimens spanning each respiratory season are tested for significant antibody rise to prevalent influenza viruses.

Houston is located on the coastal plain of Texas about 60 miles from the Gulf of Mexico. The climate is mild and the average wintertime low temperature is 7°C. During the nine years from 1974 to 1983 the population of Harris County increased rapidly from about 2·0 to 2·5 million people largely due to an influx of young adults seeking job opportunities. The 1980 census revealed that 20·7% of the population was in the 25 to 34 year age group and only 6·1% was 65 years or older.

Influenza epidemics have been observed during each respiratory disease season (Fig. 1). Although the intensity of the epidemics has varied, the peak occurrence of respiratory illnesses which cause patients to seek medical care has coincided with the peak of influenza virus activity for each season. The less intense epidemics were not apparent in the community by some of the usual measurements such as increased school absenteeism, employee absenteeism or emergency room visits. For example, school absenteeism did not exceed an average of 8% for any week during the indolent influenza B epidemic of 1979–80 but averaged 12% for four consecutive weeks during the intense epidemic of 1976–7. Despite this, the infection rates for persons observed in the Houston Family Study were not different for the two epidemics suggesting that overall consequences may have been the same but extended over a longer period of time in 1979–80 (Frank et al., 1983).

In Fig. 1 only the predominant virus for each epidemic is indicated but more than one type or sub-type was detected during each season. Table I shows the total number of viruses isolated for each epidemic year and the proportion for each type or sub-type. Infections with influenza A (H3N2) viruses were detected in six of nine seasons and predominated in five. Influenza B viruses produced three epidemics and were detected in each year but 1980–1. Influenza A (H1N1) viruses were active during every season since their re-emergence in early 1978 but were predominant only during 1978–9.

Table II shows the distribution of the major H3N2 variants after the initial epidemic caused A/Port Chalmers/1/73-like viruses in 1974–5. Retrospective analysis of a representative sample of viruses isolated early in 1976 showed that almost 98% were similar to A/Victoria/3/75 but 2.2% carried antigens of the A/Texas/1/77 virus which was isolated in San Antonio one year later (Velazco et al., 1983). During the "herald wave" of 1976–7, 32% of the H3N2 viruses were antigenically related to A/Texas and during the epidemic of 1977–8 viruses with A/Texas antigens produced 70.0% of the infections. The proportions with A/Texas antigens through 1978 include viruses that were "intermediate" between A/Victoria and A/Texas and reacted equally to antisera to the two prototype strains. Our

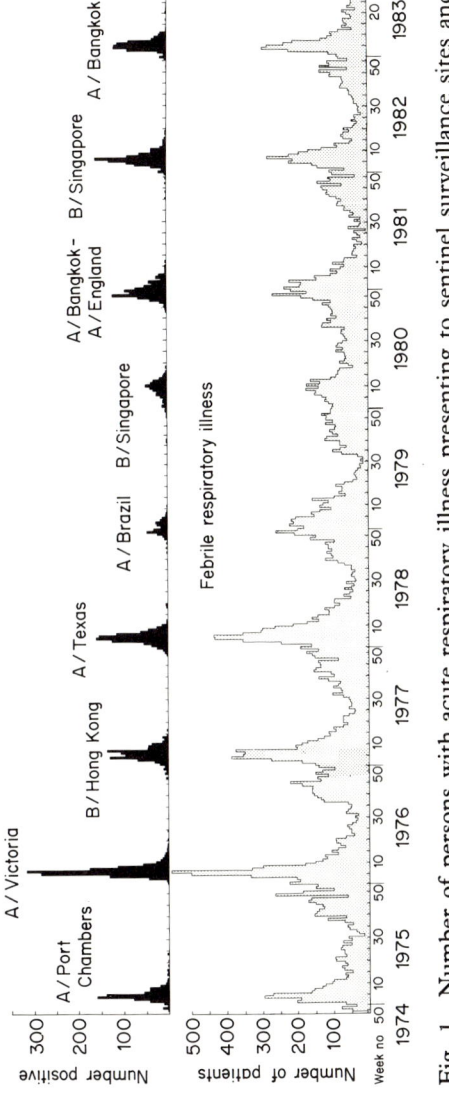

Fig. 1. Number of persons with acute respiratory illness presenting to sentinel surveillance sites and number with positive cultures for influenza viruses by week, Houston, Texas, 1974–83.

TABLE I
Distribution of influenza virus isolates from community surveillance, Houston, 1974–83

Epidemic year	Number of isolates	Percent of each influenza virus type or sub-type		
		A (H3N2)	B	A (H1N1)
1974–5	649	99·8	0·2	0
1975–6	1231	97·2	2·8	0
1976–7	774	6·2	93·8	0
1977–8	822	84·0	0·7	15·3
1978–9	255	0	0·4	99·6
1979–80	348	0	98·3	1·7[a]
1980–1	692	60·1	0	39·9
1981–2	768	0	85·3	14·7
1982–3	689[b]	85·1	4·6	10·3

[a] Includes one swine-like virus. [b] Preliminary estimate from an 80% sample

TABLE II
Distribution of major antigenic variants of sub-type influenza A (H3N2) by year, Houston, 1976–83

Antigenic variant	Percent of H3N2 isolates by year				
	1976 (N=1197)	1976–77 (N=48)	1977–78 (N=690)	1980–81 (N=416)	1982–83 (N=506)
A/Victoria/3/75	97·8	68·0	30·0		
A/Texas/1/77	2·2[a]	32·0[a]	70·0[a]	9·6	5·4
Intermediate strains				47·9[b]	53·6[c]
A/Bangkok/1/79				42·5	30·0
Others[d]					10·9[d]

[a] Includes strains sharing antigens with A/Victoria/3/75; many similar to A/Brazil/53/76 (H3N2). [b] Heterologous group sharing antigens of A/Texas/1/77 and A/Bangkok/1/79; many similar to A/Taiwan/1/79 and A/Arizona/2/80. [c] Heterologous group sharing antigen of A/Bangkok/1/79 and A/Texas/1/77; many similar to A/Oregon/4/80. [d] Includes A/Philippines/2/82 (6·4%), A/Bangkok/2/79 (2·7%) and unclassified (1·8%).

ability to classify H3N2 variants improved during the two recent epidemics by the availability of a battery of monoclonal antibodies raised against A/Texas/1/77 (kindly provided by Dr Robert Webster, Memphis, Tennessee).

After an absence of almost three years, H3N2 viruses reappeared in 1980–1 and, although A/Bangkok/1/79 was the most common single variant, A/Texas-like viruses were present and almost half of the viruses were a heterologous group of intermediate strains that reacted equally by hemagglutination inhibition with ferret antisera against A/Texas/1/77 and A/Bangkok/1/79. Many of the intermediate strains resembled A/Taiwan/1/79 or A/Arizona/2/80 and were antigenically closer to A/Texas than to A/Bangkok. After another two-year hiatus, H3N2 viruses returned in the winter of 1982–3 and, surprisingly, A/Texas-like viruses were again detected. A majority of the viruses again fell into a heterologous group of intermediate strains, but many were antigenically closer to A/Bangkok/1/79 and resembled the A/Oregon/4/80 prototype. Seven viruses similar to the A/Philippines/2/82 strain were detected; these viruses made up one-third of viruses tested during the month of March, 1983 as the epidemic waned. An overlapping progression of antigenic drift has been demonstrated from A/Victoria to A/Texas to A/Bangkok/1/79 and our data would concur with evidence from world-wide surveillance that A/Philippines-like viruses will be the next major H3N2 variant.

The major variants of influenza A (H1N1) have not overlapped in the same manner as the H3N2 variants (Table III). Although viruses like A/Brazil/11/78 were present at the end of the initial A/USSR/92/77 outbreak in early 1978, viruses like A/USSR/77 were not detected in 1978–9

TABLE III
Distribution of major antigenic variants of sub-type influenza A (H1N1) by year, Houston, 1977–83

Antigenic Variant	Percent of H1N1 isolates by year					
	1977–78 (N=126)	1978–79 (N=254)	1979–80 (N=6)	1980–81 (N=276)	1981–82 (N=113)	1982–83 (N=62)
A/USSR/92/77	74.1	0	0	0	0	0
A/Brazil/11/78[a]	8.2	91.7	83.3	0	0	0
A/England/333/80	0	0	0	62.6	82.9	67.0
Other[b]	17.7	8.7	16.7	37.4	17.1	33.0

[a] All of the isolates tested from 1978–9 had 4 internal genes from A/Texas/1/77 (H3N2); none did from 1977–8 and only 2 of 6 from 1979–80. [b] Heterologous groups of viruses none of which has demonstrated epidemic potential to date.

when A/Brazil was the major variant (Six *et al.*, 1983). Only six H1N1 viruses were detected the following year and all were antigenically similar to A/Brazil except for a single swine-like virus. In 1980–1, 107 of 276 H1N1 viruses were tested with the battery of monoclonal antibodies against A/USSR/77 (kindly provided by Dr Robert Webster) and none of the viruses reacted with antibodies produced by clone 110 which inhibited hemagglutination by the A/USSR/77 and A/Brazil/78 viruses. Most of the H1N1 viruses for 1980–1 resembled the A/England/333/80 prototype. Viruses like A/England/333/80 have continued to be active during the past two seasons but the total number of H1N1 infections has decreased by about one-half each succeeding year. A number of other variants have been detected but none have demonstrated epidemic potential thus far.

On three occasions infections with the predominant virus of an epidemic have been detected in appreciable numbers during the latter half of the epidemic of the previous season. This observation suggested that infections with these viruses might have continued to occur throughout the late spring, summer and early autumn at a rate undetectable by our virologic surveillance. During the intervals between the last virus isolation of the "herald wave" and first isolation of the epidemic of the following year (an interval of about six months), no influenza virus was isolated from over 10 000 cultures of patients presenting to surveillance sites and family study members cultured with or without respiratory illnesses (Glezen *et al.*, 1982). In addition, off-season infection could not be confirmed by serologic tests in family study members. Furthermore, reintroduction of the epidemic virus in the autumn is supported by the fact that the A/Brazil/11/78 (H1N1)-like viruses detected in February and March, 1978 contained a full complement of H1N1 genes while those that produced the epidemic during the following season were "recombinants" that included four internal genes from A/Texas/1/77 (H3N2) viruses. Of the six A/Brazil viruses isolated in Houston in early 1980 only the first two which were isolated from siblings were "recombinants" while the four viruses isolated later were not. The more likely explanation of these findings is that viruses carrying the Brazil-like haemagglutinin were being reintroduced into the Houston conurbation at the beginning of each season rather than the possibility that two reassortment events occurred during continuous transmission in Houston in parallel with similar events in other geographic locations (Cox *et al.*, 1983).

CONSEQUENCES OF INFLUENZA EPIDEMICS

Various measurements have been used to assess the consequences of influenza epidemics. Those commonly reported include school and employee absenteeism, emergency room visits, physician reports of clinically-diagnosed "influenza", and determination of excess mortality attributed to pneumonia, influenza and other causes from death certificates. The numbers of cases attributed to influenza are usually those above an arbitrarily designated threshold (Table IV).

These indicators, although usually specific for influenza activity when elevated, are relatively insensitive and underestimate considerably the impact upon the community of influenza virus epidemics (Glezen, 1982). One reason for underestimation is the failure to recognize that the agents which are responsible for most acute respiratory illnesses before and after influenza epidemics are relatively inactive during the period when influenza virus infections are epidemic. Therefore, most of the acute respiratory illnesses that occur during the most intense period of influenza virus activity can be attributed to influenza virus infection and the common practice of attributing to influenza only those illnesses above some threshold estimated without virologic data is questionable.

This can be illustrated by examination of the frequency of visits for acute respiratory disease (ARD) to a prepaid health maintenance organization* in Houston. Figure 2 shows the rate of visits for each two-week period during 1981–2. A sharp peak of visits coincided precisely with the peak of influenza virus activity for the year. Virologic surveillance for that season had shown that epidemics caused by parainfluenza virus types 1 and 2 and respiratory syncytial virus had preceded the influenza B epidemic while activity of

TABLE IV
Frequency of visits by age for acute respiratory disease (ARD) for members of a health maintenance organization[a] during the epidemic period for influenza B/Singapore, Houston, weeks 2–11, 1982

Age (years)	Number of persons enrolled	Number (rate per 100) of ARD visits	Number (rate per 100) of LRD[b] visits
<5	6687	1776 (26·6)	414 (6·2)
5–14	11 928	2202 (18·5)	347 (2·9)
15–24	13 690	1060 (7·7)	125 (0·9)
25–44	26 547	3169 (11·9)	532 (2·0)
>45	5210	561 (10·8)	148 (2·8)
Totals	64 062	8768 (13·7)	1566 (2·4)

[a] A prepaid insurance programme providing total health care. [b] Lower respiratory disease.

* The health maintenance organization is a prepaid insurance programme providing total health care for the panel of members.

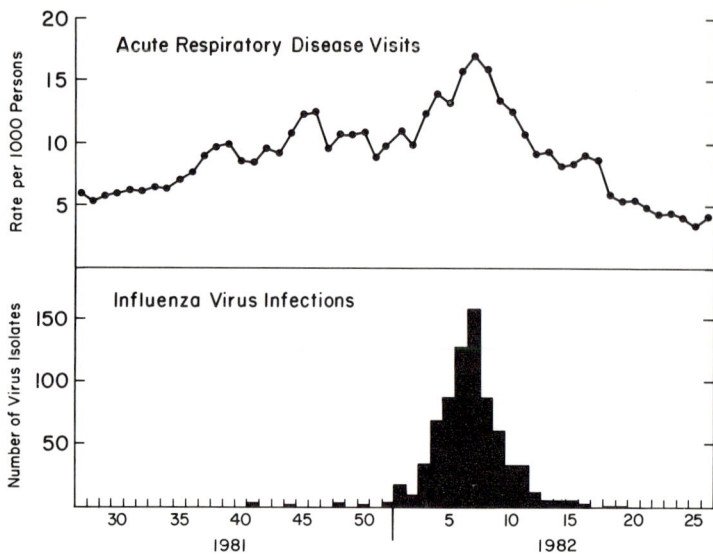

Fig. 2 Rate for patient visits for acute respiratory disease by two-week periods for members of a health maintenance organization, and the temporal relation to the influenza B/Singapore epidemic defined by the community surveillance programme of the Influenza Research Center, Houston, Texas, 1981–2.

parainfluenza virus type 3 followed as illustrated in Fig. 3. Visits for preschool children reflected activity of all the major viruses but visits for school-aged children and adults were increased only during the influenza epidemic (Fig. 4). The risk of a visit for medical care during the ten-week epidemic period is shown in Table V. The overall risk of a visit was 13·7 per 100 persons for this population of employed persons and their families. Even though the ARD visit rate for school children aged 5 to 14 years was 18·5 per 100 children, school absenteeism reached only 9% during the peak week of influenza virus activity. No cultures for influenza virus infections were obtained from persons presenting for care at the health maintenance organization, but the illness rates associated with documented infections of persons followed longitudinally in the Houston Family Study supports our contention that the high rates for ARD visits can be attributed to influenza virus infection (Glezen et al., 1983). Antibody tests of serum specimens are incomplete for 1981–2 but influenza virus was isolated from 45 family members with acute respiratory illness; this number is 13·6% of the 330 persons followed for that year. For the five years prior to this the illness rate associated with influenza virus infection evidenced by antibody rise as well as by virus isolation has been 25·6 per 100 person-years for persons in these

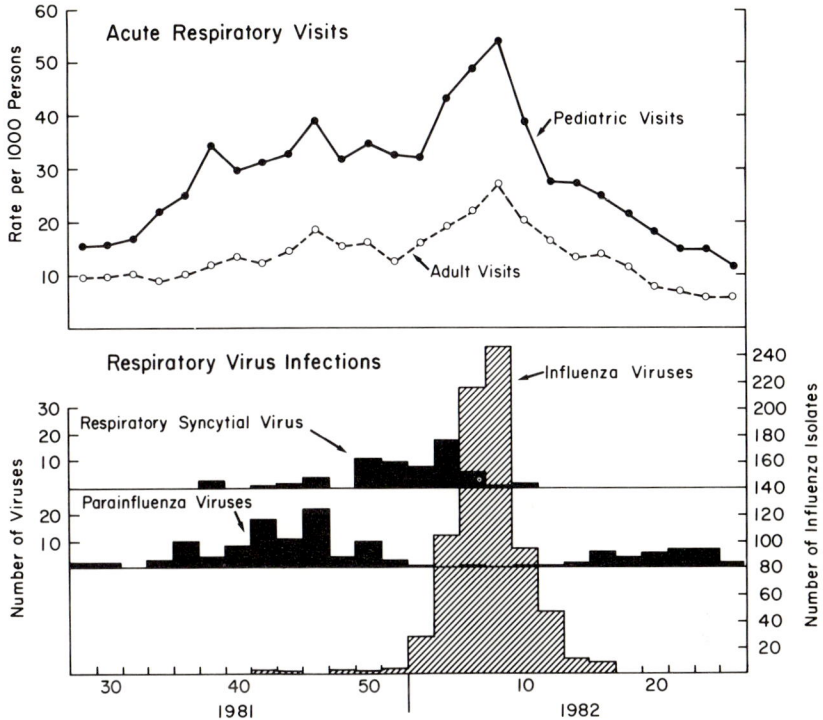

Fig. 3 Rate for pediatric (< 15 years old) visits and for adult visits for acute respiratory disease by two-week periods for members of a health maintenance organization; and the temporal relation to epidemics caused by major respiratory viruses as defined by virologic surveillance at the Influenza Research Center, Houston, Texas, 1981–2.

families (Table V). The average influenza-associated illness rate in our families is about twice the rate for ARD visits to the prepaid clinic including only the visits which occurred during the most intense period of influenza virus activity.

An estimate of serious morbidity and mortality associated with epidemic influenza has been obtained by a survey of hospitalizations with acute respiratory disease (ARD). The first survey was performed by hand tabulation of computer-generated line listings of all patients discharged with an ARD final diagnosis for the period from July 1, 1975 through June 30, 1978 (Glezen, 1982). This survey included hospitals with 17% of the available beds in Harris County and was expanded for 1977–8 to include hospitals with 23% of the beds. Sharp increases in ARD hospitalizations occurred during influenza epidemics—particularly the A/Victoria epidemic

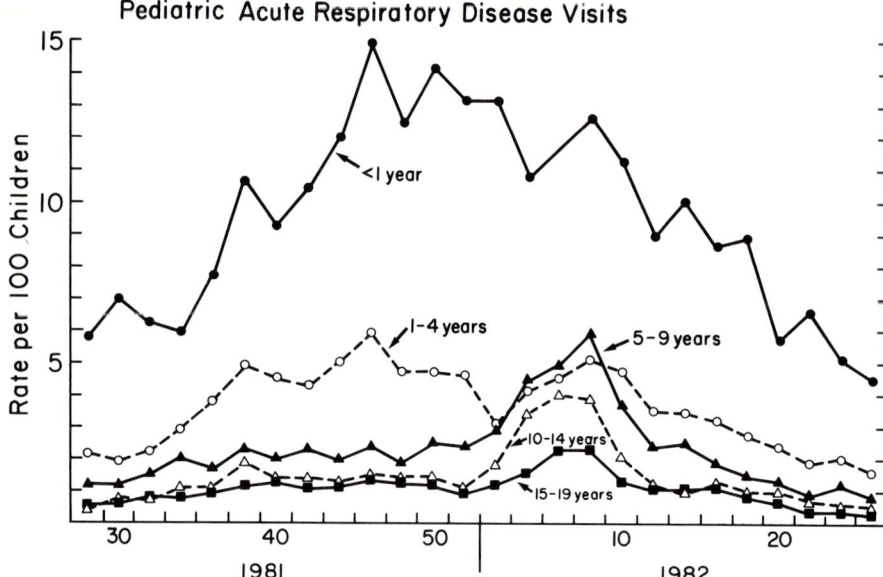

Fig. 4 Rates of visits for acute respiratory disease by two-week periods by members of a health maintenance organization for each pediatric age group, Houston, Texas, 1981–2.

TABLE V
Influenza infection and illness rates[a] for persons followed longitudinally during a five-year period, Houston Family Study, 1976–81

Age (years)	Number of person-years	Number (rate) of infections	Number (rate) of illnesses	Number (rate) LRD[b]
< 6	503	194 (38·6)	162 (32·2)	22 (4·4)
6–17	208	103 (49·5)	76 (36·5)	2 (1·0)
18–24	133	32 (24·1)	29 (21·8)	3 (2·3)
25–34	395	84 (21·2)	59 (14·9)	2 (0·5)
> 35	95	22 (23.2)	16 (16·8)	0
Totals	1334	435 (32·6)	342 (25·6)	29 (2·2)

[a] Per 100 person-years. [b] Lower respiratory disease.

TABLE VI
Survey of hospitalizations with acute respiratory disease (ARD) in Houston and Harris County, Texas, July 1, 1978–June 30, 1982

	ARD hospitalizations	
Age (years)	Number in survey	Estimated number for county
< 5	5778	10613
5–19	2186	4119
> 20	9400	22293
Totals	17364	37025

early in 1976 and the A/Texas epidemic of 1977–8. A second survey was performed by Dr Dennis Perrotta (1982) with improved methodology and has now been extended. This survey included hospitals containing about 45% of all hospital beds in Harris County and was accomplished by obtaining a computer-generated line listing of all ARD hospitalizations on a magnetic tape. In addition to the ARD diagnosis, age, sex, date of admission and length of stay, the new data base included other discharge diagnoses accompanying the ARD diagnosis and the patient's place of residence. The merged data base including only Harris County residents was established and analysed at the University of Texas Education and Research Computer Center. Table VI shows the number of hospitalizations in the survey and the number estimated for all the hospitals in Harris County for a four-year period. The bi-weekly rate of ARD hospitalizations for the four-year period from July 1, 1978 to June 30, 1982 showed that hospitalization for persons older than 5 years of age appreciably increased only during influenza virus epidemics (Fig. 5). The peak number of hospitalizations was shown to lag about one week after the peak of influenza virus morbidity by cross-correlation analysis. Hospitalizations of preschool children demonstrated multiple peaks which coincided with known activity of the major respiratory viruses as illustrated above for outpatient visits. The age distribution of patients hospitalized during influenza epidemic periods is shown in Table VII. Only one-quarter of the patients hospitalized were 65 years of age or older. The age specific hospitalization rates reflected the known susceptibility of the population to specific influenza viruses (Table VIII). The lowest overall hospitalization rate and the lowest rates in adults occurred during the A/Brazil (H1N1) epidemic of 1978–9. The impact of the indolent influenza B epidemic for 1979–80 was lower than that of 1981–2 but the former may

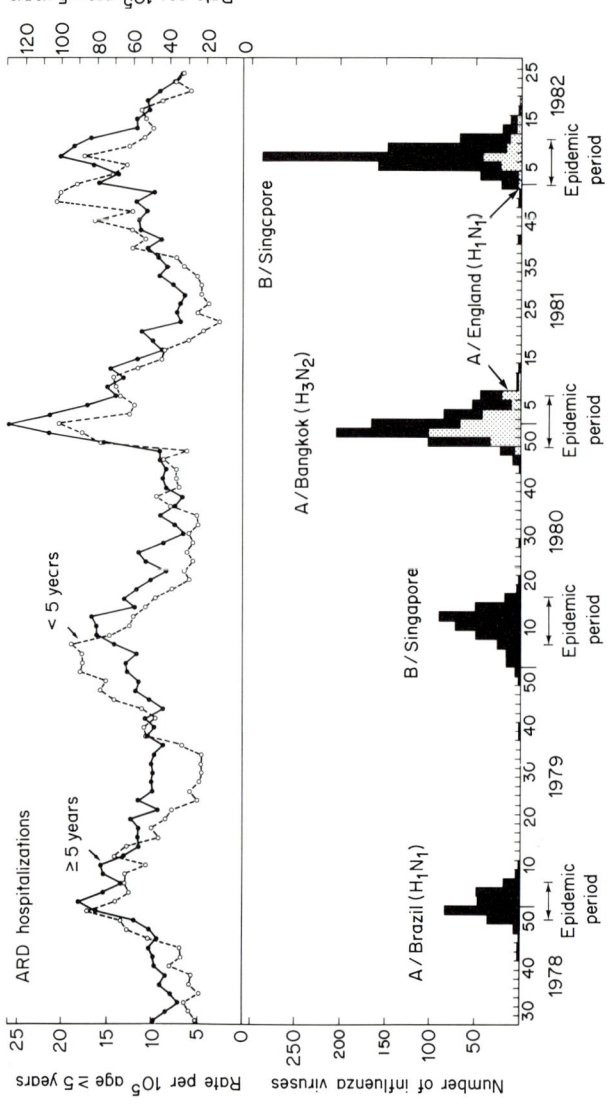

Fig. 5 Estimated rates of hospitalizations for acute respiratory disease for children less than five years of age and for persons five years and older of Harris County, Texas by two-week periods, and the temporal relation to influenza virus epidemics defined by virologic surveillance at the Influenza Research Center, Houston, Texas, 1978–82.

TABLE VII
Estimated number of hospitalizations with acute respiratory disease (ARD) during influenza epidemic periods, Houston and Harris County, Texas, 1978–82

Age (years)	ARD hospitalizations	
	Number	Percent
< 1	1188	11·6
1–4	1601	15·7
5–19	1059	10·4
20–24	476	4·7
25–34	968	9·5
35–44	632	6·2
45–54	783	7·7
55–64	946	9·3
> 65	2542	24·9
Total	10195	100·0

TABLE VIII
Risk of hospitalization with acute respiratory disease during influenza epidemic periods, Houston and Harris County, Texas, 1978–82

Age (years)	Rate per 10 000 persons by year			
	1978–9 A/Brazil	1979–80 B/Singapore	1980–1 A/Bangkok	1981–2 B/Singapore
< 5	28·7	31·9	40·9	35·1
5–19	4·3	4·2	4·6	4·2
20–44	4·1	4·3	6·8	4·4
45–54	6·1	7·5	12·3	8·0
55–64	7·5	14·4	17·6	15·8
> 65	27·7	35·2	55·7	52·0
Totals	8·1	9·5	13·3	11·0

have been underestimated because hospitalization rates for 10-week periods are compared even though the virus was active continuously for over five months in 1979–80. The epidemic of 1980–1 caused by co-circulation of A/Bangkok/1/79 (H3N2) and A/England/333/80 (H1N1) viruses produced the greatest serious morbidity. Over 3000 persons were hospitalized with highest rates among preschool children and persons over 45 years of age.

Because recommendations for influenza vaccine use in the United States are based on data derived from death certificates, it is important to compare characteristics of patients hospitalized with ARD during influenza epidemics with those who die. Over 60% of pneumonia and influenza deaths occur among persons aged 65 years or older while only about 25% of persons hospitalized are older adults. Almost all persons who die have chronic underlying conditions while only 60% to 70% of persons hospitalized had any chronic illness recorded on their discharge record. Some of these chronic conditions are not included in the high risk categories for which vaccine is indicated. Therefore, at least one-third of patients hospitalized with ARD during influenza epidemics of the past four years would not have been recommended for prophylaxis before the epidemic.

SUMMARY AND CONCLUSIONS

Influenza epidemics have occurred annually in Houston over the past nine years and have been the major determinant of acute respiratory illnesses which cause patients to seek medical care. During the same period similar patterns of influenza virus activity with high infection rates for families under continuous surveillance have been demonstrated in Seattle, Washington (Fox et al., 1982) and Tecumseh, Michigan (Longini et al., 1982). Systematic virologic surveillance has provided earliest warning of influenza activity and has defined the period of the epidemic for each season (Glezen et al., 1982 ; Foy et al., 1983). The epidemics have varied in intensity and, in Houston, have caused illnesses in 10 to 25% of persons which disrupted their usual activity or caused those persons to seek medical care. On an average, one of every 1000 persons was hospitalized with acute respiratory disease during the epidemic period. At least one-third of the patients hospitalized would not be candidates for vaccine prophylaxis under the current recommendations in the United States. This coupled with the low acceptance ($<20\%$) of available vaccines by persons recommended to receive them dictates that new approaches to control of epidemic influenza are indicated. The consistently high morbidity experienced by all segments of the population warrants efforts to inhibit spread of influenza viruses among school children and healthy working persons in addition to protection of persons at special risk for serious complications or death.

ACKNOWLEDGMENTS

The authors are grateful for the assistance of the following persons and groups: the medical staff of the sentinel clinics of the Influenza Research

Center including those of the neighbourhood clinics of the Harris County Hospital District headed by Dr Carlos Vallbona; the medical staff of the Baylor Family Practice Center headed by Dr Harold Brown; the practicing pediatricians and family physicians, who so generously participate in the surveillance program; Mr Ray Mercready, Jr., Computer Center, MacGregor Medical Association/Prucare; and our colleagues in the Influenza Research Center, Dr Arthur Frank, Dr Larry Taber, David Joyner, Janet Wells, Barbara Baxter, Nina Pruitt, Scott Kerns, Sandra Rivera and Kay Brown.

Support for these studies was provided by contract No. AI 32685 awarded by the Development and Applications Branch, National Institute for Allergy and Infectious Diseases, N.I.H.

REFERENCES

Cox, N. J., Bai, Z. S. and Kendal, A. P. (1983). Laboratory-based surveillance of influenza A (H1N1) and A (H3N2) viruses in 1980–81: antigenic and genomic analyses. *Bull. WHO* **61**, 143–152.

Fox, J. P., Hall, C. E., Cooney, M. K. and Foy, H. M. (1982). Influenza virus infections in Seattle families, 1975–1979. *Am. J. Epidemiol.* **116**, 212–227.

Foy, H. M., Hall, C. E., Cooney, M. K., Allan, I. D. and Fox, J. P. (1983). Influenza surveillance in the Pacific Northwest 1976–1980. *International J. Epidemiol.* **12**, 353–356.

Frank, A. L., Taber, L. H., Glezen, W. P., Geyer, E. A., McIlwain, S. and Paredes, A. (1983) Influenza B virus infections in the community and in families: The epidemics of 1976–1977 and 1979–1980 in Houston. *Am. J. Epidemiol.* **118**, 313–325.

Glezen, W. P. (1982). Serious morbidity and mortality associated with influenza epidemics. *Epidemiol. Rev.* **4**, 25–44.

Glezen, W. P. and Couch, R. B. (1978). Interpandemic influenza in the Houston area, 1974–1976. *N. Engl. J. Med.* **298**, 587–592.

Glezen, W. P., Couch, R. B., Taber, L. H., Paredes, A., Allison, J. E., Frank, A. L. and Aldridge, C. (1980). Epidemiologic observations of influenza B virus infections in Houston, Texas, 1976–1977. *Am. J. Epidemiol.* **111**, 13–22.

Glezen, W. P., Couch, R. B. and Six, H. R. (1982). The influenza herald wave. *Am. J. Epidemiol.* **116**, 589–598.

Glezen, W. P., Frank, A. L., Taber, L. H., Tristan, M. P., Vallbona, C., Paredes, A. and Allison, J. E. (1983). Influenza in childhood. *Pediatr Res* **17**, 1029–1032.

Longini, I. M., Koopman, J. S., Monto, A. S. and Fox, J. P. (1982). Estimating household and community transmission parameters for influenza. *Am. J. Epidemiol.* **115**, 736–751.

Perrotta, D. M. (1982). Serious morbidity due to acute respiratory disease associated with epidemic influenza. A doctoral dissertation presented to the faculty of the School of Public Health, University of Texas Health Science Center at Houston.

Six, H. R., Webster, R. G., Kendal, A. P., Glezen, W. P., Griffis, C. and Couch, R.

B. (1983). Antigenic analysis of H1N1 viruses isolated in the Houston metropolitan area during four successive seasons. *Infect. Immun.* **42**, 453–458.

Taber, L. H., Paredes, A., Glezen, W. P. and Couch, R. B. (1981). Infection with influenza A/Victoria virus in Houston families, 1976. *J. Hyg., Camb.* **86**, 303–313.

Velazco, J. G., Couch, R. B., Six, H. R. and Glezen, W. P. (1983). Surveillance of influenza in Houston, Texas, USA: gradual transition from A/Victoria/75 (H3N2) to A/Texas/77 (H3N2) predominance and antigenic characterization of "intermediate" strains. *Bull. WHO* **61**, 345–352.

DISCUSSION

Murphy Do you have any idea of the death-rate from influenza in children less than one year of age after exposure to influenza virus? How many children who have underlying disease as well as normal children will die from their first contact with influenza virus?

Glezen We did have an estimate of about 32 in 100 000 for infants for the 1976 epidemic. That was from our hospital survey but we have to realize that that would then include an estimate only of children who were hospitalized. First, let me say that mortality from influenza, pneumonia or acute respiratory disease in children between 28 days and one year of age is still very high and would still be considered one of the most important causes of death. That, coupled with the sudden infant death syndrome, or cot death syndrome as it is called here in Great Britain, are the two leading causes of death for infants after the newborn period.

I think it is important to remember that many of the infants who die do not reach the hospital. In a survey we did of infants examined by the medical examiner in Houston in the early years of the Influenza Research Center, approximately half of the babies who died suddenly at home had a pneumonitis. This was probably viral although we were not able to prove this from the autopsy specimens. Therefore, the estimate that we might make from the hospital data is low and many of those deaths did occur during influenza epidemics.

Of course, there has been a suggestion—particularly in the work of Dr Aherne and Dr Gardner at Newcastle-upon-Tyne—that some of the sudden infant deaths might also be associated with respiratory viruses, particularly RS virus and influenza viruses. At least a portion of those deaths are in some way or other associated with respiratory virus infection.

So, I think that there probably is significant mortality. Those numbers also probably include babies who are normal healthy babies at birth. Once an infant arrives at the hospital with the modern techniques we have now, the house staff is very able in managing severe respiratory distress because they are all trained in the neonatal intensive care units; they can readily intubate the small infants with pneumonia, put them on a respirator and maintain them. So that survival once an infant reaches the hospital is good now and they are not likely to die. The infants that do die in hospital are, again, those with severe congenital heart defects or with broncho-pulmonary dysplasia resulting from their neonatal intensive care experience earlier. In other words, these are babies that were premature to start with. So that the babies that actually die now are, once they reach the hospital, again, babies that have high-risk conditions. I think there is still an undefined quantity of infants dying that do not reach the hospital and these are the ones that we must also be concerned about.

Murphy Would you be willing to make an estimate of the number of influenza-specific deaths per 100 000 in children aged between 28 days and one year?

Glezen I have a slide which shows our previously published rates. My recollection is that this is approximately 32 in 100 000. That is much lower than the death-rate for persons over 65, for instance, in that age group, which would be more like 1:1000 or 2:1000.

Webster Based on this, do you have any recommendations for the vaccination of children if there was a suitable vaccine?

Glezen We should have to have a suitable vaccine. I would not recommend particularly trying to approach the problem in early infancy because I think that the infants are the victims of the spread of influenza viruses in the community. There are probably easier ways to protect the infants, one of which would be to immunize their older siblings and the people who are more responsible for disseminating the virus in the community. Also you have to remember that, since this is a continuing problem, you need an accessible population. The population currently recommended for vaccine is not particularly accessible year after year for prophylactic measures, whereas school children would be more accessible if we had a readily available, inexpensive, safe and effective prophylactic method.

J. W. G. Smith Could I just clarify the figure? We have looked for evidence of infant deaths from influenza in the United Kingdom using excess mortality estimates and have failed to find—I think from the period of 1968 up to about 1976—any excess mortality under the age of one year in association with influenza outbreaks. Excess mortality is not a sensitive way of looking for death, but I was trying to relate the high figure of 32 in 100 000 that you quoted for the Houston area to the sort of mortality you would expect in that age group anyway. Have you got the general mortality background rate?

Glezen I am sorry, I do not have that with me right now. The problem with trying to determine excess mortality is that, of course, infants are vulnerable to several respiratory viruses including respiratory syncytial virus particularly, and parainfluenza viruses. It would be our observation that their risk remains relatively constant because of the sort of reciprocal fluctuations of the intensity of epidemics caused by these viruses. We tend to see more severe RS and parainfluenza epidemics in years when influenza may not be as severe. Their risk then remains relatively constant, so I think it is very difficult to associate this risk specifically with influenza epidemics as they occur by determining "excess mortality". You would have to use more direct methods to try to determine this.

Tyrrell Can I answer Dr Smith's questions? In Britain the sudden infant death syndrome occurs in approximately 1 in 500 children. That usually occurs in the first year of life, which gives you a figure of about 200 in 100 000 as the frequency of the most important single cause of death within which, if the figures were the same here, 32 would be rather lost. There are no accurate data on what proportion of sudden infant deaths there is active influenza virus infection. Certainly the overall frequency of that syndrome is going to swamp the figure that you are talking about now.

Kilbourne There is a striking epidemiological phenomenon revealed by your slides and that is the concordance of infection with different agents, the sharp peaks you get with two different types of influenza. That was something that piqued my curiosity first back in 1950 when we studied it in an institutional population with simultaneous A and B epidemics. It is telling us something about the biology of the disease which is very important and I would welcome any speculation anyone wants to make about it. Certainly if one invokes ideas about latency of the agent, for example, one has to explain the simultaneous emergence then of the A and B together, or H1 and H3 at the same time. This directs our attention back to the host or to the ecological circumstances. Since this is a symposium on epidemiology as well as molecular virology I thought I would point that out. It is a fascinating phenomenon.

Mahy I would like to ask a question about influenza virus C. Clearly there are difficulties in recognizing and looking at the amount of influenza virus C infection in the population but talking to Dr Flewett in Birmingham his opinion was that if one took the trouble to look for influenza virus C, there was a large amount of infection particularly in young children and this was a continuous circulation perhaps with less pathogenicity. Have you had an opportunity to look at this in Houston?

Glezen No, we have not. But we did see that recent study from Japan where, with continuous surveillance in a day-care population, they were able to identify an outbreak of acute respiratory illness in the children associated with acute influenza C infection. Serological surveys in the United States show that infection is very common and probably occurs at an early age but we would have to suspect that it does not cause serious morbidity.

Lambert Taking this question of the change in age distribution during the course of the epidemic, presumably if you analysed the data within the families themselves, as opposed to within the population at large, you would show the same phenomenon. I wonder if you could take that a bit further and tell us anything about the relative importance of different age groups as introducers of influenza into their family groups.

Glezen The number of persons included in our families is relatively small and since our families are all recruited at the time of birth of a newborn infant, these are also relatively young families and do not include large numbers of school-aged children. It is interesting that when you look at the family studies that address this problem their findings vary. One of the major factors in this variance is the type of families recruited. Some investigators have recruited families with at least one school age child; some have recruited families with younger children. They agree that children in the families are important for spread and that infection rates in families with children are much higher than in families without children. We found that the presence of a school-aged child certainly increases the risk for influenza virus infection for the family for that year. Much of our data is based on antibody rises, so we do not have precise timing by direct observation of the introducer.

There is a new mathematical model for this now published from the United States that Dr Longini from Ann Arbor has adapted to the Tecumseh data and to Dr Fox's family study data in Seattle. These studies would, if I remember correctly now, or at least their latest studies would indicate that in families with a pre-school child, many times the pre-school child is the introducer rather than the school child. But there are some changing social customs, I think, that might be associated with this. One, of course—and a very important one—is the frequent use of daycare for pre-school children so that pre-school children often have very continuous contact with the community and the daycare centres obviously represent a very important place for spread of respiratory viruses.

Brownlee I wondered if Dr Glezen had had an opportunity, or whether it is possible, to extend his studies to estimate the risks to the foetus.

Glezen No, I do not really think that we have examined, say, excess foetal loss or perinatal problems in relation to influenza epidemics. That information is included in our hospitalization data. We have perinatal events recorded. They did not appear to be excessive, though.

Kilbourne Has anyone considered immunization of pregnant women for taking care of the problem of deaths in the first year of life? Are there any reliable data on the transfer of influenza antibody transplacentally and its survival in the infant?

Glezen You may be aware of one study we have performed, looking at maternal antibody levels in relation to the age of infants at the time of infection. Our studies showed that there was a direct correlation between the level of maternal antibody at birth and the age at which the infant became infected with an H3N2 virus—specifically A/Victoria virus. The higher the maternal antibody level was at the time of birth, the older the infant was when infected with influenza virus. This was a relatively small study but it suggested then, of course, that the antibody transferred from the mother to the infant was protective. Interestingly enough that protection appeared to be relatively absolute because we were able to get early acute specimens on 14 infants who were infected before five months of age and by the sensitive RIA (radio-immuno-precipitation) antibody test, Dr Six could not detect any influenza antibody at the time of infection. This showed that the antibody which the infants had received from their mothers had essentially disappeared by the time of infection. We did not find that any of those infants had detectable antibody at the time we isolated the virus. These were infants who were ill enough to be admitted to the hospital. I would not say that babies with maternal antibody are never infected but it appears that it protects against serious illness.

Murphy Have you seen this association in subsequent epidemics or just the one epidemic you reported?

Glezen We really have not studied it since then. This requires saving large numbers of cord-blood samples as the babies were born and then monitoring babies that were hospitalized. We have not been able to pursue that.

Couch In subsequent years in the family members the attack rate in infants has been low compared with what it was that year, and while we do not have direct data on passive immunity protection the immunity of mothers is much greater to these related viruses. The data at least fits with continued passive immunity but there is no direct data other than that mentioned.

Klenk What is the latest state of the correlation of influenza infections and Reye syndrome?

Glezen We have tried to maintain surveillance of Reye syndrome in children in Houston. Our rate of Reye syndrome associated with influenza is about seven cases per million children under 19 years of age each year. That is the average for a six year period. That rate is about the same as that determined nationally by surveillance reporting to the Centre for Disease Control for the large influenza B epidemics. It is close to one per 100 000 school children. The risk has been slightly greater during influenza B epidemics, but there is an appreciable risk during influenza A epidemics too. In reviewing world-wide data there is a suggestion that probably Reye syndrome will occur more frequently with influenza A when a new type or a new sub-type or a relatively new and different variant emerges. Murphy called our attention to the paper reported from India in 1957 which may be the earliest report of Reye syndrome entitled neurologic and hepatic disorders associated with the Asian influenza epidemic. Certainly in our country when the A/USSR/77 (H1N1), swept through there were many cases of Reye syndrome and this has not occurred subsequently. Influenza B seems to be able to trigger this problem on a fairly regular basis when it is epidemic.

Klenk Your data if I recall correctly showed three years of particularly high influenza B incidence. Would they support this correlation?

Glezen Yes, they certainly would. We do find an increased risk for Reye syndrome during the influenza B epidemics. That is right. It is a little higher than with the influenza A epidemic. The problem was less severe with only four cases reported during the most recent influenza B epidemic of 1981–2—about half of that seen with the previous influenza B epidemics. Concurrently, the possible association of aspirin ingestion has arisen and this may be another risk factor for the development of Reye syndrome. The use of aspirin for children with febrile respiratory illness has also decreased. The likelihood that school children will receive aspirin with febrile respiratory illness is now half what it was in 1980–1. So in just two years, with the publication of this warning, the use of aspirin has dropped considerably. Last year I think CDC had the lowest reporting of Reye syndrome since surveillance was initiated.

Dowdle I should like to follow up those comments. First, the Reye syndrome is associated not only with influenza but with varicella as well. Secondly, the question of association with aspirin has been a subject of great controversy in the United States. The Public Health Service is planning a major study of the association of aspirin and Reye syndrome, beginning this year. The study protocol is now under review by the Institute of Medicine and a report should be issued within the next week. It will probably take two or three years to do the study. At the same time, the Public Health Service is committed to providing information which warns parents of the reported association. Labelling will not be required but rather information to parents will be provided in all sorts of ways, including in drug stores and grocery stores. How this will affect the study I do not know. We may never know but at least we are committed to trying.

Shortridge Dr Glezen, you drew attention to the fact that maternal antibodies played some protective role in infants in moderating infection. I wondered whether those infants were breast-fed or not? I say this against the background that colostrum and early milk contains quite a wealth of antibodies, and also a spectrum of non-specific inhibitors, whose role, of course, is somewhat questionable.

Glezen Dr Frank has looked at breast-feeding practised by the mothers in the Houston family study, but it is important first to recognize that our families were not chosen with this particular matter in mind. As you know, breast-feeding is much more likely to be practised in the United States by middle income or upper income mothers than by low income mothers. Obviously, if you start with an unselected group of families where breast-feeding practices are not controlled for socioeconomic factors, you may have difficulty in drawing conclusions.

We did not find that breast-fed infants had fewer respiratory virus infections than did infants that were not breast-fed. Overall respiratory illness morbidity appeared to be the same for breast-fed and bottle-fed infants. Our population is very small. There is a suggestion that breast-fed infants are unlikely to have serious morbidity resulting from these infections. In other words, the breast-fed infant seemed to be less likely to develop lower respiratory illness, bronchiolitis and pneumonia, than the bottle-fed babies. This would then conform to larger clinical studies that have suggested that breast-fed infants were less likely to develop bronchiolitis or pneumonia. There is no evidence that breast-feeding prevents infection with any of the respiratory viruses. The infants seem to acquire them readily.

Palese Do you have any hard data concerning neurological disorders, Parkinsonism etc. which are possibly caused by influenza virus infections?

Glezen No, we do not.

H. Smith It is a little early to bring in ferrets—I shall be talking about them tomorrow—and I shall be saying something about the increased susceptibility in neonates, but there are two points in our recent ferret work that are apt in regard to what has been said.

The first point is that in recent work we have immunized ferrets by live infection and the neonates are protected against challenge. In fact, it is strain-specific when two strains are used.

The second point is that about two years ago we showed that if we took down the temperature of ferrets by salicylate—not acetyl salicylate, as aspirin is—it increased the persistence of influenza virus over quite a few days.

Pandemics and Animal Influenza Viruses

R. G. WEBSTER, V. S. HINSHAW, C. W. NAEVE, and
W. J. BEAN

Department of Virology and Molecular Biology, St Jude Children's Research Hospital, Memphis, Tennessee, USA

INTRODUCTION

There is a considerable body of evidence which suggests that the H3N2 viruses may have originated by genetic reassortment between the currently circulating H2N2 virus and a virus antigenically related to A/Duck/Ukraine/63. There is ample evidence for genetic reassortment between influenza A viruses from humans and lower animals *in vivo* (Webster et al., 1971). Genetic and biochemical studies have suggested that the 1957 and 1968 strains have arisen by a process of genetic reassortment (Scholtissek, 1979; Laver and Webster, 1973). The 1957 strain contained the HA, NA, and two polymerase genes that differed significantly in nucleic acid sequence from the preceding H1N1 strains. In 1968, the shift virus contained the NA (and all other) genes from an Asian (H2N2) strain of human influenza and a HA which is antigenically related to that of A/Duck/Ukraine/63 (H3N8) and A/Equine/1/Miami/63 (H3N8) viruses (Fang et al., 1981; Ward and Dopheide, 1982). The amino acid sequence homology between the haemagglutinins of A/Duck/Ukraine/63 and A/Aichi/2/68 viruses (both of

"The Molecular Virology and Epidemiology of Influenza" (Eds Sir Charles Stuart-Harris and Professor C.W. Potter). Academic Press, London, New York and Orlando, 1984

sub-type H3) is 96%. We do not know if an animal or bird virus donated the HA gene during the recombination event that led to the formation of the Hong Kong strain, but the sequence homology suggests that the virus was closely related to A/Duck/Ukraine/63 (H3N8).

The purpose of this report is to review recent developments concerning the host range of influenza A viruses, and to examine some of the genetic properties required for replication in different tissues.

Influenza A viruses infect swine, horses, seals, and a great variety of different birds, as well as humans. Influenza B viruses, on the other hand, infect only humans. Representatives of each of the known sub-types of influenza A viruses have been isolated from birds (Hinshaw and Webster, 1982). These viruses have been isolated in many countries from both domestic and wild species. The largest number of viruses have been isolated from feral water birds including ducks, geese, terns, shearwaters, and gulls, as well as from a wide range of domestic avian species, including turkeys, chickens, quail, pheasants and geese, along with ducks (Easterday, 1975).

In water birds, the majority of influenza viruses are enterotropic, are shed in faeces, and are transmitted through water. The hypothesis is that influenza A viruses in avian species are the primordial source of all influenza A viruses. Three recent outbreaks of disease in mammalian species have been associated with influenza A viruses that probably originated from avian species or lower animals. These include:

(1) Outbreaks of influenza in seals associated with mortality.
(2) Outbreaks of disease in turkeys associated with classical swine (H1N1) influenza viruses.
(3) An epidemic of swine influenza in European pigs caused by a virus antigenically similar to influenza viruses from avian species.

INFLUENZA VIRUSES IN SEALS

In 1979–80, approximately 20% of the harbour seal (*Phoca vitulina*) population of the northeast coast of the United States died of a severe respiratory infection with consolidation of the lungs, typical of primary viral pneumonia (Geraci *et al.*, 1982). Influenza virus particles were found in high concentrations in the lungs and brains of the dead seals. Antigenic analysis showed that this virus was closely related to fowl plague virus [A/FVP/Dutch/27 (H7N7)], a highly lethal influenza virus of chickens not previously found in mammals (Webster *et al.*, 1981). Analysis of the RNAs of the seal virus by competitive RNA–RNA hybridization showed that all of the genes were closely related to those from different avian influenza strains, but the virus replicated poorly in avian species, produced no disease signs and was not shed in the faeces. Biologically, the virus behaved more like a mammalian strain of influenza, replicating to high titres in ferrets, cats and pigs. The A/Seal/Mass/1/80 influenza virus also replicates in the eyes of humans and causes conjunctivitis. In humans, the infection is confined to the conjunctiva and infected persons recovered without complications and no antibodies to the virus were found in the sera from infected individuals.

In squirrel monkeys, the seal influenza virus replicates in the lungs and nasopharynx after intratracheal administration (Murphy *et al.*, 1982a and b) and in the conjunctiva after administration in the eye. In one monkey that died of pneumonia, the seal influenza virus was recovered from the spleen, liver and muscles, as well as the lung, indicating that this virus has the capability for systemic spread in primates.

It is not known whether the A/Seal/Mass/1/80 virus originated by transmission from birds or whether influenza in seals has previously escaped detection. Serological and biological information favours the former explanation—no serological evidence for seal influenza was obtained except in the surviving animals on the New England coast, and since 1980 there has been no further evidence of this virus in seals.

The A/Seal/Mass/1/80 (H7N7) influenza virus provides the first evidence suggesting that a strain deriving all of its genes from one or more avian influenza virus can be associated with severe disease in a mammalian population in nature. Whether this breach of species specifically represents a unique event in influenza evolution remains to be determined, but raises the possibility that human or animal influenza viruses may be derived directly from avian strains. If this event had occurred in humans instead of seals, the resulting pandemic might have been similar to that in 1918–9.

A second influenza virus was isolated from common seals (*Phoca vitulina*) in 1982. Influenza A viruses of the H4N5 sub-type (which has previously been detected only in birds) were recovered from harbour seals dying of viral pneumonia on the New England coast from June 1982 through August 1983. Comparisons of these seal isolates with other mammalian and avian viruses in serological assays and RNA–RNA competitive hybridization indicated that the seal viruses were most closely related antigenically and genetically to recent avian strains and were readily distinguishable from mammalian viruses, including H7N7 isolates from seals in 1980 (Table I). Unlike any previous isolate from mammals, these recent seal viruses replicate in the intestinal tracts of ducks—a characteristic of avian viruses. The association of avian viruses with influenza outbreaks in seals suggests that transmission of avian viruses to seals is occurring in nature. Potentially, this may be an example of adaptation of avian viruses to mammals—an intermediate step in the evolution of new mammalian strains.

TABLE I
Comparison of disease outbreak associated with influenza virus in common seals on the New England coast, USA from 1979–83

Properties	Time of disease outbreaks	
	1979–80	1982–83
Antigenic sub-type of virus isolates	H7N7	H4N5
Estimated mortality	500	50
Histopathology	Bronchopneumonia	Bronchopneumonia
Virus titres (EID_{50}/g) in tissues of dead seals	Lung $10^{7.8}$ Brain $10^{1.5}$ Hilar node ND^a	Lung $10^{5.5}$ Brain $10^{3.5}$ Hilar node $10^{3.3}$
Virus recovery from experimentally inoculated animals: (EID_{50}/g)		
Seals (nasal passages and eyes)	+	+
Ferrets (nasal passages)	+ ($10^{8.0}$)	+ ($10^{6.0}$)
Ducks (intestinal tract)	−	+ ($10^{5.5}$)
Human infections (conjunctivitis)	+	−
RNA homologies between:		
Seal isolates	−	−
Other avian strains	+	+
Mammalian strains	−	−
Time course of epidemic	Limited	Continuing

^{a} ND = not determined.

SWINE INFLUENZA VIRUSES IN TURKEYS

Swine influenza-like viruses (sub-type H1N1) are periodically isolated from humans (Dowdle and Hattwick, 1977). There is no doubt that in some cases the viruses in humans originate from pigs. For example, viruses isolated from sick pigs and humans on farms in Wisconsin were antigenically and genetically indistinguishable (Hinshaw et al., 1978). However, there is not always a clear connection between human infections and contact with pigs. The outbreak of swine influenza in soldiers at Fort Dix, New Jersey, in 1976 was not preceded by such contact, nor was the influenza in a leukaemia patient who died of viral pneumonia in Nevada (CDC Report, 1982). This raises the question of whether other sources of swine influenza viruses exist.

Two viruses were isolated from six adult female turkeys that showed a sudden drop in egg production in Missouri in 1981. In a separate laboratory other H1N1 viruses were recovered from turkeys that had similar problems with egg production in Missouri, Colorado, and Kansas in 1980 and 1981.

TABLE II

Antigenic characterization of influenza A viruses from turkeys

Virus	Ferret antiserum to			HI titres with the following antibodies Monoclonal antibodies to the haemagglutinin of A/NJ/11/76 (X-53a)	
	NJ/8/76 (post-infection)	Dk/Alb/35/76 (hyperimmune)	Ty/Mo/1/81 (post-infection)	6/1	30/2
Human					
NJ/8/76	640	80	320	51 200	3 200
Nev/101/82	640	160	320	12 800	800
Mem/4/82	1 280	320	640	51 200	1 600
Swine					
Sw/Ia/15/30	40	20	80	51 200	<100
Sw/Wis/8/80	320	40	160	6 400	400
Avian					
Ty/Ks/4880/80	1 280	320	640	51 200	1 600
Ty/Mo/1/81	320	160	320	102 400	3 200
Dk/Alb/35/76	<40	320	<40	<100	<100

Sera and antibodies were treated with receptor-destroying enzyme before their use in the assays. Each value is the reciprocal of the serum dilution inhibiting four agglutinating doses of virus.

The viruses were grown in 10- to 11-day-old chick embryos and characterized serologically as H1N1 with hyperimmune goat and rabbit antiserum.

Influenza A viruses (sub-type H1N1) were isolated from the turkeys in different areas of the United States and were determined to be closely related to strains typically associated with pigs. This conclusion was based on comparisons of H1N1 isolates from pigs, humans, ducks, and turkeys with polyclonal and monoclonal antibodies (Table II), RNA–RNA competitive hybridization, and replication studies. One of the H1N1 isolates from turkeys caused influenza in a laboratory technician who displayed fever, respiratory illness, virus shedding, and seroconversion (Hinshaw et al., 1983). These studies raise the question as to how the viruses were introduced into the turkeys. It is possible that humans were the source, having acquired the viruses while slaughtering pigs. Since swine viruses infect humans, it is possible that infected farm personnel transmitted the viruses to the turkeys. The reverse is also possible, i.e. that the turkeys transmit these viruses to other hosts, particularly humans in close contact with them. The infection of the laboratory technician by one of the turkey isolates establishes the potential for such an event. Whether such transmission occurs in nature is not known; however, in cases of human infection with swine viruses, epidemiologists should consider birds as well as pigs as a potential source.

SWINE INFLUENZA VIRUSES IN EUROPEAN PIGS

Influenza disease outbreaks in pigs involving H1N1 viruses represent a significant problem in these animals. Although pigs in the USA have experienced a high incidence of influenza for many years, this has not been the case in other areas of the world. In Europe, there had been little indication of swine influenza until 1977 (Nardelli et al., 1978); since then, disease outbreaks in European pigs have increased in severity and frequency. Although some outbreaks have been associated with the importation of US pigs, this is not always the case. In view of the increased circulation of H1N1 viruses in pigs in different countries, an international collaborative effort was undertaken to examine the distribution of these viruses and to characterize the isolates from these animals.

Antigenic characterization of the H1N1 viruses was of particular interest because previous studies had suggested that isolates from pigs in Belgium were more closely related to avian H1N1 viruses, whereas viruses from pigs in France were more like human H1N1 strains. Since antigenically related viruses exist in humans and birds, it is possible that these H1N1 viruses in pigs originated from other sources. Recent studies also suggested that the

European swine isolates were antigenically (Aymard, M., personal communication) and genetically (Scholtissek, C., personal communication) different from the viruses from US pigs.

An international collaborative study on H1N1 isolates from pigs, birds and humans in 12 different countries was done using haemagglutination-inhibition assays with post-infection ferret sera and monoclonal antibodies to H1N1 strains. The results (Table III) indicate that recent swine isolates from several European countries (Belgium, Denmark, France, Germany and Spain) possess a haemagglutinin antigenically distinguishable from the H1N1 viruses typically associated with pigs as represented by swine isolates from Hong Kong, Italy, Japan and the United States. In serological assays, the viruses from the European pigs were antigenically similar to avian H1N1 viruses. These studies suggest that the H1N1 viruses in pigs are antigenically heterogeneous and the circulation of particular strains is associated with the geographical location of the animals. These results raise the question as to whether the European swine influenza viruses originate from avian sources.

The likelihood of interspecies transmission of viruses between birds and pigs in nature cannot be predicted; however, laboratory studies (Hinshaw and Webster, 1982) have demonstrated that avian viruses, including H1N1 strains, are capable of infecting and replicating in pigs, and even being

TABLE III
H1N1 influenza viruses currently circulating in pigs and birds

Virus	Country	Ferret antisera to A/NJ/8/76	Five different monoclonal antibodies to A/NJ/8/76 (HA)
Swine/Tn/1/75	US, Hong Kong Italy, Japan	1·0	+
Swine/Belgium/426/79	Belgium, Denmark, Germany, France, Spain	0·1	−
Duck/Bavaria/2/77	Germany, France, US, Hong Kong, USSR, China	0·1	−

1·0 indicates that the viruses were not significantly different from A/NJ/8/76. 0·1 indicates that the HI titres were 10-fold below those obtained with A/NJ/8/76. + indicates that the viruses reacted with the monoclonal antibodies to the same titres as the parental A/NJ/8/76 strain. − greater than 10-fold different from A/NJ/8/76.

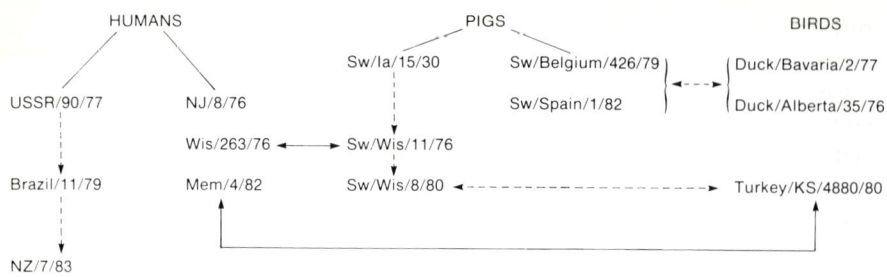

Fig. 1 Interspecies transmission of H1N1 influenza A viruses.
⟵⟶ Antigenic and genetic identity between isolates.
⟵--⟶ Antigenic relationships between isolates.
↓ Antigenic drift.

transmitted to other pigs. It is also known that swine influenza viruses infect birds, e.g. the swine-influenza-like viruses in turkeys in the US are apparently of swine origin and they have been associated with disease outbreaks in turkeys (see above). Recent disease outbreaks in turkeys in France involve viruses very similar to the European swine viruses and the birds are located in close proximity to swine herds. These findings lend support to the possibility that H1N1 viruses are being exchanged between birds and pigs and, therefore, antigenically related viruses may be detected in both groups (Fig. 1).

THE ROLE OF THE HAEMAGGLUTININ IN ENTEROTROPISM

In addition to the ability of influenza viruses to undergo antigenic drift and shift, the spread of the virus requires the proper gene constellation for the interrelated properties of virulence, host range, and tissue tropism. Little is known of the genetic factors responsible for these biological attributes. Many studies have examined the properties of infectivity, pathogenicity, and neurovirulence of reassortant avian strains and suggest that these attributes are polygenic and that the required gene combinations may differ from strain to strain (Rott, 1979; Rott et al., 1976; Scholtissek et al., 1979). Cleavage activation of the haemagglutinin (HA) has been shown to be a key determinant for infectivity and virulence (Lazarowitz and Choppin, 1975), while other studies suggest that additional genes are required: the neuraminidase (NA) and matrix (M) genes (Ogawa et al., 1981), or the nucleoprotein (NP) gene (Bean and Webster, 1978). The genetic determinants of host range have also been examined through the use of reassortants. Almond (1978) provided evidence suggesting that the gene coding for one of the polymerase proteins, P3, is the sole determinant of host range in a tissue culture system. The property of tissue tropism has also been addressed through investigation of neurovirulent mammalian strains of influenza. The neurotropism of A/WSN in mice has been shown to be a property of the NA gene although the M and nonstructural (NS) proteins may also be involved (Sugiura and Ueda, 1980). NA is thought to facilitate cleavage activation of the HA polypeptide while NS and M are required to keep growth rate or yield to a sufficiently high level (Nakajima and Sugiura, 1980).

The interpretation of reassortant studies is complicated by what has been referred to as clonal phenotypic variation, i.e., mutations occurring during virus passage which give rise to phenotypic variation among viruses having the same genotype as determined by hybridization analysis (Ogawa et al., 1981). The occurrence of point mutations, undetected by hybridization studies, could easily be sufficient to alter virulence, host range, or tissue tropism.

To determine which gene segments of influenza A viruses are responsible for the property of tissue tropism, reassortants were produced between the avian influenza strain, A/Mal/NY/6750/78 [H2N2] (Mal/NY), and a human strain, A/Udorn/307/72 [H3N2] (Udorn). The avian strain replicates in the intestinal tract of ducks and the human strain does not. Eight reassortants were shown by hybridization analysis to have the same gene constellation, having received haemagglutinin gene segment 4 from Udorn and the remaining seven gene segments from Mal/NY (Naeve et al., 1983). With one exception, all reassortants containing the Udorn HA were restricted in their ability to traverse the digestive tract of ducks and replicate therein (Table IV). The exception, reassortant R2, replicated to high titres in the intestinal tract. The R2 virus was shown to possess a haemagglutinin molecule that was antigenically distinguishable from the Udorn parent with polyclonal and monoclonal antibodies.

Results of HI tests with antisera specific to the haemagglutinin of Aichi/2/68 or England/42/72 indicated that the reactivity of R2 virus was at least 10-fold different from the parental virus. Analysis with monoclonal antibodies specific for the haemagglutinin of Mem/1/71 showed that the R2 virus was not inhibited at all in HI tests (Table V). These results indicate that the haemagglutinin of R2 virus is still of the H3 sub-type but is antigenically different from the parental Udorn strain. Monoclonal and polyclonal antibodies to the H2 haemagglutinin of Mal/NY did not react with the R2 virus in either HI or ELISA assays (results not shown).

TABLE IV
Replication of parental and reassortant viruses in the intestinal tract of ducks

Virus	No. animals infected/No. animals inoculated	Peak virus titre ($\log_{10}EID_{50}/G$)	
		Faeces	Rectum
Parental			
A/Udorn/307/72	0/4	0	0
A/Mallard/NY/6870/78	4/4	7·0	5·5
Reassortants			
R1, R3-R6, R8, R9	0/21	0	0
R2	6/7	6·0	5·8

[a] Pekin ducks were inoculated orally with 10^7 EID_{50} of virus. Tissues were collected at three days post-infection and titrated for infectious virus (Webster et al., 1978). [b] Number of animals infected is based on virus recovery from cloaca, bursa, rectum, or faeces from inoculated birds.

Monoclonal antibodies specific for the different antigenic regions on the haemagglutinin of Mem/1/71 (H3) were tested in HI assays with the reassortant viruses in an attempt to determine which antigenic region of the HA molecule on R2 was altered. Monoclonal antibody to site A (138/1) did not react with either the parental virus Udorn HA or with the reassortants so that no information could be obtained about this region (Table V). Antibody to site B (4/1) reacted strongly to Udorn and reassortants R1 and R3 to R6

TABLE V
Antigenic analysis of reassortant influenza viruses

	HI titres to the following influenza viruses:		
	Udorn/307/72	R2	R1 and R3-R6
Polyclonal antisera to:			
Aichi/2/68 (H3N2)	8 100[a]	140	8 100
Eng/42/72 (H3N2)	24 000	4 000	24 000
R2	10 000	1 500	10 000
Monoclonal antibodies to:			
Mem/1/71 (H3)			
138/1 (Site A)	<[b]	<	<
4/1 (Site B)	50 000	<	50 000
H14/A2 (Site C)	900	<	900

[a] The values give the reciprocal of the dilution inhibiting 4 HA units of virus. [b] < = Less than 50.

but did not react with R2. Monoclonal antibodies to site C (H14/A2) reacted with the parental Udorn strain and reassortants R3 to R6, but only reacted with the R2 strain after the virus had been disrupted with ether indicating that this antigenic site is probably present but is masked in some way in the intact R2 virion. These results indicate that an antigenic change has occurred in site B of the R2 virus, that site C is still present but perhaps masked, and that site A in the parental virus is changed so that no information could be obtained about this region.

The results suggest that the R2 haemagglutinin has undergone mutation(s) altering tissue tropism and antigenic properties of the virus. These studies illustrate the importance of the haemagglutinin gene in determining tissue tropism and present an example of phenotypic variation in a virus population with the same gene constellation but do not exclude a requirement for other gene products.

To determine the location of mutations in the R2 haemagglutinin, the RNA genes coding for the HA1 of both the parental Udorn and the tissue tropism mutant R2 were sequenced. These were obtained by making synthetic oligodeoxynucleotides and using them to prime dideoxynucleotide chain termination sequencing reactions containing total virus RNA, reverse transcriptase and ^{32}P-labelled deoxynucleotides (Air, 1979). Only two amino acid changes are present in the R2 HA molecule at residues 226 and 228, both in the receptor binding site. The leucine at residue 226 in Udorn was changed to glutamine in R2 as a result of a codon change from CTG to CAG, while the serine at 228 in Udorn was changed to glycine in R2 as a result of a codon change from AGT to GGT.

Studies by Rogers *et al.* (1983) demonstrated that the change at residue 226 from leucine to glutamine correlated with sensitivity to neutralization by an inhibitor present in horse serum and furthermore, this change correlated with altered sialic acid binding specificities, i.e. those HAs with leucine at 226 bind SAα2;6, Gal-linkages, while those with glutamine bind SAα2,3 Gal-linkages. To determine if only the change at 226 was required for the altered tissue tropism of R2, additional reassortants with the same genotype were sequenced through the receptor binding site and were tested for sensitivity to the horse serum inhibitor (data not shown). Those reassortants with leucine at 226 are sensitive to the inhibitor, those with glutamine are insensitive in agreement with Rogers *et al.* (1983). However, the change at 226 did not correlate with tissue tropism, since examples of reassortants with either leucine or glutamine at 226 but with serine at 228 did not replicate in the intestinal tract of ducks. Only R2 with the serine to glycine mutation at 228, along with glutamine at 226, exhibits avian enterotropism.

Examination of the published sequences of 28 HA1 molecules reveals only four that can be considered avian strains: A/Duck/Ukraine/1/63 (Ward and Dopheide, 1982), fowl plague virus (Porter *et al.*, 1979), A/Seal/Mass/1/80 (Naeve and Webster, 1983), and now reassortant R2. All have the same amino acid sequence in the receptor binding site—gly-gln-ser-gly-arg-ile-.

As a result of these studies, we suggest that (1) mutation in the influenza haemagglutinin receptor binding site can alter the important biological property of tissue tropism, (2) the change at 226 correlates with horse serum inhibitor sensitivity and sialic acid binding specificity but an additional change at 228 is required for altered tissue tropism, and (3) all avian strain receptor binding sites are likely to have the same amino acid sequences.

ACKNOWLEDGMENTS

This work is supported by Grants AI 08831 and AI 02649 from the National Institute of Allergy and Infectious Diseases, by Childhood Cancer Center Support Grant CA 21765 from the National Cancer Institute, and by ALSAC.

The authors acknowledge the excellent technical assistance of Mary Ann Bigelow, Ken Cox, Lisa Newberry and Deanna Williams.

REFERENCES

Air, G. M. (1979). Nucleotide sequence coding for the "signal receptor" and N terminus of the haemagglutinin from an Asian (H2N2) strain of influenza virus. *Virology* **97**, 468–472.

Almond, J. W. (1978). A single gene determines the host range of influenza virus. *Nature* (Lond.), **270**, 617–618.

Baez, M., Zazra, J. J., Elliott, R. M., Young, J. F. and Palese, P. (1981). Nucleotide sequences of the influenza A/Duck/Alberta/60/76 virus NS RNA: conservation of the NS1/NS2 overlapping gene structure in a divergent influenza virus RNA segment. *Virology* **113**, 397–402.

Bean, W. and Webster, R. G. (1978). Phenotypic properties associated with influenza genome segments. *In* "Negative Strand Viruses and Host Cells". (Eds B. W. J. Mahy and R. D. Barry) pp. 685–692. Academic Press, London and New York.

CDC Influenza Surveillance Report (1982). 23rd April, 1982, pp. 195–197. Communicable Disease Centers, Atlanta.

Dowdle, W. R. and Hattwick, M. A. W. (1977). Swine influenza virus infection in humans. *J. Infect. Dis.* **136**, (Suppl.) 386–389.

Easterday, B. C. (1975). Animal influenza. *In* "The Influenza Viruses and Influenza". (Eds E. D. Kilbourne) pp. 449–481. Academic Press, New York and London.

Fang, R., Min Jou, W., Huylebroeck, D., Devos, R. and Fiers, W. (1981). Complete structure of A/Duck/Ukraine/63 influenza haemagglutinin gene: animal virus as progenitor of human H3 Hong Kong 1968 influenza haemagglutinin. *Cell* **25**, 315–323.

Geraci, J. R., St Aubin, D. J., Barker, I. K., Webster, R. G., Hinshaw, V. S. Bean, W. J., Ruhnke, H. L., Prescott, J. H., Early, G., Baker, A. S., Madoff, S. and Schooley, R. T. (1982). Mass mortality of harbor seals: Pneumonia associated with influenza A virus. *Science* **215**, 1129–1131.

Hinshaw, V. S. and Webster, R. G. (1982). The natural history of influenza A viruses. *In* "Basic and Applied Influenza Research". (Ed A. S. Beare) pp. 79–104. CRC Press, Florida.

Hinshaw, V. S., Bean, W. J. Jr., Webster, R. G. and Easterday, B. C. (1978). The prevalence of influenza viruses in swine and the antigenic and genetic relatedness of influenza viruses from man and swine. *Virology* **84**, 51–62.

Hinshaw, V. S., Webster, R. G., Bean, W. J. Jr., Downie, J. and Senne, D. A. (1983). Swine influenza-like viruses in turkeys: potential source of virus for humans? *Science* **220**, 206–208.

Laver, W. G. and Webster, R. G. (1973). Studies on the origin of pandemic influenza. III. Evidence implicating duck and equine influenza viruses as possible progenitors of the Hong Kong strain of human influenza. *Virology* **51**, 383–391.

Lazarowitz, S. C. and Choppin, P. W. (1975). Enlargement of the infectivity of influenza A and B viruses by proteolytic cleavage of the haemagglutinin polypeptide. *Virology* **69**, 440–454.

Murphy, B. R., Hinshaw, V. S., Sly, D. L., London, W. T., Hosier, N. T., Wood, F. T., Webster, R. G. and Chanock, R. M. (1982a). Virulence of avian influenza A viruses for squirrel monkeys. *Infect. Immun.* **37**, 1119–1126.

Murphy, B. R., Sly, D. L., Tierney, E. L., Hosier, N. T., Massicot, J. G., London W. T., Chanock, R. M., Webster, R. G. and Hinshaw, V. S. (1982b). Reassortant virus derived from avian and human influenza A viruses is attenuated and immunogenic in monkeys. *Science* **218**, 1330–1332.

Naeve, C. W. and Webster, R. G. (1983). Sequence of the haemagglutinin gene from influenza virus, A/Seal/Mass/1/80. *Virology* **129**, 298–308.

Naeve, C. W., Hinshaw, V. S. and Webster, R. G. (1983). Phenotypic variation in influenza virus reassortants with identical gene constellations. *Virology* **128**, 331–340.

Nakajima, S. and Sugiura, A. (1980). Neurovirulence of influenza virus in mice. II. Mechanism of virulence as studied in a neuroblastoma cell line. *Virology* **101**, 450–457.

Nardelli, L., Pascucci, S., Gualandi, G. L. and Loda, P. (1978). Outbreaks of classical swine influenza in Italy in 1976. *Zentralbl Veterinarmed.* (B) **25**, 853–857.

Ogawa, T., Ueda, M. and Sugimura, A. (1981). Genes involved in the virulence of an avian influenza virus. *In* "Genetic Variation Among Influenza Viruses". (Ed. D. P. Nayak) pp. 387–397. Academic Press, New York and London.

Porter, A. G., Barber, C., Carey, N. H., Hallewell, R. A., Threlfall, G. and Emtage, J. S. (1979). Complete nucleotide sequence of an influenza virus haemagglutinin gene from cloned DNA. *Nature* (Lond.) **282**, 471–477.

Rogers, G. N., Paulson, J. C., Daniels, R. S., Skehel, J. J., Wilson, I. A. and Wiley, D. C. (1983). Single amino acid substitutions in influenza haemagglutinin changes receptor binding specificity. *Nature* (Lond.) **305**, 76–78.

Rott, R. (1979). Molecular basis of infectivity and pathogenicity of myxovirus *Arch. Virol.* **59**, 285–298.

Rott, R., Orlich, M. and Scholtissek, C. (1976). Attenuation of pathogenicity of fowl plague virus by recombinations with other influenza A viruses non-pathogenic for fowl: Non-exclusive dependence of pathogenicity on haemagglutinin and neuraminidase of the virus. *J. Virol.* **19**, 54–60.

Scholtissek, C. (1979). Influenza virus genetics. *Adv. Genet.* **20**, 1–36.

Scholtissek, C., Vallbracht, A., Flehmig, B. and Rott, R. (1979). Correlation of pathogenicity and gene constellation of influenza viruses. II. Highly neurovirulent recombinants derived from non-neurovirulent or weakly neurovirulent parent strains. *Virology* **95**, 492–500.

Sugiura, A. and Ueda, M. (1980). Neurovirulence of influenza virus in mice. I. Neurovirulence of recombinants between virulent and avirulent virus strains. *Virology* **101**, 440–449.

Ward, C. and Dopheide, T. (1982). The Hong Kong haemagglutinin. Structural relationships between the human (H3) haemagglutinins and the haemagglutinin from the putative progenitor strain A/Duck/Ukraine/1/63 (Hav 7). *In* "Genetic Variation Among Influenza Viruses". (Eds D. P. Nayak and C. F. Fox) pp. 323–340, ICN-UCLA Symposia on Molecular and Cellular Biology, Vol. XXI. Academic Press, New York and London.

Webster, R. G., Campbell, C. H. and Granoff, A. (1971). The "in vivo" production of "new" influenza A viruses. *Virology* **44**, 317–328.

Webster, R. G., Yakhno, M., Hinshaw, V. S., Bean, W. J. and Murti, K. G. (1978). Intestinal influenza: Replication and characterization of influenza viruses in ducks. *Virology* **84**, 268–278.

Webster, R. G., Hinshaw, V. S., Bean, W. J. Jr., van Wyke, K. L., Geraci, J. R., St Aubin, D. J. and Petursson, G. (1981). Characterization of an influenza A virus from seals. *Virology* **113**, 712–724.

DISCUSSION

Palese Do you have any monoclonal antibody which recognizes the amino acid 228 of the R1 haemagglutinin? If a site B specific monoclonal antibody recognizes 228, would you be able, by passaging the R1 virus in the presence of the amino acid antibodies, to get out a virus which has R2 properties?

Webster The answer is "no". So far we do not have a monoclonal antibody that specifically recognizes 228.

Palese What do you get if you passage the virus in the presence of the site B antibody which you mentioned in your talk?

Webster This is being done now. You will have to wait for the answer. There is one thing I can tell you that we can readily isolate variants at 226 by passaging in the presence of horse serum. We have not yet been successful in selection of variants with changes only at 228.

Schild You mentioned an association between the antigenic character of nucleoprotein and host range, at least for avian viruses. Have you done this for the two seal viruses?

Webster This has been done with the seal virus and the seal virus nucleoprotein is grouped with the avian viruses and is the odd man out. In every way it is avian and yet it replicates in seals.

Schild This is based on using monoclonal antibodies?

Webster No. This is based on Dr Bean's RNA–RNA competitive hybridization studies. It is not based on antigenic analysis.

Scholtissek I want to make one comment and then I have one question. The comment is this: we have studied these different swine isolates from Europe and compared them with the United States' isolates and those from other parts of the world by hybridization. We found that the haemagglutinin of the European strains is quite different from that of the United States' isolates but genetically highly related with the bird isolates. We think that the haemagglutinin of the European swine viruses is not derived just by a few point mutations, it is not just a variant but must come from a new reservoir. There are reassortants involved because the duck/Bavaria strain, for example, carries a segment 8 which is genetically little related to segment 8 of the other swine viruses of Northern Europe. So there must also be a reassortant involved, if the virus went from one species to the other.

Webster Have you looked at the other genes?

Scholtissek Not yet. Only at the neuraminidase, but not the other genes. That was my comment, and now my question: when you studied the variant which has a mutation in the pocket, did you also find changes in the affinity to specific substrates, according to the method Dr Paulson is using—erythrocytes which he could load with neuraminic acid-containing substrates which have different linkages, let us say 2–3 linkages or 2–6 linkages of the neuraminic acid to the corresponding substrate?

Webster I skipped over this because I knew John Skehel would be dealing with it later. I will leave that for him to answer. In relation to the avian–human reassortant viruses, they correlate exactly with what Dr J. Paulson has been finding namely, that the R3, the horse serum sensitive strain, combines with the 2–6 Gal-linkage, and R34, the inhibitor resistant virus, combines specifically with the 2–3 Gal-linkage.

Mahy Does the ability of the R2 variant to grow in ducks correlate with its growth in colon organ culture? Have you looked at this property?

Webster No. We are working on the development of this system.

Murphy Do you have any explanation for isolating a haemagglutinin variant with two amino acid changes? Theoretically you should have detected this in one in 10^{10} but you were able to do it in one in 34. I have heard of the luck of the Irish but I was wondering how you might explain this!

Webster I do not think it is so much luck other than the luck of the New Zealanders! When we make these reassortants we use rabbit antiserum in selection. Rabbit antiserum may select variants with the change at 226 readily and this leaves the selection of a variant at 228—and here we were lucky.

Chu May I show a few slides on the viruses from ducks and pigs in China? We chose ducks and pigs for obvious reasons, because the influenza viruses are most abundant amongst these species. These animals and birds are very abundant in China and, in certain circumstances, they live in very close contact with man.

I have compared our data, which consists of about 250 strains of viruses from ducks over three years with that of Dr Shortridge in Hong Kong: presumably he was working with ducks mostly imported from China. I think you can see from the slide that there is very good agreement. The highly prevalent haemagglutinins and neuraminidases are almost the same. In mainland China, H4 occurs in over 20% and in Hong Kong H4, H3, and H6—that is for the haemagglutinin—and for neuraminidase they are all the same, N6, N2 and N8. The least frequent ones with the haemagglutinin are H1, H2, H7, H8 and H12. There is a little difference between Hong Kong and mainland China data, because some are absent in the mainland China series which are present in the Hong Kong series—but these are the infrequent ones. For neuraminidase, N1 is also quite infrequent in our series. In spite of the fact that you can find all sub-types of haemagglutinin and neuraminidase among ducks, there is a definite difference in the distribution of the sub-types. These are the results in about 700 strains altogether over three to five years of time. We see that it is quite representative.

Coming to the isolations in pigs. The black ones and the first two columns represent H3N2 barriers in 77 and 78. The first one is Victoria/75-like, the second column is Texas/77-like. All the blank ones represent influenza C viruses. They are drawn by month of isolation. You can see that they are absent during the summertime and are most prevalent in the winter and spring. Those with horizontal bars are from H1N1 strains. Then again we have more H3N2. We also reckon the isolation from the sea as well. By virological evidence, we have influenza A, all the variants, from Victoria to Texas, now more akin to Bangkok and Shanghai 31/81 so that obviously the viruses from pigs are following the antigenic drifts in man.

What is interesting is that the influenza C viruses are very close to a strain called New Jersey/76, which is the most recent influenza C virus we have. They are quite remote from earlier strains. Speaking of recent assays of pig sera against influenza B, out of about 1300 sera from Guo Yuanji in Southwest China, we had 10 sera which were positive by SRH single radial haemolysis test. We tested them again with haemagglutinin-inhibition, neuraminidase-inhibition, complement fixation and neutralization. As you can see, some of these are definitely positive by all tests, for instance 209 and 923. These sera are positive by all tests, and some of them are positive by complement fixation, so there is very little doubt about the authenticity of the antibody there.

Our conclusion is that pigs can be infected with all types of influenzas A, B and C. We have not got definite virological results yet with B, but we are continuing the study.

Another thing is that the pigs probably got the infection from men, because in all three cases the virus or the antibody resembled the most recent one prevalent in man, so the pigs probably got the infection from man.

That raises a question. We have no classical swine virus in China, but H3N2 is certainly very prevalent and influenza C is very prevalent, and now it seems that we also have influenza B. It seems to me that pigs, besides, may not be a dead-end host, because pigs usually mix very much with ducks, so it is possible that reassortment, if it does not occur in man, probably occurs in pigs, so we are looking for avian antibody in pigs now.

Shortridge Animal influenza is an incredibly complex field and I think it will be a long time before we really understand its relationship to human influenza. But I did wonder, in the light of Dr Webster's talk and the general comments, whether he might have any views on the role of the duck as a source of human influenza. The duck is an abundant source of virus which primarily multiplies asymptomatically in the intestine. Could therefore the avian (duck) virus be one that merely is denied access to the human intestinal tract but is able to multiply in the respiratory tract in an imperfectly adapted way so that it gives rise to disease?

Webster From a very general point of view, the information we have so far is that perhaps the haemagglutinin and/or neuraminidase of human strains may be derived from influenza viruses in lower animals, but I do not believe that the replicating complex from the avian virus is likely to be involved. At least, we have no information on this at the moment, and the indications from Dr Bean's work is that the nucleoprotein is restricted to a particular species. The seal virus is the exception.

Shortridge Having dealt with the duck, what do you think might be the role of the pig in influenza ecology? I have often felt that the pig, by virtue of the fact that it lives close to man and also to ducks particularly in China and in the Southeast Asia is generally nothing more than a recipient of virus following mammalian adaptation in man.

Webster There is no doubt that the pig also has resident viruses, and your own work shows that in some cases the human H3N2 viruses continue to circulate in pigs for rather a long time. Whether or not they can persist in the pig long enough to be important on reintroduction into man is not known.

Kilbourne   Webster has ducked this issue, and I would like to talk turkey for a moment. We have been interested, as all of you know, in some swine mutants, haemagglutinin mutants, with different pathogenic properties and have recently, in collaboration with Both, been able to pinpoint their difference to a single base change, but I do not intend to discuss that now.

What I wanted to bring out is that inadvertently we did preliminary work relevant to what Webster just told us about in terms of the turkey/swine viruses. Easterday and I were anxious to find out whether the phenomenon of this sort of allelic dimorphism of the haemagglutinin variants of swine was also more generally applicable. I got from Webster his turkey/swine viruses. From them we selected the same types of mutants. We looked for a role for the so-called H mutant, which replicates very poorly in swine and therefore seems to have no reason for existing in nature. We had surmised that perhaps what this does is to replicate in fowl more efficiently. Accordingly, with Easterday we looked at the relative replication rates in turkeys—before the turkey data came out from Webster—of the swine variants. The important bit of information was that these mutants which were derived from the A/New Jersey/76, and PR8, the swine variants replicated practically not at all, neither the L nor H variant, except to the extent that they had reassorted PR8 genes in them, which is probably not surprising in view of the long egg passage history of the PR8. They were essentially avianized and took off very well in the birds.

The important base line to Webster's observation is that the viruses of either human or swine origin, depending on the point of view, intrinsically with identical gene constellations, do not replicate in the turkey. I think that makes his observations of the fact that he has strains in nature that do so very important and implies once again that very minor changes may have occurred to cause this adaptation.

Webster   Could you tell us the base change that is involved?

Both   It appears to be the mass of residue 158 and I just forget the precise base number for it.

Kilbourne   It is 155, but you know better than I.

Both   The H nomenclature I used relates to the structural information of haemagglutinin. It is residue 155 if you are just looking at HI amino acids but in relation to the H structure it is 158. The change is from glycine to glutamic acid.

Kilbourne   The mutation changes from G to A is at base 547.

Skehel   Is there any correlation with the binding activity?

Kilbourne   I thought this discussion might be more relevant later but we have looked very, very hard for any evidence of differences in binding activity. At the moment there seems to be different elution patterns from sheep erythrocytes of the L and H haemagglutinins, but it has been a very tenuous kind of a handle. We have looked very hard for differences in absorption to cell monolayers and absorption kinetics and the like, and anything that can credibly be associated with what the haemagglutinin does. We have not been able to get that kind of non-molecular biology done.

Brownlee I have a very detailed point which again may be appropriate to a later talk. You raise the difficulty, Dr Webster, that you had a mutant R2, distinct from R3, and the other variants which differed in replication properties. You postulated that the critical mutation was at glycine 228, but you wondered why it caused such large effects on the binding of specific antibodies.

Webster I think the change that is important is at 226, and this comes out from John Skehel's work as well; a single change at 226 will markedly affect the combination of monoclonal antibodies that recognize the B determinant. We do not know how a change at 228 affects antigenic determinants.

Brownlee Whether it is 226 or 228 I was going to suggest a possible reason. In the work we have done in the past in collaboration with Dr Gerhart and indeed yourself in isolating mutants of HA1. This showed quite clearly that one antigenic site, the Ca site, could be characterized by mutants of residue 224 and 225. Residue 225 is sufficiently close to this site that one could make the postulate that there is a very small change in the tertiary structure of the molecule and it is this that is affecting the binding to monoclonal antibodies.

Webster It could well be.

Skehel Obviously it is possible, but I do not think Dr Brownlee has sequenced the variant to map the monoclonals that he is talking about yet. We have seen in both cases differences of reactivity with monoclonals and the binding mutants. They certainly are not in a cleft, in fact, they are on the helix at the top of the molecule. So in these cases they are not involved in sub-unit interaction, but, of course, that does not mean that in other cases they could not be.

Mahy I would like to ask one more general question of Dr Webster before leaving the animal question. We have heard about the virus isolation from seals and also the large amount of influenza activity in avians, but I wonder to what extent we know about the animal population as a whole. When you say "exhaustively looked", presumably you are looking in other animal species and would you perhaps think this was exemplified by the seal example, which is something that was not looked at before?

Webster There may be more examples of influenza in species not yet studied, e.g. as in seals, but over the last ten years, WHO has had a major programme to look for influenza viruses in lower animals. Dr M. Kaplan and

Dr Assaad have emphasized the need for these studies. The only thing I can say is that studies in many countries have not resulted in the detection of many new sub-types or in the detection of virus in different species. We cannot rule out the possibility of influenza in animal species that are not economically relevant and we might miss them; but at this stage I do not think there are an unlimited number of influenza virus subtypes.

Kilbourne It seems that we now have five haemagglutinins that are undeniably associated with mammalian disease, H1, H2, H3, H4 as you just told us, and H7. Is that a fair summary?

Webster That would be a fair summary.

Scholtissek I have one question concerning the seal virus. Is this virus very contagious? Fowl plague virus is not very contagious. However, both viruses are very pathogenic and I could imagine from the teleological point of view that it is not very advantageous for a virus to kill its host so rapidly.

Webster The epidemiology of the H7N7 incident in seals in the United States would suggest just that. It initially killed about 25% of the seals and it has now disappeared from seals whereas the recent H4N5, that is killing fewer animals, is continuing.

Skehel Did you do any laboratory studies on this?

Webster It is not easy to do work on seals in the United States. We have had to go to Iceland to do experimental studies where common seals are not protected by the law. Marine biologists (Dr Geraci) predict an outbreak of influenza in seals next year. Since legislation was introduced in the United States in 1972 to totally protect seals, the population has increased remarkably. In the next year seals on the coast of north America are probably going to experience another epidemic of influenza.

Schild I would like to know what your reaction is to the Chinese studies. During all of the animal and avian investigations that you listed, was it common practice to look for Bs and Cs at the same time?

Webster We certainly looked for the viruses but found no type B or C viruses. We have stayed away from serological studies because there is always this problem of non-specific inhibitors.

Schild There have been several unconfirmed reports, for example, from east Europe, of influenza B infections in various species. There was a great explosion at one time of such unconfirmed reports, for example, isolation of H1N1 virus in whales and so on. This caused WHO to suggest rigid guidelines which had to be fulfilled before you accepted that a virus isolated was of authentic origins. This concerned serologic data, isolation and other confirmatory evidence. It is important that these guidelines are adhered to when we are considering strong evidence of involvement of a particular species.

Chu I think one has to take into consideration the breeding practice in different countries; for instance, in China pigs are reared in individual families and sometimes they are free-ranging and they have much more contact with man than in a big pig farm, say, in the United States. You have to consider these social and breeding practices.

Studies on the Haemagglutinin

J. J. SKEHEL[a], R. S. DANIELS[a], A. R. DOUGLAS[a], M. WANG[a], M. KNOSSOW[b], I. A. WILSON[b] and D. C. WILEY[b]

[a]Division of Virology, National Institute for Medical Research, London, UK, [b]Department of Biochemistry and Molecular Biology, Harvard University, Cambridge, Mass., USA

The haemagglutinin of the 1968 Hong Kong virus A/Aichi/2/68 (X-31, Kilbourne, 1969) has a molecular weight of about 225 000 and is a trimer of identical sub-units each consisting of two polypeptide chains, HA1 and HA2 (Wiley et al., 1977). HA1 contains 328 amino acids and HA2 221 and the two polypeptides are linked in each sub-unit by a single disulphide bond between residues 14 of HA1 and 137 of HA2. The amino acid sequences of both chains are known (Verhoeyen et al., 1980; Ward and Dopheide, 1980) and are summarized in Fig. 1. Both polypeptides are glycosylated: at six sites in HA1, at asparagine residues 8, 22, 38, 81, 165 and 285; and at one site in HA2, asparagine 154. In virus particles the molecule is associated with the lipid membrane by a hydrophobic region near the carboxyl terminus of HA2 between residues 185 and 210; the projecting portion of the molecule consisting of the HA1 polypeptides and the HA2 (residues 1–175) polypeptides, of molecular weight about 210 000 is released as a soluble glycoprotein, BHA, by digesting viruses with bromelain.

"The Molecular Virology and Epidemiology of Influenza" (Eds Sir Charles Stuart-Harris and Professor C.W. Potter). Academic Press, London, New York and Orlando, 1984.

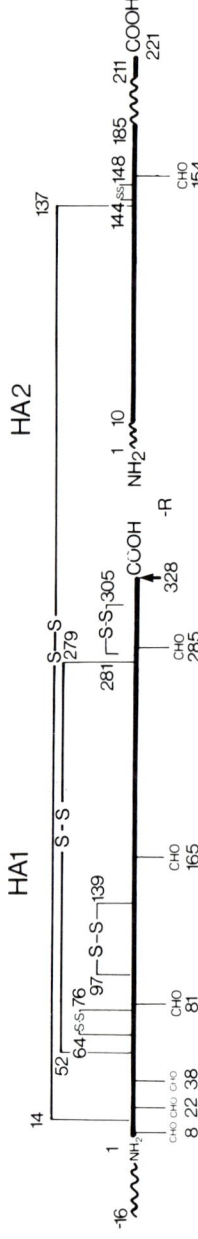

Fig. 1 A summary of the primary structure of the X-31 haemagglutinin. The initial biosynthetic product is depicted to show three important hydrophobic sequences: the 16 residue amino terminal "signal" sequence; the site of proteolytic cleavage which removes an arginine, generates the amino terminus of HA2 and potentiates fusion activity; and the membrane associated carboxyl-terminus of HA2. The asparagine residues which are glycosylated and disulphide bonds are also shown.

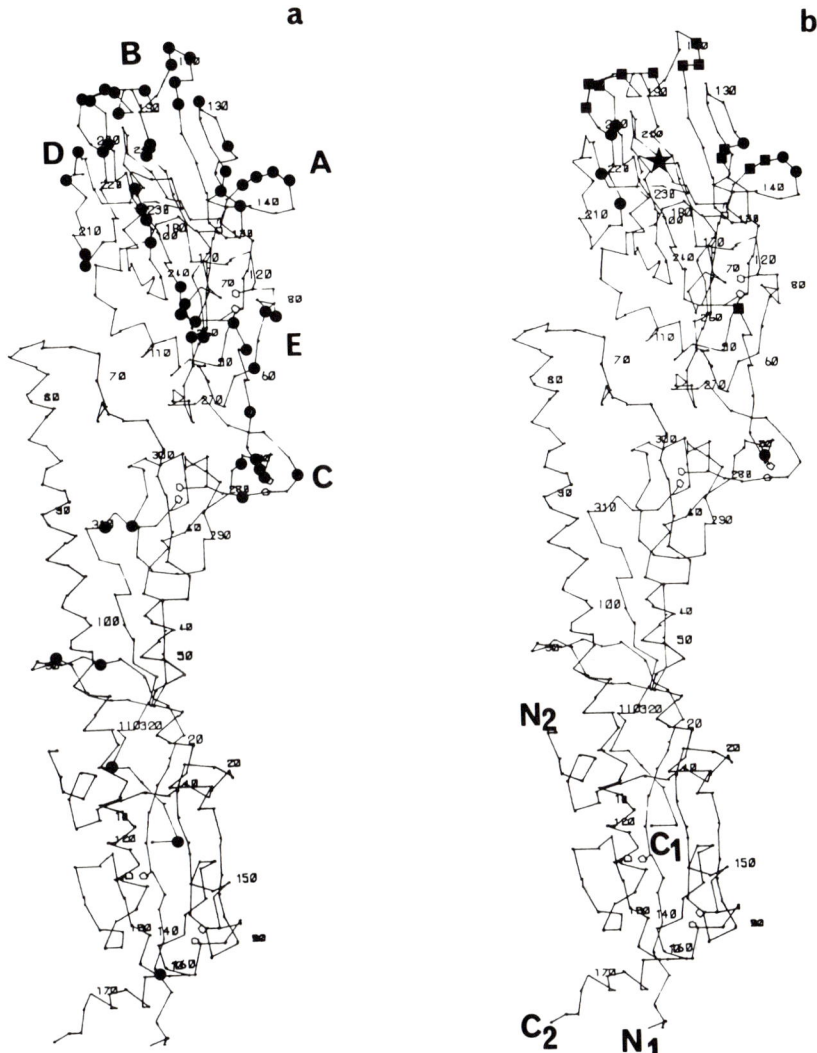

Fig. 2 Tracings of the α-carbon co-ordinates of X-31 haemagglutinin sub-unit to show (a) the amino acid residues in HA1 which have changed during the Hong Kong era between 1968 and 1983 (information from Both and Sleigh (1981), Laver et al. (1980) and Skehel et al. (1983)). The antigenic sites A, B, C, D and E are also indicated. (b) The sites of amino acid substitutions in monoclonal antibody selected variants of ● A/Memphis/71 (Laver et al., 1979) and ■ A/Aichi/68 (Daniels et al., 1983b). In addition ★ indicates residue 226 in the sialic acid binding site and the amino- and carboxyl- termini of HA1 and HA2 are also shown.

X-ray crystallographic analyses of BHA crystals indicate that the amino terminus of HA1 is also near the lipid membrane of the virus. The HA1 chain extends from the base of the molecule through a fibrous stem into a peripheral β-structure-rich region, and then returns to the fibrous region and terminates about 30 Å from the virus membrane. The most prominent features of the part of the sub-unit composed of HA2 residues are two antiparallel α-helices, one 29 Å long which proceeds distally from the membrane end of the molecule to connect through an extended chain with the other helix which stretches 76 Å back towards the membrane. Tracings of the α-carbon atoms of a sub-unit are shown in Fig. 2. Details of the structure have been published (Wilson et al., 1981) and this contribution summarizes their use in attempts to understand the functions of the molecule in receptor binding and membrane fusion and the molecular basis of its antigenicity.

RECEPTOR BINDING

It has been known for some time that influenza viruses bind to cells by interacting with membrane receptor molecules containing sialic acid (see Gottschalk, 1959) and that the virus component involved is the haemagglutinin. This interaction varies in detailed specificity for different influenza viruses and comparative analyses of the haemagglutinins of viruses which demonstrate preferences for binding to carbohydrate side chains containing neuraminic acid in either $\alpha 2,6$ or $\alpha 2,3$ linkage with penultimate residues have been used to obtain information concerning the location of the receptor binding site on the haemagglutinin. The haemagglutinin of X-31 virus recognizes sialyloligosaccharides with the terminal sequence SA $\alpha 2,6$ Gal-, and variants selected for their ability to grow in the presence of non-immune horse serum, a rich source of SA $\alpha 2,6$ Gal- containing glycoprotein inhibitors of haemagglutinin-cell membrane interaction, specifically recognize sialyloligosaccharides with the sequence SA $\alpha 2,3$ Gal-. Comparisons of the amino acid sequences of wild type and variant haemagglutinins deduced from the nucleotide sequences of their RNA genes indicate that they differ only at residue 226 of the HA1 polypeptide chain (Rogers et al., 1983). At this position the wild type haemagglutinin contains leucine (codon CUG) variants which recognize SA $\alpha 2,3$ Gal- linkages contain glutamine (codon CAG), and a variant which bound to sialyloligosaccharides with either SA $\alpha 2,6$ Gal- or SA $\alpha 2,3$ Gal- linkages contained methionine (codon AUG) at residue 226. These observations of changes in receptor binding specificity as a consequence of amino acid substitutions at residue 226 support the proposition that the sialic acid binding site is a surface pocket at the distal end of the haemagglutinin molecule (Wilson et al., 1981). This proposal was originally based on the presence of the conserved residues tyrosine 98, tryptophan 153, histidine 183, glutamic acid 190, and leucine 194, in this pocket and the location of amino acid 226 in this site (Fig. 2) is consistent with a role for this residue in receptor binding.

MEMBRANE FUSION

Binding of virus particles to their receptors is followed by endocytosis and fusion of virus and endosomal membranes. *In vitro*, haemolysis and membrane fusion by influenza viruses have been found to be optimum at about pH 5·0, the pH of endosomes, and also to involve the haemagglutinin. The mechanism of haemagglutinin-mediated fusion is not known but a number of observations indicate that at pH 5·0 haemagglutinin structure is modified and the molecule displays properties which suggest that in the process of fusion it may interact directly with the endosomal membranes. Specifically, on incubation at pH 5·0, soluble haemagglutinin released from virus particles by bromelain digestion, acquires the ability to bind to lipid vesicles, to bind detergent, or to aggregate in lipid and detergent-free solutions. The molecule also becomes susceptible to proteolysis but CD analyses indicate that the structural modifications which these observations imply, do not involve gross conformational changes; they are more consistent with the relative movement of molecular domains which retain their individual secondary structure. The region of the molecule responsible for the pH 5·0-specific aggregation and lipid interactions appears to be the NH_2-terminus of HA2 (Fig. 2). This is the site at which the proteolytic processing of the haemagglutinin precursor, necessary for fusion activation, occurs (see Rott and Klenk, 1977). It is highly conserved, hydrophobic and is released from pH 5·0-haemagglutinin aggregates by thermolysin digestion which reverses the aggregation. For these reasons it is considered that the fusion which initiates virus replication may involve the direct interaction of the HA2 amino terminal region with the endosomal membrane (Skehel *et al.*, 1982; Daniels *et al.*, 1983b).

ANTIGENIC VARIATION IN THE HONG KONG (H3) VIRUSES

Since the initial pandemic of 1968 caused by the influenza virus A/Hong/Kong/1/68, epidemics have occurred in 1972–3, caused by viruses similar to A/England/42/72, in 1975–6 caused by viruses similar to A/Victoria/3/75, and in America in 1979–80 caused by viruses similar to A/Bangkok/1/79. The amino acid sequences of these haemagglutinins and of the haemagglutinins of more recently isolated viruses have been determined by protein and nucleic acid sequencing techniques and the amino acid substitutions were located in the three-dimensional structure of the molecule (Fig. 2). Fourteen amino acid substitutions were detected in the HA1 polypeptide chain of A/England/42/72 compared with that of the A/Aichi/2/68 virus, a further 13 in HA1 of A/Victoria/1/75, and a further 14 in HA1 of A/Bangkok/1/79. A detailed summary of the structural locations and possible stereochemical consequences of these substitutions has been presented before (Wiley et al., 1981).

Further definition of the regions of the 1968 haemagglutinin, which may be involved in antibody binding, is provided by studies of antigenic variants selected by growth in the presence of monoclonal antibodies against the haemagglutinin. Figure 2 shows the locations of single amino acid substitutions in the haemagglutinins of eight variants of the A/Memphis/1/71 virus and 12 antigenic variants of A/Aichi/1/68 (Laver et al., 1980; Daniels et al., 1983b).

From the data summarized in Fig. 2 it is evident that amino acid substitutions on a large fraction of the surface of the globular domain of HA1 appear to affect antibody binding. On the basis of small cross-reactivity among classes of monoclonal antibodies with the antigenic variants and on the basis of the clustering of amino acid substitutions in the natural strains, it is possible to separate the antigenic surface into regions labelled by five different symbols in Fig. 2. Each one of the proposed antigenic sites A, B, C, D and E is identified by a monoclonal antibody-selected variant and each site has accumulated at least one amino acid substitution between each reoccurrence of epidemic influenza since 1968.

Site A includes part of an unusual protruding loop of amino acids (140–146) and the adjacent surface of HA1. The amino acids ALA 138, CYS 139, PHE 147 and PHE(tyr) 148 occurring at each end of this loop are conserved in all haemagglutinins sequenced, including those from viruses from all three pandemic eras and avian and equine viruses. Thus the structural foundation of this antigenic site is conserved.

Site B is centred on a loop of amino acids 155–160 and the region 188–198 which includes an α helix, both located at the distal tip of the HA1 domain. This site was originally defined on the basis of amino acid changes in the natural epidemic viruses of 1972 and 1975. However, more recent data from antigenic variants selected by monoclonal antibodies indicate that it can be split into two partially overlapping sites B1 and B2, which comprise opposite sides of the region (Daniels et al., 1983b). Like site A, the structural potential for site B is conserved in other haemagglutinins.

Site C is a bulge in the tertiary structure of the haemagglutinin, 60 Å from the distal tip in a region containing a highly conserved disulphide bond. Although a few substitutions have been observed in this region in natural isolates, its definition relies heavily on the partial sequence of a single variant selected with monoclonal antibodies against A/Memphis/1/71 (Laver *et al.*, 1980).

Site D In the first three sites, the amino acid substitutions which are suggested to cause antigenic changes are external and, in principle, directly recognizable by molecules of the immune system. Parts of site D depart from this apparently simple situation. Again as in site C, a single monoclonal antibody-selected variant defines this region, along with a number of naturally occurring amino acid substitutions. The only amino acid substitution reported for a monoclonal antibody-selected variant is at serine 205, which is found in the trimer interface between adjacent globular HA1 domains. Whether this substitution is recognized directly as a result of a relative movement of the globular domains or indirectly at a nearby surface is unknown.

Site E On the basis of natural variation, site E was not convincingly defined, although single substitutions have occurred in that region in each epidemic virus since 1968. The subsequent discovery of an antigenic variant selected by monoclonal antibodies which resulted in the single amino acid substitution ASP-63 to ASN-63, further characterized this site and led to an interesting observation. The amino acid substitution found in the antigenic variant creates a new oligosaccharide attachment site ASN-63 CYS-64 THR-65, which is glycosylated. Immunoprecipitation experiments with extracts from variant virus-infected cells prepared in the presence or absence of tunicamycin, which inhibits glycosylation of the haemagglutinin, demonstrate that the addition of the new oligosaccharide chain is required to escape reaction with the monoclonal antibodies. Thus the ASP to ASN change is not recognized directly, but instead the new oligosaccharide chain on the variant haemagglutinin must interfere with antibody binding to a nearby region of the haemagglutinin surface. This is a direct indication that carbohydrate can alter the antigenic structure of the molecule by effectively covering some region of its surface, an idea that became apparent when the positions of oligosaccharide attachment sites from fowl plague virus and the Asian strain A/Japan/305/57 haemagglutinin sequences were noted to occur in the regions A, B, and D described as antigenic sites in the 1968 structure (Wiley *et al.*, 1981).

Similar immunoprecipitation experiments with the site E monoclonal antibodies on two viruses in the Hong Kong pandemic era A/England/878/69 and A/Victoria/3/75, which are glycosylated at position 63 also indicate that the oligosaccharide is required to prevent reaction with the antibodies, providing evidence for the epidemiological significance of carbohydrate-mediated modifications of haemagglutinin antigenicity.

ACKNOWLEDGMENTS

We thank David Stevens, Rose Gonsalves and Gary White for assistance, and acknowledge support from the National Institutes of Health, Grant No. AI-13654, and from Nato Research Grant No. 0222215/83.

REFERENCES

Both, G. W. and Sleigh, M. J. (1981). Conservation and variation in the haemagglutinins of Hong Kong subtype influenza viruses during antigenic drift. *J. Virol.* **39**, 663–672.

Daniels, R. S., Douglas, A. R., Skehel, J. J., Waterfield, M.D., Wilson, I. A. and Wiley, D. C. (1983a). Studies of the influenza virus haemagglutinin in the pH 5 conformation. *In* "The Origins of Pandemic Influenza". (Ed. W. G. Laver) (in press).

Daniels, R. S., Douglas, A. R., Skehel, J. J. and Wiley, D. C. (1983b). Analysis of the antigenicity of influenza haemagglutinin at the pH optimum for virus-mediated membrane fusion. *J. Gen. Virol.* **64**, 1657–1662.

Gottschalk, A. (1959). Chemistry of virus receptors. *In* "The Viruses" Vol. 3 (Eds F. M. Burnet and W. M. Stanley) Academic Press, London and New York, pp. 51–61.

Kilbourne, E. D. (1969). Future influenza vaccines and the use of genetic recombinants. *Bull. WHO* **41**, 643–645.

Laver, W. G., Air, G. M., Webster, R. G., Gerhard, W., Ward, C. W. and Dopheide, T. A. (1979). Antigenic drift in type A influenza virus: sequence differences in the haemagglutinin of Hong Kong (H3N2) variants selected with monoclonal hydridoma antibodies. *Virology* **98**, 226–237.

Laver, W. G., Air, G. M., Dopheide, T. A. and Ward, C. W. (1980). Amino acid sequence changes in the haemagglutinin of A/Hong Kong (H3N2) influenza virus during the period 1968–77. *Nature* (Lond.) **283**, 454–457.

Rogers, G. N., Paulson, J. C., Daniels, R. S., Skehel, J. J., Wilson, I. A. and Wiley, D. C. (1983). Single amino acid substitutions in influenza haemagglutinin change receptor binding specificity. *Nature* (Lond.) **304**, 76–78.

Rott, R. and Klenk, H.-D. (1977). Structure and assembly of viral envelopes. *In* "Cell Surface Reviews" (Eds G. Poste and G. L. Nicolson) North-Holland, Amsterdam, pp. 47–81.

Skehel, J. J., Bayley, P. M., Brown, E. B., Martin, S. R., Waterfield, M. D., White, J. M., Wilson, I. A. and Wiley, D. C. (1982). Changes in the conformation of influenza virus haemagglutinin at the pH optimum of virus-mediated membrane fusion. *Proc. Natl. Acad. Sci. USA* **79**, 968–972.

Skehel, J. J., Daniels, R. S., Douglas, A. R. and Wiley, D.C. (1983). Antigenic and amino acid sequence variations in the haemagglutinins of type A influenza viruses recently isolated from humans. *Bull. WHO* **61**, 671–676.

Verhoeyen, M., Fang, R., Min Jou, W., Devos, R., Huylebroeck, D., Saman, E. and Fiers, W. (1980). Antigenic drift between the haemagglutinin of the Hong Kong influenza strains A/Aichi/2/68 and A/Victoria/3/75. *Nature* (Lond.) **286**, 771–776.

Ward, C. W. and Dopheide, T. A. G. (1980). Completion of the amino acid sequence of a Hong Kong influenza haemagglutinin heavy chain: Sequence of cyanogen bromide fragment CNI. *Virology* **103**, 37–53.

Wiley, D. C., Skehel, J. J. and Waterfield, M. D. (1977). Evidence from studies with a cross-linking reagent that the haemagglutinin of influenza virus is a trimer. *Virology* **79**, 446–448.

Wiley, D. C., Wilson, I. A. and Skehel, J. J. (1981). Structural identification of the antibody-binding sites of Hong Kong influenza haemagglutinin and their involvement in antigenic variation. *Nature* (Lond.) **289**, 373–378.

Wilson, I. A., Skehel, J. J. and Wiley, D. C. (1981). The haemagglutinin membrane glycoprotein of influenza virus: structure at 3 Å resolution. *Nature* (Lond.) **289**, 366–373.

DISCUSSION

Murphy Have you any idea how the N terminus of the HA 2 polypeptide could get into approximation with the cellular membrane if it is 100 angstroms away from it?

Skehel There are at least two possibilities. One is that if you try to look at the structure of the haemagglutinin after incubation at pH5, the HA 1 regions of the molecule have come apart. So far—this is just by microscopy so the resolution is nothing compared with crystallography—you do not see anything of HA 2 and do not know whether it is pushed forward as a result. The second possibility is that, as another consequence of the structural change which happens at pH5, the molecule becomes susceptible to proteolysis. The first clip which happens—and it happens extremely simply—is at residue 27 of HA 1 and it leads to the whole of HA 1 floating off the molecule. It floats off not as a trimer of HA 1 but as HA 1 in monomers. That is because the junction between the HA 1 regions at the head have been broken by acid incubation. The possibility exists that that also happens in endosomes. There is no evidence for that but it is a possibility.

Kilbourne Before calling on anyone else, it seems to me that the weight of current evidence is against glycosylation as being terribly important in mediating significant antigenic differences.

Skehel Why do you say that?

Kilbourne Why do I summarize it in that way? Well, I am thinking of Compan's recent studies, where he has looked at variance in different glycosylation sites, and drew such conclusions from those data. I wanted to ask Dr Both if he would comment on his recent findings with the swine haemagglutinin, because there are significant differences there in terms of glycosylation from some of the other HA1s that have been looked at.

Both I happen to have a slide of that.

Skehel While Dr Both is getting his slide ready, may I say that in this position 63, there have also been substitutions for an asparagine in natural isolates of the Hong Kong series, one in 1969, England/878/69 and also in the Victoria/75 virus. If you do the same experiment with either the 69 or the Victoria virus—that is, grow the virus in the presence of tunicamycin and then see if it will react with the monoclone antibody which recognizes residue 63, it does. So it seems that in those natural isolates the carbohydrate is also preventing that antibody from interacting. Therefore, although we could go through the evidence against it, I suspect that the presence of carbohydrate side chains is going to be highly significant and in fact comparative analysis of the haemagglutinins from all the sub-types suggests that in some cases where particular regions of the molecule in one sub-type do not appear to be antigenic, a carbohydrate side chain can be found.

Kilbourne I just want to say that this does not reflect any personal position on my part.

Skehel It is an interesting question. The monoclonal antibody is the first direct evidence that it might be involved. The importance of it is something else.

Both This slide is a comparison of the amino acid sequences for the WSN strain, PR8 and swine influenza (New Jersey/11/76) which has been recently sequenced. Wherever there is a letter change it indicates an amino acid difference between WSN and the other two strains. The carbohydrate sites are indicated by the black boxes. The point you can take from this is that there are certainly differences in glycosylation between these three H1 haemagglutinins. In particular you can see that PR8 and swine viruses have lost the site at position 56–59, and that carbohydrate was likely to mask the area called antigenic site E. Some of these amino acids (68–75) would be included in that region and you can see that where these two strains have lost the carbohydrate site there are a significant number of amino acid changes in that region, particularly for the New Jersey swine. Similarly, in the region at 125, you can see there is actually an amino acid deletion in the WSN strain relative to the other two, but in the PR8 strain the carbohydrate site is retained while it is lost in the New Jersey swine strain. Again, there is significant amino acid variations in this strain. There is one other carbohydrate site down in the so-called C-antigenic region and again there are a significant number of amino acid changes which occur in the swine 'flu strain which is the only one to have lost the glycosylation sites.

This is circumstantial evidence that is entirely consistent with Brownlee's interpretation that carbohydrates can mask particular areas of the protein and when the carbohydrate is missing those areas are susceptible to antibody pressure.

Kilbourne   Does Brownlee have anything to add to Dr Both's comments?

Brownlee   Only that I would emphasize what Skehel said. Perhaps we have all underestimated the possible role of carbohydrate. First we must distinguish suggestions and evidence. We derived good circumstantial evidence that carbohydrate was involved in antigenicity from a detailed study of many point mutations involved in the antigenicity of H1 sub-type field strains. We arrived at an antigenic map of four major antigenic sites and then noticed that those were not the same as the four proposed for the haemagglutinin of the H3 sub-types. Only two are common the H1 and H3; two are different.

In seeking an explanation for this surprising observation, it became obvious that carbohydrate was involved. Simply, where there was a carbohydrate one did not have an antigenic site. We proposed that carbohydrate could modulate antigenicity by masking regions of the haemagglutinin which would otherwise be antigenic.

Scholtissek   We have recently isolated a mutant of fowl plague virus which has lost by mutation one of the carbohydrate side chains and we have studied this with three monoclonal antibodies provided by Skehel. We did not find significant changes in the reaction of monoclonal antibodies when compared with wild type virus. However, this carbohydrate side chain was on the HA 2. It is important to look at where the carbohydrate side chains are bound to the protein backbone, whether its removal might change the antigenicity or not.

Skehel   It is not the suggestion that the carbohydrate chain is antigenic or would be an antibody-binding site?

Couch   This may be just a related question and it may be naive but have any of these strains with the carbohydrates been used to immunize ferrets and then see how they react with different viruses? Does this alter that kind of reactivity?

Skehel   By and large single monoclone-selected variants do not respond differently with ferret sera than do the wild type because the sera contain antibodies with many different kinds of specificity. But the England/878 virus, for example, which was published some time ago, had I suppose, changes in two important regions, one at residue 144 and one at the site at 63. If you compare the reaction with ferret sera against X-31 virus of the monoclonal antibody-selected mutant which has just a change at 144, with the England/878 virus which has a change at both 144 and 63, then there is a bigger difference between England/878 and X31 than there is between the 144 mutant and the X-31 virus. As far as I know, that is all that is available. It is hardly evidence, but it is in the right direction.

Klenk It is very important to do all of these studies with monoclonal antibodies as Skehel has done and not with polyclonal antibodies. If you use polyclonal antibodies you do not see significant differences in the interaction with glycosylated haemagglutinin and with completely unglycosylated haemagglutinin that has been obtained in the presence of tunicamycin or other glycosylation inhibitor. So you really have to have specific monoclonal antibodies.

Couch You have to modify more of the active sites on HA 1, that was my interpretation of what Skehel was just telling us. That has been demonstrated to alter reactivity with ferret sera.

Skehel The evidence with ferret sera is that you get a bigger difference with England/878 with ferret sera against X31 wild type than you do with a monoclonal antibody-selected variant which only has a change at 144.

Kendal Would you care to speculate after viewing the total sequence data now available within and between sub-types as to what portions of the HA are responsible for sub-type specific antigenic determinants within the molecule?

Skehel I did not know that those actually existed.

Kendal Do you feel the fact that two viruses can be typed as H3, that might show no reactions or cross-reactions whatsoever in H1 tests, result from a variety of different types of antigenic determinants within the sub-type, or that there are one or more that are conserved throughout the sub-type and which vary between sub-types.

Skehel We certainly could not. The only way to do it is to get monoclonal antibodies which are cross-reacting. What Kendal refers to is the basis for classification of viruses into sub-types, that is the reaction in immuno-diffusion with hyperimmune rabbit sera. Webster probably has antibodies which react with quite a lot of the human H3s. Do you know what they recognize?

Webster We do not know the sequence change of those monoclonal variants.

Laver How do you think that antibodies to the HA neutralize infectivity?

Skehel Simply it could prevent binding to sialic acid. I imagine it could do other things too. I imagine it could just bind and not affect either activity and be recognized by a cell which contains an Fc receptor. I also imagine that certain antibodies could prevent the molecule from being involved in its fusion activity, e.g. by preventing the conformational change. But I do not know how it actually happens. I do not believe it affects transcriptase activity.

Palese I would like to add to the comment about cross-reactivity of haemagglutinins. We have been able to obtain antibody preparations made against the HA2 portion of influenza A viruses and then one can find cross-reactivity among sub-type haemagglutinins. This is not surprising because the sequence of the HA2 is very similar from one sub-type to another. One can also detect slight cross-reactivity going from A to B viruses.

Kilbourne Before we get on to that point, I want to make an amendment to this discussion. That is at the meeting at WHO at Geneva some three years ago, when we were considering classification and division of sub-types, in a working paper I did go through the literature as well as some of my own experiments and I came up with some examples of cross-reactivity amongst sub-types which are antibody-mediated, not T-cell mediated. That has to be kept in mind as a background. It is perhaps not surprising that a molecule with so many shared residues would have some kind of potential cross-reactivity. Peter, you have some data referring to the haemagglutinin structure of yet another subtype.

Palese We have recently obtained the complete sequence of an influenza B virus haemagglutinin and I have some slides comparing this sequence with that of an influenza C virus haemagglutinin.

This slide shows an amino acid sequence comparison of the B/Lee/40 and the A/PR8/34 haemagglutinins. We are using the single letter code for the different sequence homology between these two haemagglutinins. The yellow areas indicate that there are identical amino acids in the B/Lee and in the PR8 sequence that are particularly interesting. I believe that the HA2 is very much conserved. You can see here many amino acids which are identical. In addition, the cysteines, which are in red, are also very much conserved in the A and B virus haemagglutinins.

One can look at this by using dot matrices. Without going into detail one uses a computer for comparison of the two sequences. When there is some homology between the two sequences one gets a diagonal on the dot matrix. We can clearly see on the slide the area of the HA2 which is conserved between the two haemagglutinins. It is quite interesting that the A and B haemagglutinins have quite a lot of sequence conservation both in the HA1 and the HA2 portions.

In contrast, we have recently obtained the sequence of the influenza C/Cal/78 virus haemagglutinin. When we do the same kind of comparison using dot matrices we can see there is practically no sequence homology between the B and the C virus haemagglutinins. When we do the same thing with the C/Cal and the A virus haemagglutinins, B and C haemagglutinin genes have common ancestors. The reason for that is that if we look specifically at conserved structural features then we can see there is some relationship between the three molecules. This is shown on the next slide, which is a complicated one. We have attempted to align the A, B and C sequences. Although there is no direct sequence homology any more, what comes out is that many of the cysteines in the three molecules are conserved. I would draw your attention to the HA 2 portions. The three internal cysteines which are conserved in the A and the B virus haemagglutinin are also found in the influenza C virus haemagglutinin with the same spacing as observed for the two other haemagglutinins. There is a conserved cysteine right at the beginning of the HA 1 which is most likely linking the HA 1 and the HA 2 together. However, beyond the conservation of the cysteines there is basically no sequence homology left. Evolution has gone to completion, as I call it; there appears to be a complete exchange of individual amino acids going from A to B to C haemagglutinins but certain structural features are conserved in particular when we look at a hydrophilic plot, we see that hydrophobic signal peptides are conserved. In addition, these are conserved hydrophobic amino terminal regions of the HA 2 region. However, precise amino acids are conserved in the A and B virus haemagglutinins but not in the C virus haemagglutinin. Finally the carboxyl terminal regions of all 3 HA 2s are hydrophobic suggesting that they have probably retained the same structure, where the haemagglutinins sit in the membrane.

In conclusion, we have completed the sequence of an influenza C virus haemagglutinin and it tells us that despite the lack of sequence homology there is still similar function and, most likely, similar structure among the A, B and C virus haemagglutinins.

Skehel Was the amino terminus of the HA 2 C lined up, irrespective of homology?

Palese We know where the HA 2 portion starts because of amino acid data obtained by Dr Compan's group.

Skehel Is it lined up there? There was a stretch of hydrophobics to the right of it.

Palese We lined it up, yes. We allowed for a few insertions and deletions and succeeded in aligning the cysteine residues. The amino terminal portion of the HA 2 has different amino acids not shared by the A and B viruses, but it is still hydrophobic.

Skehel It is not. It has two aspartic acids right in there.

Palese If you plot it, using the computer program, the first fifteen are as hydrophobic as those of the A or B virus HA 2s.

Skehel Because the next 11 are, but the actual amino terminal ones are not.

Palese Maybe we can discuss this later.

Brownlee When you have sequences so dissimilar, one of the problems is alignment. How do you know that you are not just forcing an artificial alignment? How do you know your alignment has any significance? If you just take any two random amino acid sequences there is, I believe, a 70% chance of homology.

Palese This is certainly a problem. As you saw, there is no detectable homology using the dot matrices. What one has to do is to weight the cysteines more heavily than the other amino acids, and if one does this then one can align it. Also, the total length of the HA 2s is practically identical for all three haemagglutinins.

Brownlee Is you optional alignment greater than 7%?

Palese Not much. I think the total is about 8–10%.

Brownlee So even with you forcing the issue you may get more than you would get if you took two random amino acid sequences.

Palese Basically, yes, that is correct, except that the conserved cysteines would not be there nor would the hydrophobic regions be conserved.

Both I wanted to make one quick comment regarding Skehel's comment on the hydrophobicity of Palese's sequence. We have recently been agonizing over a functional region of one of the Rotavirus proteins, whether it is a trans-membrane region or not, and it also has a charged residue in the middle of it. Someone pointed out to me that in the bacterial rhodopsin situation there are multiple charged residues in the membrane. It does not rule out the HA 2 region of the influenza virus which can still interact with membranes.

Skehel They clearly interact with each other in the model of the rhodopsin molecule. Where there is a single chain going across the membrane it might not be easy. In rhodopsin charges are compensated by charged residues on neighbouring chains.

Influenza Virus Neuraminidase: Structure and Variation

W. G. LAVER,[a] P. M. COLMAN, C. W. WARD,
J. M. VARGHESE,[b] G. M. AIR,[c] R. G. WEBSTER,
V. HINSHAW, L. BROWN,[d] and D. JACKSON[e]

[a]John Curtin School of Medical Research, Canberra City, Australia; [b]CSIRO Division of Protein Chemistry, Melbourne, Australia; [c]Laboratory for Special Cancer Research, University of Alabama in Birmingham, Birmingham, Alabama, USA, [d]Division of Virology, St Jude Children's Research Hospital, Memphis, Tennessee, USA, [e]Department of Microbiology, University of Melbourne, Melbourne, Australia

Two glycoproteins are embedded in the membrane of influenza virus, a neuraminidase and a haemagglutinin (Laver and Valentine, 1969). Haemagglutinin mediates attachment of the virus to host cells, (Hirst, 1941) via a sialic acid-containing glycoconjugate receptor (Gottschalk, 1966) and the subsequent fusion of viral and host cell membranes (Skehel, see p. 65, this volume). A number of roles have been suggested for the neuraminidase (acylneuraminyl-hydrolase, EC 3.2.1.18). The enzyme catalyses cleavage of the α-ketosidic linkage between terminal sialic acid and an adjacent sugar

"The Molecular Virology and Epidemiology of Influenza" (Eds Sir Charles Stuart-Harris and Professor C.W. Potter). Academic Press, London, New York and Orlando, 1984.

residue (Gottschalk, 1957; Drzeniek, 1972). This reaction permits transport of the virus through mucin and destroys the haemagglutinin receptor (Burnet and Stone, 1947) on the host cell, thus enabling elution of progeny virus particles from infected cells. The removal of sialic acid from the carbohydrate moiety of newly synthesized haemagglutinin and neuraminidase is also necessary to prevent self-aggregation of the virus (Palese et al., 1974). In general, then, the role of neuraminidase may be one of permitting mobility of the virus both to and from the site of infection.

The neuraminidase exists as a mushroom-shaped spike on the surface of the virion. It has a box-like head made out of four co-planar and roughly spherical sub-units and a centrally attached stalk containing a hydrophobic region by which it is embedded in the viral membrane (Fig. 1) (Laver and Valentine, 1969; Wrigley et al., 1973; Wrigley, 1979).

The neuraminidase molecule is composed of a single polypeptide chain coded by gene segment 6 and is oriented in the virus membrane in the opposite way to the haemagglutinin (Fig. 2). No post-translational cleavage of the NA polypeptide occurs, no signal peptide is split off and even the initiating methionine is retained (Blok et al., 1982). No processing at the C-terminus takes place—the C-terminal sequence, -MET-PRO-ILE predicted from the N2 gene sequence, is found in intact NA molecules isolated from virus, and in the pronase-released NA heads (Blok et al., 1982). A sequence of six polar amino acids at the N-terminus of the NA polypeptide, which are totally conserved in the nine different NA sub-types, is followed by a sequence of hydrophobic amino acids which probably represent the transmembrane region of the NA stalk (Blok and Air, 1982).

This sequence is not conserved at all between sub-types (apart from conservation of hydrophobicity). Pronase cleaves the polypeptide in the positions shown (Figs 1 and 2), removing the stalk and releasing the enzymically and antigenically active head of the NA which, in some cases, can be crystallized (Fig. 3).

ANTIGENIC VARIATION IN THE NEURAMINIDASE

Antigenic shift and antigenic drift occur in the NA; among the human influenza viruses antigenic shift occurred in 1957, with the emergence of the H2N2 sub-type and the replacement of N1 by N2.

Gene sequences (and the deduced amino acid sequences) of the NA from five N2 strains (Elleman et al., 1982; Ward et al., 1982; Bentley and Brownlee, 1982; van Rompuy et al., 1982) and two N1 strains (Fields et al., 1981; Hiti and Nayak, 1982) have been obtained. The overall homology

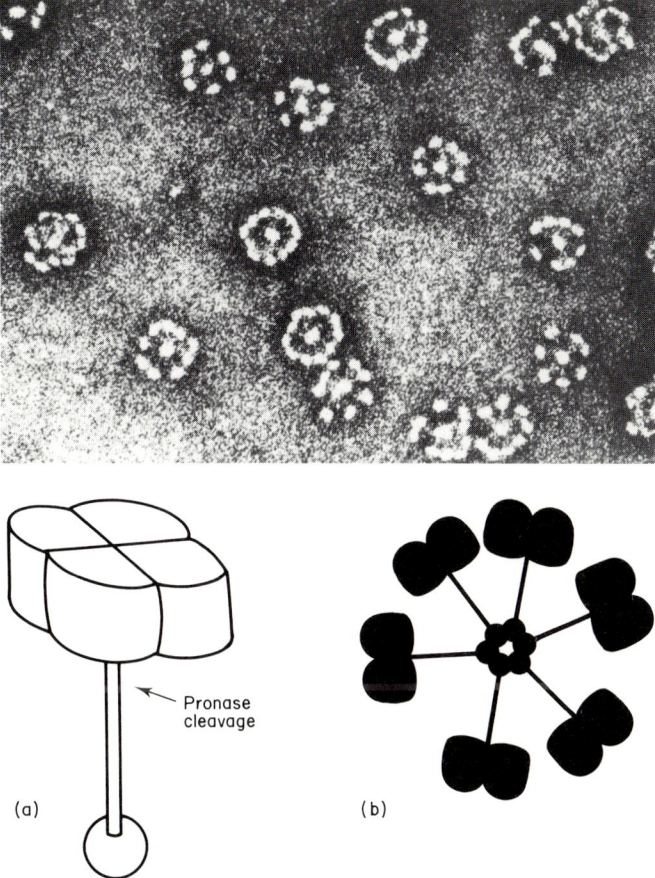

Fig. 1 Electron micrograph and diagram showing detergent-released neuraminidase molecules from which the detergent has been removed. The NA molecules have aggregated by the hydrophobic region near the end of the stalk which serves to attach the NA to the lipid of the virus envelope. Treatment of virus particles with pronase releases the head of the NA which carries the enzymic and antigenic activities of the molecule and, in some cases, can be crystallized. Electron micrograph was taken by N. Wrigley.

between the amino acid sequences of the N1 and N2 neuraminidase was estimated to be 39%.

Antigenic drift in N2 neuraminidase has been investigated most extensively. Neuraminidase-inhibition tests using polyclonal hyperimmune rabbit antisera showed that the neuraminidases of the 1957 and 1975 H2N2 and H3N2 strains were antigenically very different (Table I).

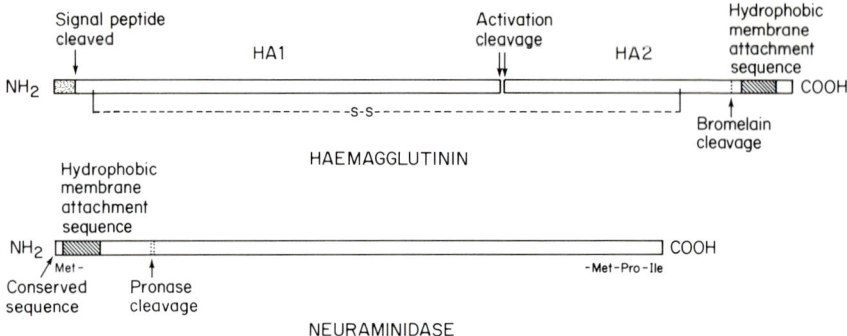

Fig. 2 Diagrammatic representation contrasting certain features of the haemagglutinin and neuraminidase polypeptides. (1) Haemagglutinin. The HA is synthesized as a single polypeptide. Following its synthesis an N-terminal signal peptide is cleaved off and the molecule is cleaved further into HA1 and HA2 with the removal of one or more intervening amino acids. This latter cleavage is necessary for the virus to be infectious. HA1 and HA2 remain linked by a single disulphide bond and each HA spike contains three of these dimers. A sequence of hydrophobic amino acids near the C-terminus of HA2 serves to anchor the HA in the lipid of the virus membrane. Treatment with bromelain removes this hydrophobic region without damaging the rest of the molecule which, in some cases, can be crystallized. (2) Neuraminidase. The neuraminidase is orientated in the virus membrane in the opposite way to the haemagglutinin. No post-translational cleavage of the NA polypeptide occurs, no signal peptide is split off and even the initiating methionine is retained. No processing at the C-terminus takes place—the C-terminal sequence -MET-PRO-ILE predicted from the N2 gene sequence is found in intact NA molecules isolated from virus and in the pronase-released NA heads. A sequence of six polar amino acids at the N-terminus of the NA polypeptide, which are totally conserved in the nine different NA sub-types, is followed by a sequence of hydrophobic amino acids which probably represent the transmembrane region of the NA stalk. This sequence is not conserved at all between sub-types (apart from conservation of hydrophobicity). Pronase cleaves the polypeptide in the positions shown, removing the stalk and releasing the enzymically and antigenically active head of the NA which, in some cases, can be crystallized.

These antigenic differences are associated with a number of sequence changes in the NA polypeptide (Fig. 4) but which of these are located in antigenic sites and which have no effect on antigenicity is not precisely known.

SEQUENCE CHANGES IN THE NEURAMINIDASE OF "MONOCLONAL VARIANTS"

Antigenic variants of neuraminidase have been selected with a frequency of approximately 10^{-5} after a single passage of A/Tokyo/3/67 influenza virus in

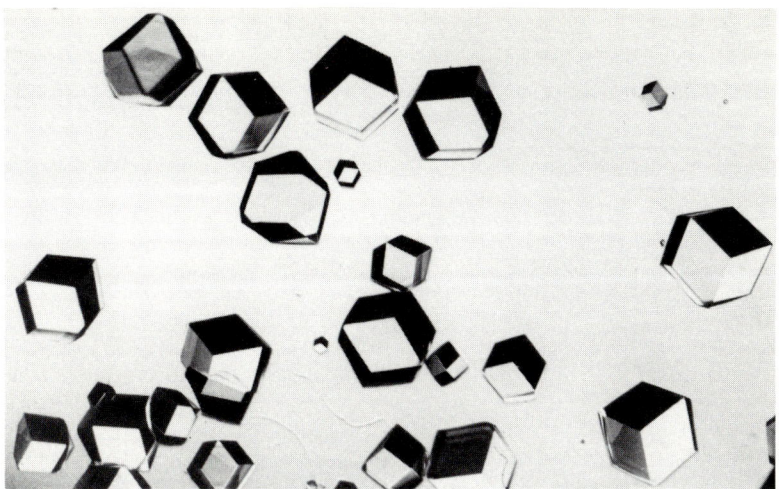

Fig. 3 Crystals of pronase-released neuraminidase heads of NA sub-type N9 (intact N9 neuraminidase molecules possess haemagglutinin activity).

The NA was crystallized by mixing equal volumes of NA solution (10–15 mg/ml in water) and potassium phosphate buffer (1·7 M pH 6·6) which was equilibrated through the vapour phase with a reservoir of 1·9 M phosphate pH 6·8. The large rhombic dodecahedral crystals grew in a few days.

TABLE I
Cross-reactions (in neuraminidase-inhibition tests) of the neuraminidase of viruses isolated in 1957 and 1975

	Virus	
Serum	X-7F1 (RI/5$^+$/57)	Vic/1/75
Anti-X-7F1 NA	1500	10
Anti-Vic/75 NA	10	5000

Note: N1 tests using fetuin substrate were done as described (Aymard-Henry et al., 1973). Hyperimmune rabbit antisera to NA heads from X-7F1 and VIC/75 viruses were made as described (Webster and Laver, 1967).

the presence of monoclonal antibody to the neuraminidase (Webster et al., 1982). These "monoclonal variants", like those of influenza virus haemagglutinin previously described (Laver et al., 1981), do not bind at all to the antibody used for their selection, and each shows a single change in the amino-acid sequence of the neuraminidase.

```
RI/5⁻/57      Met Asn Pro Asn Gln Lys Thr Ile Thr Ile Gly Ser Val Ser Leu Thr Ile Ala Thr Val
Tokyo/3/67    Met Asn Pro Asn Gln Lys Ile Ile Thr Ile Gly Ser Val Ser Leu Thr Ile Ala Thr Val
NT/60/68      Met Asn Pro Asn Gln Lys Ile Ile Thr Ile Gly Ser Val Ser Leu Thr Ile Ala Thr Val
Udorn/307/72  Met Asn Pro Asn Gln Lys Ile Ile Thr Ile Gly Ser Val Ser Leu Thr Ile Ala Thr Ile
Vic/3/75      Met Asn Pro Asn Gln Lys Ile Ile Thr Ile Gly Ser Val Ser Leu Thr Ile Ala Thr Ile
                                      10                                              20

RI/5⁻/57      Cys Phe Leu Met Gln Ile Ala Ile Leu Ala Thr Thr Val Thr Leu His Phe Lys Gln His
Tokyo/3/67    Cys Phe Leu Met Gln Ile Ala Met Leu Val Thr Thr Val Thr Leu His Phe Lys Gln His
NT/60/68      Cys Phe Leu Met Gln Thr Ala Ile Leu Val Thr Thr Val Thr Leu His Phe Lys Gln Tyr
Udorn/307/72  Cys Phe Leu Met Gln Ile Ala Ile Gln Val Thr Thr Val Thr Leu His Phe Lys Gln Tyr
Vic/3/75      Cys Phe Leu Met Gln Ile Ala Ile Leu Val Thr Thr Val Thr Leu His Phe Lys Gln Tyr
                                      30                                              40

RI/5⁻/57      Glu Cys Asp Ser Pro Ala Ser Asn Gln Val Met Pro Cys Glu Pro Ile Ile Ile Glu Arg
Tokyo/3/67    Asp Cys Asp Ser
NT/60/68      Glu Cys Asp Ser Pro Ala Ser Asn Gln Val Met Pro Cys Glu Pro Ile Ile Ile Glu Arg
Udorn/307/72  Glu Cys Asp Ser Pro Ala Asn Asn Gln Val Met Pro Cys Glu Pro Ile Ile Ile Glu Arg
Vic/3/75      Glu Cys Asp Ser Pro Ala Asn Asn Gln Val Met Pro Cys Glu Pro Ile Ser Ile Glu Arg
                                      50                                              60

RI/5⁻/57      Asn Ile Thr Glu Ile Val Tyr Leu Asn Asn Thr Thr Ile Glu Lys Glu Ile Cys Pro Glu
Tokyo/3/67                                                      Glu Lys Glu Ile Cys Pro Lys
NT/60/68      Asn Ile Thr Glu Ile Val Tyr Leu Asn Asn Thr Thr Ile Glu Lys Glu Ile Cys Pro Lys
Udorn/307/72  Asn Ile Thr Glu Ile Val Tyr Leu Thr Asn Thr Thr Ile Glu Lys Gly Ile Cys Pro Lys
Vic/3/75      Asn Ile Thr Glu Ile Val Tyr Leu Thr Asn Thr Thr Ile Glu Lys Gly Ile Cys Pro Lys
                                      70                                              80

RI/5⁻/57      Val Val Glu Tyr Arg Asn Trp Ser Lys Pro Gln Cys Gln Ile Thr Gly Phe Ala Pro Phe
Tokyo/67      Val Val Glu Tyr Arg Asn Trp Ser Lys Pro Gln Cys Gln Ile Thr Gly Phe Ala Pro Phe
NT/60/68      Val Val Glu Tyr Arg Asn Trp Ser Lys Pro Gln Cys Gln Ile Thr Gly Phe Ala Pro Phe
Udorn/72      Leu Val Glu Tyr Arg Asn Trp Ser Lys Pro Gln Cys Lys Ile Thr Gly Phe Ala Pro Phe
Vic/3/75      Leu Val Glu Tyr Arg Asn Trp Ser Lys Pro Gln Cys Lys Ile Thr Gly Phe Ala Pro Phe
                                      90                                             100

RI/5⁻/57      Ser Lys Asp Asn Ser Ile Arg Leu Ser Ala Gly Gly Asp Ile Trp Val Thr Arg Glu Pro
Tokyo/3/67    Ser Lys Asp Asn Ser Ile Arg Leu Ser Ala Gly Gly Asp Ile Trp Val Thr Arg Glu Pro
NT/60/68      Ser Lys Asp Asn Ser Ile Arg Leu Ser Ala Gly Gly Asp Ile Trp Val Thr Arg Glu Pro
Udorn/72      Ser Lys Asp Asn Ser Ile Arg Leu Ser Ala Gly Gly Asp Ile Trp Val Thr Arg Glu Pro
Vic/3/75      Ser Lys Asp Asn Ser Ile Arg Leu Ser Ala Gly Gly Asp Ile Trp Val Thr Arg Glu Pro
                                     110                                             120

RI/5⁻/57      Tyr Val Ser Cys Asp Pro Gly Lys Cys Tyr Gln Phe Ala Leu Gly Gln Gly Thr Thr Leu
Tokyo/67      Tyr Val Ser Cys Asp Pro Val Lys Cys Tyr Gln Phe Ala Leu Gly Gln Gly Thr Thr Leu
NT/60/68      Tyr Val Ser Cys Asp His Gly Lys Cys Tyr Gln Phe Ala Leu Gly Gln Gly Thr Thr Leu
Udorn/72      Tyr Val Ser Cys Asp Pro Gly Lys Cys Tyr Gln Phe Ala Leu Gly Gln Gly Thr Thr Leu
Vic/75        Tyr Val Ser Cys Asp Pro Arg Lys Cys Tyr Gln Phe Ala Leu Gly Gln Gly Thr Thr Leu
                                     130                                             140

RI/5⁻/57      Asp Asn Lys His Ser Asn Gly Thr Ile His Asp Arg Ile Pro His Arg Thr Leu Leu Met
Tokyo/67      Asp Asn Lys His Ser Asn Asp Thr Val His Asp Arg Ile Pro His Arg Thr Leu Leu Met
NT/60/68      Asp Asn Lys His Ser Asn Asp Thr Ile His Asp Arg Ile Pro His Arg Thr Leu Leu Met
Udorn/72      Asp Asn Lys His Ser Asn Asp Thr Ile His Asp Arg Thr Pro His Arg Thr Leu Leu Met
Vic/75        Glu Asn Lys His Ser Asn Asp Thr Ile His Asp Arg Thr Pro His Arg Thr Leu Leu Met
                                     150                                             160

RI/5⁻/57      Asn Glu Leu Gly Val Pro Phe His Leu Gly Thr Lys Gln Val Cys Val Ala Trp Ser Ser
Tokyo/67      Asn Glu Leu Gly Val Pro Phe His Leu Gly Thr Arg Gln Val Cys Ile Ala Trp Ser Ser
NT/60/68      Asn Glu Leu Gly Val Pro Phe His Leu Gly Thr Arg Gln Val Cys Ile Ala Trp Ser Ser
Udorn/72      Asn Glu Leu Gly Val Pro Phe His Leu Gly Thr Arg Gln Val Cys Ile Gly Trp Ser Ser
Vic/75        Asn Glu Leu Gly Val Pro Phe His Leu Gly Thr Arg Gln Val Cys Ile Ala Trp Ser Ser
                                     170                                             180

RI/5⁻/57      Ser Ser Cys His Asp Gly Lys Ala Trp Leu His Val Cys Val Thr Gly Asp Asp Arg Asn
Tokyo/67      Ser Ser Cys His Asp Gly Lys Ala Trp Leu His Val Cys Ile Thr Gly Asp Asp Asp Asn
NT/60/68      Ser Ser Cys His Asp Gly Lys Ala Trp Leu His Val Cys Ile Thr Gly Asp Asp Lys Asn
Udorn/72      Ser Ser Cys His Asp Gly Lys Ala Trp Leu His Val Cys Val Thr Gly Tyr Asp Lys Asn
Vic/3/75      Ser Ser Cys His Asp Gly Lys Ala Trp Leu His Val Cys Val Thr Gly Tyr Asp Lys Asn
                                     190                                             200

RI/5⁻/57      Ala Thr Ala Ser Phe Ile Tyr Asp Gly Arg Leu Val Asp Ser Ile Gly Ser Trp Ser Gln
Tokyo/67      Ala Thr Ala Ser Phe Ile Tyr Asp Gly Arg Leu Val Asp Ser Ile Gly Ser Trp Ser Gln
NT/60/68      Ala Thr Ala Ser Phe Ile Tyr Asp Gly Arg Leu Val Asp Ser Ile Gly Ser Trp Ser Gln
Udorn/72      Ala Thr Ala Ser Phe Ile Tyr Asp Gly Arg Leu Val Asp Ser Ile Gly Ser Trp Ser Gln
Vic/3/75      Ala Thr Ala Ser Phe Ile Tyr Asp Gly Arg Leu Val Asp Ser Ile Gly Ser Trp Ser Gln
                                     210                                             220

RI/5⁻/57      Asn Ile Leu Arg Thr Gln Glu Ser Glu Cys Val Cys Ile Asn Gly Thr Cys Thr Val Val
Tokyo/67      Asn Ile Leu Arg Thr Gln Glu Ser Glu Cys Val Cys Ile Asn Gly Thr Cys Thr Val Val
NT/60/68      Asn Ile Leu Arg Thr Gln Glu Ser Glu Cys Val Cys Ile Asn Gly Thr Cys Thr Val Val
Udorn/72      Asn Ile Leu Arg Thr Gln Glu Ser Glu Cys Val Cys Ile Asn Gly Thr Cys Thr Val Val
Vic/3/75      Asn Ile Leu Arg Thr Gln Glu Ser Glu Cys Val Cys Ile Asn Gly Thr Cys Thr Val Val
                                     230                                             240
```

Fig. 4 Amino acid sequence changes associated with antigenic drift in the N2 neuraminidase. The data sources are A/RI/5⁻/57 (Elleman et al., 1982), A/Tokyo/3/67 (Ward et al., 1982), NT/60/68 (Bentley and Brownlee, 1982),

```
RI/5⁻/57    Met Thr Asp Gly Ser Ala Ser Gly Arg Ala Asp Thr Arg Ile Leu Phe Ile Lys Glu Gly
Tokyo/67    Met Thr Asp Gly Ser Ala Ser Gly Arg Ala Asp Thr Arg Ile Leu Phe Ile Glu Glu Gly
NT/60/68    Met Thr Asp Gly Ser Ala Ser Gly Arg Ala Asp Thr Arg Ile Leu Phe Ile Glu Glu Gly
Udorn/72    Met Thr Asp Gly Ser Ala Ser Gly Arg Ala Asp Thr Lys Ile Leu Phe Ile Glu Glu Gly
Vic/3/75    Met Thr Asp Gly Ser Ala Ser Gly Arg Ala Asp Thr Lys Ile Leu Phe Ile Glu Glu Gly
                                              250                                    260

RI/5⁻/57    Lys Ile Val His Ile Ser Pro Leu Ser Gly Ser Ala Gln His Ile Glu Glu Cys Ser Cys
Tokyo/67    Lys Ile Val His Ile Ser Pro Leu Ala Gly Ser Ala Gln His Val Glu Glu Cys Ser Cys
NT/60/68    Lys Ile Val His Ile Ser Pro Leu Ser Gly Ser Ala Gln His Val Glu Glu Cys Ser Cys
Udorn/72    Lys Ile Val His Ile Ser Pro Leu Ser Gly Ser Ala Gln His Val Glu Glu Cys Ser Cys
Vic/3/75    Lys Ile Val His Ile Ser Pro Leu Ser Gly Ser Ala Gln His Val Glu Glu Cys Ser Cys
                                              270                                    280

RI/5⁻/57    Tyr Pro Arg Tyr Pro Asp Val Arg Cys Ile Cys Arg Asp Asn Trp Lys Gly Ser Asn Arg
Tokyo/67    Tyr Pro Arg Tyr Pro Gly Val Arg Cys Ile Cys Arg Asp Asn Trp Lys Gly Ser Asn Arg
NT/60/68    Tyr Pro Arg Tyr Pro Gly Val Arg Cys Ile Cys Arg Asp Asn Trp Lys Gly Ser Asn Arg
Udorn/72    Tyr Pro Arg Tyr Pro Gly Val Arg Cys Ile Cys Arg Asp Asn Trp Lys Gly Ser Asn Arg
Vic/3/75    Tyr Pro Arg Tyr Pro Gly Val Arg Cys Ile Cys Arg Asp Asn Trp Lys Gly Ser Asn Arg
                                              290                                    300

RI/5⁻/57    Pro Val Ile Asp Ile Asn Met Glu Asp Tyr Ser Ile Asp Ser Ser Tyr Val Cys Ser Gly
Tokyo/67    Pro Val Val Asp Ile Asn Met Glu Asp Tyr Ser Ile Asp Ser Ser Tyr Val Cys Ser Gly
NT/60/68    Pro Val Val Asp Ile Asn Met Glu Asp Tyr Ser Ile Asp Ser Ser Tyr Val Cys Ser Gly
Udorn/72    Pro Val Val Asp Ile Asn Val Lys Asp Tyr Ser Ile Asp Ser Ser Tyr Val Cys Ser Gly
Vic/3/75    Pro Val Val Asp Ile Asn Val Lys Asp Tyr Ser Ile Asp Ser Ser Tyr Val Cys Ser Gly
                                              310                                    320

RI/5⁻/57    Leu Val Gly Asp Thr Pro Arg Asn Asp Asp Ser Ser Asn Ser Asn Cys Arg Asp Pro
Tokyo/67    Leu Val Gly Asp Thr Pro Arg Asn Asp Asp Arg Ser Ser Asn Ser Asn Cys Arg Asn Pro
NT/60/68    Leu Val Gly Asp Thr Pro Arg Asn Asp Asp Arg Ser Ser Asn Ser Asn Cys Arg Asn Pro
Udorn/72    Leu Val Gly Asp Thr Pro Arg Asn Asn Asp Arg Ser Ser Asn Ser Tyr Cys Arg Asn Pro
Vic/3/75    Leu Val Gly Asp Thr Pro Arg Lys Asn Asp Arg Ser Ser Ser Ser Tyr Cys Arg Asn Pro
                                              330                                    340

RI/5⁻/57    Asn Asn Glu Arg Gly Asn Pro Gly Val Lys Gly Trp Ala Phe Asp Asn Gly Asp Asp Val
Tokyo/67    Asn Asn Glu Arg Gly Thr Gln Gly Val Lys Gly Trp Ala Phe Asp Asn Gly Asn Asp Leu
NT/60/68    Asn Asn Glu Arg Gly Asn Gln Gly Val Lys Gly Trp Ala Phe Asp Asn Gly Asn Asp Val
Udorn/72    Asn Asn Glu Lys Gly Asn His Gly Val Lys Gly Trp Ala Phe Asp Asp Gly Asn Asp Val
Vic/3/75    Asn Asn Glu Lys Gly Ile His Gly Val Lys Gly Trp Ala Phe Asp Asp Gly Asn Asp Val
                                              350                                    360

RI/5⁻/57    Trp Met Gly Arg Thr Ile Asn Lys Glu Ser Arg Ser Gly Tyr Glu Thr Phe Lys Val Ile
Tokyo/67    Trp Met Gly Arg Thr Ile Ser Lys Asp Leu Arg Ser Gly Tyr Glu Thr Phe Lys Val Ile
NT/60/68    Trp Met Gly Arg Thr Ile Ser Lys Asp Leu Arg Ser Gly Tyr Glu Thr Phe Lys Val Ile
Udorn/72    Trp Met Gly Arg Thr Ile Ser Glu Asp Ser Arg Ser Gly Tyr Glu Thr Phe Lys Val Ile
Vic/3/75    Trp Met Gly Arg Thr Ile Ser Glu Asp Ser Arg Ser Gly Tyr Glu Thr Phe Lys Val Ile
                                              370                                    380

RI/5⁻/57    Gly Gly Trp Ser Thr Pro Asn Ser Lys Ser Gln Val Asn Arg Gln Val Ile Val Asp Asn
Tokyo/67    Gly Gly Trp Ser Thr Pro Asn Ser Lys Ser Gln Ile Asn Arg Gln Val Ile Val Asp Ser
NT/60/68    Gly Gly Trp Ser Thr Pro Asn Ser Lys Ser Gln Ile Asn Arg Gln Val Ile Val Asp Ser
Udorn/72    Gly Gly Trp Ser Thr Pro Asn Ser Lys Leu Gln Ile Asn Arg Gln Val Ile Val Asp Ser
Vic/3/75    Gly Gly Trp Ser Thr Pro Asn Ser Lys Leu Gln Ile Asn Arg Gln Val Ile Val Asp Ser
                                              390                                    400

RI/5⁻/57    Asn Asn Trp Ser Gly Tyr Ser Gly Ile Phe Ser Val Glu Gly Lys Ser Cys Ile Asn Arg
Tokyo/67    Asp Asn Arg Ser Gly Tyr Ser Gly Ile Phe Ser Val Glu Gly Lys Ser Cys Ile Asn Arg
NT/60/68    Asp Asn Arg Ser Gly Tyr Ser Gly Ile Phe Ser Val Glu Gly Lys Ser Cys Ile Asn Arg
Udorn/72    Asp Asn Arg Ser Gly Tyr Ser Gly Ile Phe Ser Val Glu Gly Lys Ser Cys Ile Asn Arg
Vic/3/75    Ala Asn Arg Ser Gly Tyr Ser Gly Ile Phe Ser Val Glu Gly Lys Ser Cys Ile Asn Arg
                                              410                                    420

RI/5⁻/57    Cys Phe Tyr Val Glu Leu Ile Arg Gly Arg Pro Gln Glu Thr Arg Val Trp Trp Thr Ser
Tokyo/67    Cys Phe Tyr Val Glu Leu Ile Arg Gly Arg Lys Gln Glu Thr Arg Val Trp Trp Thr Ser
NT/60/68    Cys Phe Tyr Val Glu Leu Ile Arg Gly Arg Lys Gln Glu Ala Arg Val Trp Trp Thr Ser
Udorn/72    Cys Phe Tyr Val Glu Leu Ile Arg Gly Arg Glu Gln Glu Thr Arg Val Trp Trp Thr Ser
Vic/3/75    Cys Phe Tyr Val Glu Leu Ile Arg Gly Arg Glu Gln Glu Thr Arg Val Trp Trp Thr Ser
                                              430                                    440

RI/5⁻/57    Asn Ser Ile Val Val Phe Cys Gly Thr Ser Gly Thr Tyr Gly Thr Gly Ser Trp Pro Asp
Tokyo/67    Asn Ser Ile Val Val Phe Cys Gly Thr Ser Gly Thr Tyr Gly Thr Gly Ser Trp Pro Asp
NT/60/68    Asn Ser Ile Val Val Phe Cys Gly Thr Ser Gly Thr Tyr Gly Thr Gly Ser Trp Pro Asp
Udorn/72    Asn Ser Ile Val Val Phe Cys Gly Thr Ser Gly Thr Tyr Gly Thr Gly Ser Trp Pro Asp
Vic/3/75    Asn Ser Ile Val Val Phe Cys Gly Thr Ser Gly Thr Tyr Gly Thr Gly Ser Trp Pro Asp
                                              450                                    460

RI/5⁻/57    Gly Ala Asn Ile Asn Phe Met Pro Ile
Tokyo/67    Gly Ala Asn Ile Asn Phe Met Pro Ile
NT/60/68    Gly Ala Asn Ile Asn Phe Met Pro Ile
Udorn/72    Gly Ala Asp Ile Asn Leu Met Pro Ile
Vic/3/75    Gly Ala Asp Ile Asn Leu Met Pro Ile
                                              469
```

A/Udorn/72 (Markoff and Lai, 1982) and A/Victoria/75 (van Rompuy et al., 1982). The amino acid substitutions that have accumulated since 1957 are shaded.

Three different neuraminidase variants, grown from Tokyo/3/67, have been partially sequenced, and they show sequence changes at residues 221, 344 and 368 (Laver et al., 1982). The latter two changes occurred in chain segments also showing high variation in field strain sequences. The other change, at residue 221, is in a segment of structure undergoing no change in the field strains. However, the three-dimensional structure shows residue 221 to be on an adjacent loop to 197–199 where variation is found in field strains (Varghese et al., 1983).

THREE-DIMENSIONAL STRUCTURE OF N2 NEURAMINIDASE HEADS

Neuraminidase from two different field strains, A/Tokyo/3/67 and A/RI/5$^+$/57, hereafter referred to as Tokyo and RI/5$^+$ respectively, have been used in this study (Varghese et al., 1983; Colman et al., 1983). The crystallization and low resolution electron density map of the Tokyo enzyme were described (Wright and Laver, 1978; Colman and Laver, 1981). The space group is I422, a = 139·6Å, c = 191·0Å with one sub-unit per asymmetric unit. The RI/5$^+$ enzyme was solubilized from X-7F1 virus (Kilbourne et al., 1968) with pronase (Laver, 1978) and crystallized by vapour diffusion against 0·75M sodium citrate at pH 7. The crystals are octohedral bipyramids with space group $P4_12_22$ or enantiomorph, a = 124·1Å, c = 181·2Å and two sub-units per asymmetric unit. Both crystal forms diffract X-radiation at Bragg spacings of 3Å.

The structure of influenza virus neuraminidase (Fig. 5) provides the first known example of a tetrameric protein with circular four-fold symmetry. The polypeptide chain folds into six, topologically identical, four-stranded, anti-parallel β-sheets which are themselves arranged like the blades of a propeller. Calcium ions are believed to be bound on the four-fold axis between a cluster of eight acidic groups. The most C-terminal of the five glycosylation sequences carries no carbohydrate.

The catalytic sites of influenza virus neuraminidase are located in a deep cleft on the upper corners of the box-shaped tetramer. These are flanked and surrounded by nine acidic residues, six basic residues and three hydrophobic residues (Fig. 5) all of which are strictly conserved in all known influenza virus neuraminidase sequences.

Amino acids which change during antigenic drift are observed to cluster preferentially into the distal surface loops which connect the various strands of β sheets. Some of these variable residues are immediately adjacent to amino acids implicated in enzyme activity (Fig. 5). The variable loops do not segregate into spatially distinct non-overlapping areas of variation. Rather

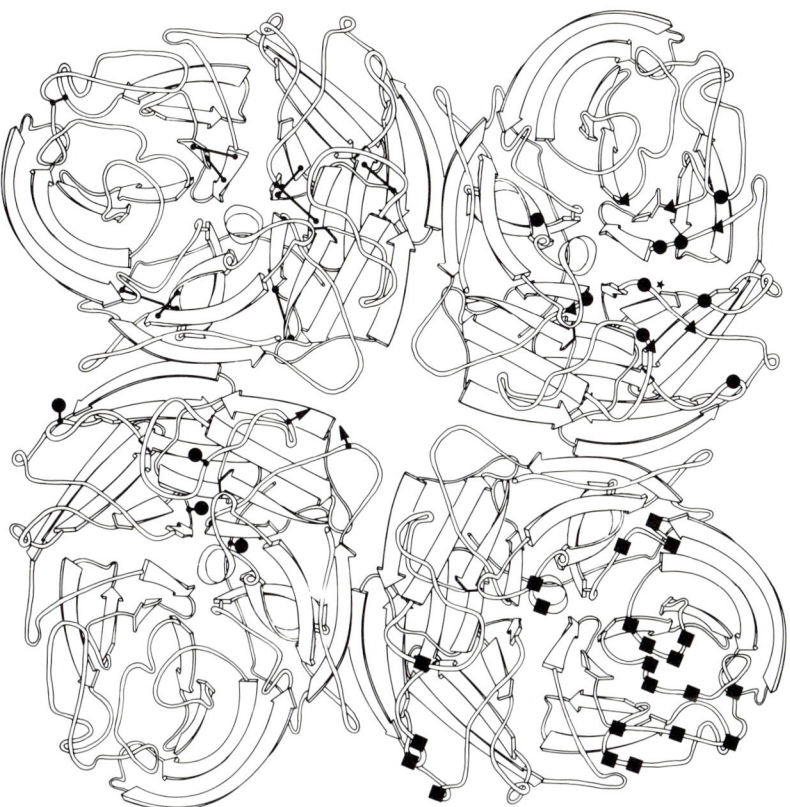

Fig. 5 Schematic of the neuraminidase tetramer viewed from above down the symmetry axis. The four sub-units highlight different features of the structure. Top left disulphide bonds. Bottom left carbohydrate attachment sites at 86, 146, 200 and 234 and metal ligands ASP 113 and ASP 114. Bottom right Residues which changed in field strains and in variants selected with monoclonal antibodies. Top right conserved acidic and basic residues in influenza A and B neuraminidase. * marks the sialic acid binding site.

they form a nearly continuous surface across the top of the sub-unit, encircling the catalytic site. It remains to be seen whether all of these variable loops can participate in forming complexes with immunoglobulins. Neuraminidase variants selected with monoclonal antibodies show that residues 221, 344 and 368 form part of antigenic determinants and it is likely that when more mutants are characterized, remaining regions of frequent field strain variation will also be seen to form sites for interaction with antibodies. Recently neuraminidase heads of sub-type N9 have been crystallized (Fig. 3). This neuraminidase possesses haemagglutinin activity and its structure is currently being determined.

EFFECT OF CHEMICAL MODIFICATION OF X-7F1 NA ON ITS ANTIGENIC ACTIVITY

Pronase released neuraminidase "heads" of X-7F1 (H1N2) virus were crystallized and the crystals dissolved in 0·15M NaCl 0·1M NaHCO$_3$. Aliquots of 2.4.6 trinitrobenzenesulphonic acid or succinic anhydride were added to the neuraminidase over a 2h period with continuous stirring. The reaction mixtures were kept in ice.

The trinitrophenylated (TNP) and succinylated neuraminidase preparations were dialysed against cold 0·15M NaCl and tested for neuraminidase and antigenic activity and analysed for amino acid composition.

NEURAMINIDASE ACTIVITY

The TNP and succinylated neuraminidase preparations possessed approximately 75% of the NA activity of the untreated material (fetuin substrate).

LYSINE CONTENT

Neuraminidase treated with TNBS had 52·6% of its lysine content converted to TNP-lysine and in neuraminidase treated with succinic anhydride, 52·0% of the lysine was succinylated.

It is not know whether the same lysine residues reacted with each reagent.

DOUBLE IMMUNODIFFUSION (ID) TESTS

In ID tests, using hyperimmune rabbit antisera to X-7F1 NA, lines of identity were obtained between untreated NA and NA in which more than half the lysine content was trinitrophenylated or succinylated (Fig. 6). With some sera, a small spur developed between the untreated NA and the derivative, suggesting that some antigenic sites may have been modified by the treatment.

REACTION OF TNP-NA WITH MONOCLONAL ANTIBODIES

Competitive radioimmunoassays using monoclonal antibodies have established that X-7F1 neuraminidase can be divided into four overlapping antigenic regions (Webster et al., 1984). Antigenic regions 1 and 4 are

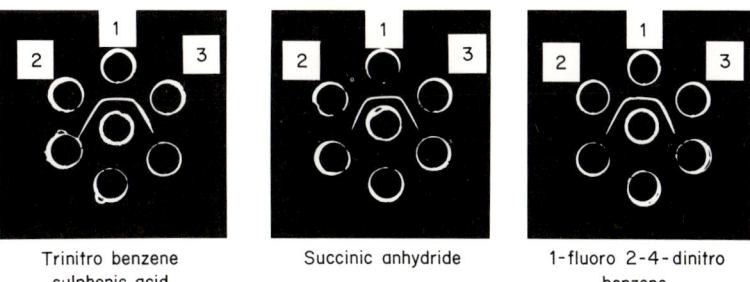

Fig. 6 Double immunodiffusion tests showing lines of identity between X-7F1 NA and NA treated with 2-4-6 trinitrobenzenesulphonic acid (52·6% of the lysine converted to TNP-lysine) or succinic anhydride (52·0% of the lysine succinylated) or 1-fluoro 2-4-dinitrobenzene. Well 1 contains untreated NA and Wells 2 and 3 treated NA in each case. Hyperimmune rabbit antisera to X-7F1 NA was in the centre well in each case.

sufficiently far apart so that antibodies to one do not affect the binding of antibodies to the other. The antibodies belonging to groups 2 and 3 inhibited catalytic activity on fetuin substrate whereas antibodies in groups 1 and 4 did not.

Using the reactivity patterns of antigenic variants, an operational antigenic map was constructed which further divided antigenic region 2 into four overlapping areas (2a, 2b, 2c, 2d). Of 18 monoclonal antibodies which recognized region 2b, 16 failed to inhibit the enzyme activity of TNP-NA. Antibodies in regions 2a, 2c and 3 inhibited the activity of TNP-NA to the same extent as the untreated enzyme (Table II). A similar pattern of inhibition was obtained with succinylated NA.

Although the amino acids which were substituted with TNP or succinate have not been identified, these results suggest that the antigenic region 2b contains one or more lysine residues which make contact with the antibodies which bind to this region. Alternatively, antibodies which recognize region 2b might bind to TNP-NA but fail to inhibit the NA activity.

A curious fact, for which there is no explanation, is that substitution of more than half of the lysine in the NA with TNP or succinate, apparently has little effect on the binding of antibody to the NA in double immunodiffusion precipitation tests using polyclonal antisera to the NA (Fig. 6). This result seems to be inconsistent with that obtained with the monoclonal antibodies.

Summary

The influenza virus neuraminidase (NA) glycoprotein is a tetramer with a box-shaped head, $100 \times 100 \times 60 Å$, attached to a slender stalk. The

TABLE II

Antibody group	Monoclonal antibody	NA inhibition with following substrates		NA inhibition using TNP substituted NA
		Fetuin	NAL	
1	254/1	−	−	
	239/3	−	−	
	552/5	−	−	
	618/1	−	−	
	562/1	−	−	
	129/2	−		
2A	81/4	+	−	+
	93/1	+	+ +	+
2B	438/1	+	−	−
	415/1	+	−	−
	443/2	+	−	−
	193/2	+	−	−
	474/1	+	−	−
	490/3	+	−	−
	220/3	+	−	−
	342/4	+	−	−
	101/5	+	−	−
	664/1	+	−	−
	513/1	+	−	−
	514/1	+	−	−
	561/3	+	−	−
	11/1	+	+/−	−
	112/2	+	+/−	−
	103/1	+	−	−
	233/3	+	−	+
	132/6	+	−	+
2C	73/1	+	−	+
	560/1	+	−	+
2D	145/1	+	+ +	+
	509/1	+	+	+
	266/4	+	+	+
	480/2	+	−	+
	307/2	+	−	+
3	72/1	+	−	+
	120/1	+	−	+
4	190/1	−	−	
	441/2	−	−	
	157/1	−	−	
	740/1	−	−	
	458/1	−	−	

neuraminidase polypeptide is coded by RNA segment 6 in the virus and is orientated in the virus membrane in the opposite way to the haemagglutinin. No post-translational cleavage of the NA polypeptide occurs, no signal peptide is split off and even the initiating methionine is retained. A sequence of six polar amino acids at the N-terminus of the NA polypeptide, which are totally conserved in the nine different NA sub-types, is followed by a sequence of hydrophobic amino acids which probably represent the transmembrane region of the NA stalk. This sequence is not conserved at all between sub-types (apart from conservation of hydrophobicity). Pronase cleaves the polypeptide at about position 75 removing the stalk and releasing the enzymically and antigenically active head of the NA which, in some cases, can be crystallized. The three-dimensional structure of N2 neuraminidase heads shows that each monomer is composed of six topologically identical β sheets arranged in a propeller formation. The tetrameric enzyme has circular four-fold symmetry stabilized in part by metal ions bound on the symmetry axis. Sugar residues are attached to four of the five potential glycosylation sequences, and in one case contribute to the interaction between subunits in the tetramer. The catalytic sites are located on the upper corners of the box-shaped tetramer. Antigenic determinants form a nearly continuous surface across the top of the monomer encircling the catalytic site. Approximately the same number of amino acid sequence changes occur in these determinants between the years 1968 and 1975 as occur in the antigenic sites of the haemagglutinin in the same period.

REFERENCES

Aymard-Henry, M., Coleman, M. T., Dowdle, W. R., Laver, W. G., Schild, G. C. and Webster, R. G. (1973). Influenza virus neuraminidase and neuraminidase-inhibition test procedures. *Bull. WHO* **48**, 199–202.

Bentley, D. R. and Brownlee, G. G. (1982). Sequence of the N2 neuraminidase from influenza virus A/NT/60/63. *Nucl. Acids Res.* **10**, 5033–5042.

Blok, J. and Air, G. M. (1982). Variation in the membrane-insertion and "stalk" sequences in eight subtypes of influenza type A virus neuraminidase. *Biochemistry* **21**, 4001–4007.

Blok, J., Air, G. M., Laver, W. G., Ward, C. W., Lilley, G. G., Woods, E. G., Roxburgh, C. M. and Inglis, A. S. (1982). Studies on the size, chemical composition and partial sequence of the neuraminidase (NA) from type A influenza viruses show that the N-terminal region of the NA is not processed and serves to anchor the NA in the viral membrane. *Virology* **118**, 109–121.

Burnet, F. M. and Stone, J. D. (1947). Receptor-destroying enzyme of *V. cholerae*. *Aust. J. Exp. Biol. Med. Sci.* **25**, 227–233.

Colman, P. M. and Laver, W. G. (1981). The structure of influenza virus neuraminidase heads at 5Å resolution. *In* "Structural Aspects of Recognition and

Assembly in Biological Macromolecules" (Ed. M. Balaban). I.S.S. Rehovot, pp. 869–872.

Colman, P. M., Varghese, J. N. and Laver, W. G. (1983). Structure of the catalytic and antigenic sites in influenza virus neuraminidase. *Nature* (Lond.) **303**, 41–44.

Drzeniek, R. (1972). Viral and bacterial neuraminidases. *Current Topics in Microbiol. Immunol.* **59**, 35–74.

Elleman, T. C., Azad, A. A. and Ward C. W. (1982). Neuraminidase gene from the early Asian strain of human influenza virus: A/RI/5⁻/57 (H2N2) *Nucl. Acid Res.* **10**, No. 21, 7005–7015.

Fields, S., Winter, G. and Brownlee, G. G. (1981). Structure of the neuraminidase gene in human influenza virus A/PR/8/34. *Nature* (Lond.) **290**, 213–217.

Gottschalk, A. (1957). Neuraminidase: the specific enzyme of influenza virus and *Vibrio cholerae*. *Biochim. Biophys. Acta* **23**, 645–646.

Gottschalk, A. (1966). "The Glycoproteins. Their Composition, Structure and Function", Vol. 5. Elsevier, Amsterdam.

Hirst, G. K. (1941). Agglutination of red cells by allantoic fluid of chick embryos infected with virus. *Science* **94**, 22–33.

Hiti, A. L. and Nayak, D. P. (1982). Complete nucleotide sequence of the neuraminidase gene of human influenza virus A/WSN/33. *J. Virol.* **41**, 730–734.

Kilbourne, E. D., Laver, W. G., Schulman, J. L. and Webster, R. G. (1968). Antiviral activity of antiserum specific for an influenza virus neuraminidase. *J. Virol.* **2**, 281–288.

Laver, W. G. (1978). Crystallization and peptide maps of neuraminidase "heads" from H2N2 and H3N2 influenza virus strains. *Virology* **86**, 78–87.

Laver, W. G. and Valentine, R. C. (1969). Morphology of the isolated hemagglutinin and neuraminidase subunits of influenza virus. *Virology* **38**, 105–119.

Laver, W. G., Air, G. M. and Webster, R. G. (1981). Mechanism of antigenic drift in influenza. Amino acid sequence changes in an antigenically active region of Hong Kong (H3N2) influenza virus hemagglutinin. *J. Mol. Biol.* **145**, 339–361.

Laver, W. G., Air, G. M., Webster, R. G. and Markoff, L. J. (1982). Amino acid sequence changes in antigenic variants of type A influenza virus N2 neuraminidase. *Virology* **122**, 450–460.

Markoff, L. and Lai, C.-J. (1982). Sequence of the influenza A/Udorn/72 (H3N2) virus neuraminidase gene as determined from cloned full-length DNA. *Virology* **119**, 288–297.

Palese, P., Tobita, K., Ueda, M. and Compans, R. W. (1974). Characterization of temperature sensitive influenza virus mutants defective in neuraminidase. *Virology* **61**, 397–410.

van Rompuy, L., Min-Jou, W., Huylebroeck, D. and Fiers, W. (1982). Complete nucleotide sequence of a human influenza neuraminidase gene of subtype N2 (A/Victoria/3/75). *J. Mol. Biol.* **161**, 1–11.

Varghese, J. N., Laver, W. G. and Colman, P. M. (1983). Structure of the influenza virus glycoprotein antigen neuraminidase at 2.9Å resolution. *Nature* (Lond.) **303**, 35–40.

Ward, C. W., Elleman, T. C. and Azad, A. A. (1982). Amino acid sequence of the Pronase-released heads of neuraminidase subtype N2 from the Asian strain A/Tokyo/3/67 of influenza virus. *Biochem. J.* **207**, 91–95.

Webster, R. G. and Laver, W. G. (1967). Preparation and properties of antibody directed specifically against the neuraminidase of influenza virus. *J. Immunol.* **99**, 49–55.

Webster, R. G., Hinshaw, V. S. and Laver W. G. (1982). Selection and analysis of antigenic variants of the neuraminidase of N2 influenza viruses with monoclonal antibodies. *Virology* **117**, 93–104.

Webster, R. G., Brown, L. E. and Laver, W. G. (1984). Antigenic and biological characterization of influenza virus neuraminidase (N2) with monoclonal antibodies. *Virology* **30**, 539–545.

Wright, C. E. and Laver, W. G. (1978). Preliminary crystallographic data for influenza virus neuraminidase "heads". *J. Mol. Biol.* **120**, 133–136.

Wrigley, N. G. (1979). Electron microscopy of influenza virus. *Brit. Med. Bull.* **35**, 35–38.

Wrigley, N. G., Skehel, J. J., Charlwood, P. A. and Brand, C. M. (1973). The size and shape of influenza virus neuraminidase. *Virology* **51**, 525–529.

DISCUSSION

Kilbourne I wonder if we could initially address any specific questions on the actual data to Graeme Laver and then generalize the discussion to include both glycoproteins.

Skehel In the variants that you generate, do any show, as does the mutant at 144 in HA, decreased reactivity with polyclonal serum?

Laver Not so far. We have not found any variants that show any change with polyclonal serum, no.

Palese You showed that your alkylating agents do not change the antigenicity of the neuraminidase or the haemagglutinin and you were surprised about this. How does formalin change the antigenicity using your test?

Laver We have not done this, but formerly it has been traditionally used. It is a reagent which attacks the amino groups and it has been used because it does not do anything to antigenicity, and this may well be the reason. We have not looked at formalin in inactivated virus.

Palese Theoretically one could use these alkylating agents in the same way as formalin.

Laver Also the alkylating agents act on the RNA and I think that is how they destroy infectivity. Also, they react with the amino groups on proteins, and because they do not do anything to antigenicity this is why they have been used. The basic action of destroying infectivity is on the RNA, is it not?

Schild They do not affect neuraminidase activity?

Laver No, for the same reason. If you can destroy the amino groups and not destroy antigenic activity, then that is fine.

Dowdle I should like to ask Graeme Laver if he has given thought to what the role of calcium might be, if it is not always required for activity?

Laver Many neuraminidases can actually be isolated in detergent containing ethylenediaminetetra-acetic acid which chelates calcium, and they are fully active, so clearly calcium is not needed for all of them, or else it is bound so strongly that the EDTA does not remove it.

Kilbourne Graeme, I do not think that kind of evidence can be definitive, because we have been interested in totally abolishing NA activity in order to be sure that some of our reactions of the HA were really HA determined; and even with EDTA present in the haemagglutinin and haemagglutination-inhibition reactions we still see evidence of elution effects. I think one would have to have more definitive evidence of lack of calcium.

Skehel In the case where you bind virus (with haemagglutinating NA) to the cells through the neuraminidase by blocking the haemagglutinin with antibody, does the virus get internalized?

Laver We do not know. Obviously that experiment has to be done. We do not even know whether the neuraminidase attaches to host cells. The experiments were done on red cells and the answers could be quite different.

Skehel But you can neutralize infectivity, you said?

Laver You can neutralize infectivity, but the question is whether the neutralized virus still attaches to the host cell. We know it attaches to the red cell, but, as people have pointed out, red cells and host cells are quite different and it may not attach to the host cell.

Tyrrell I should like to make a point which I was going to have made in the previous discussion, but I think it refers to both of them. I am very anxious that we do not make the mistake of thinking that neutralization always means the same thing. A neutralized virus is no more specific than a dead virus. There are all sorts of ways to get to the neutralized state, I suspect. I think the sort of localization of function at the molecular level which we have been talking about could mean that in some circumstances neutralization takes place by blocking a different function. I do not know whether people who understand these things think that is a nonsense idea. It does seem to me that it is worth looking on how an antibody neutralizes in terms of what function is blocked.

Kilbourne I certainly agree. I think that the work with the synthetic peptide antigens now is bringing out the fact that there are many antigens which can stimulate the formation of antibody which can bind to viruses and not neutralize. One would have to take it a further step to see whether they affected biologic activity. That would be another kind of definition of neutralization. I think the point is well made.

Schild I should like to mention the polio virus for which we have been studying neutralization. I think it is quite clear that neutralization of poliovirus requires antibody-binding to a small specific antigenic site on the virus. There are a lot of restrictions about what an antibody must do before it will neutralize, and I suspect the same thing is true for influenza. I am not prepared to say exactly what those restrictions are, but I think we are beginning to understand them.

Kilbourne It depends how broadly we define neutralization, I guess.

Skehel This relates to what I asked Graeme Laver about whether neuraminidase-bound virus was internalized. It seems to me that work in your laboratory suggested that uncleaved haemagglutinin also bound but viruses containing uncleaved haemagglutinin did not get internalized. Do you know of that, or of any more details?

Palese The experiment performed by Dr Schulman and myself is the following. If one takes influenza virus with uncleaved haemagglutinin and lets it attach to the cell, one can take it off with antibody until about four hours after infection. Virus with cleaved haemagglutinin is internalized after half an hour at the longest, I would say. But when it has an uncleaved haemagglutinin virus remains probably at the cell surface, or at least it can be inactivated by antibody. I think that might indicate that virus with uncleaved haemagglutinin cannot be internalized.

Klenk What is the interpretation of this?

Palese That you need a cleaved haemagglutinin to get internalized.

Klenk I am just wondering if it may tell you something about where fusion takes place.

Palese It may take place at the cell surface or in the endosome.

Klenk I wonder whether this observation of yours may allow some conclusion to this question.

Kilbourne Would you like to draw the conclusion?

Klenk Only that this observation as such would be compatible with the view that the virus may normally fuse at the cell surface. If it is not fusing because it does not have a cleaved haemagglutinin, it may be accessible to and taken off by the antibody. It would be difficult to explain this observation if the virus were to be taken up in the endocytotic vesicles.

Tyrrell I would like to mention some work done by Dr Dourmashkin and myself about ten years or so ago, which was morphological, in which we showed that the addition of antibody prevented adsorbed influenza virus from being taken up from the cell surface in vesicles. We interpreted that as meaning that in some way there was an interaction between the virus and the surface of the cell, which triggered the formation and entry or the movement of something that was essential in order for the virus to get taken up into a vesicle. So it could be a phenomenon of that sort. I do not understand how it would work, but if the haemagglutinin had not been cleaved, could it fail to give a signal to the surface of the cell to take it inside? In other words, it need not mean it had to be entering by direct fusion at cell surface, there are other possibilities.

H. Smith I have a question which relates to this and the change in haemagglutinin function which occurs under the influence of pH. As I understand it, the haemagglutinin adheres to the surface of a susceptible cell at neutral pH. Then a vacuole might start forming in the cell which would result in a change of pH to acid. Due to transformational changes in the haemagglutinin or possibly break away of haemagglutinins fusion would occur and the virus would go into the cell. Is that right?

Skehel Except for the time of the cleavage.

H. Smith What would happen in an environment of pH 5 as happens in an inflammatory exudate? Would the preliminary adherence go on at pH 5?

Skehel Yes, pH 5 treatment does not destroy sialic acid binding activity but it inactivates the virus presumably because instead of the amino terminus interacting with the lipid of the membrane—if that is what it has to do—it interacts with itself or a neighbouring molecule.

H. Smith So you can get binding and fusion at pH 5.

Skehel If you drop the pH to 5 before binding, as you suggest, in such an exudate, you may well get binding but you probably would not get fusion. You would have inactivated virus infectivity, just as you do if you incubate virus at pH 5 before sticking it into an egg.

H. Smith I just wondered whether that might well be one of the protective effects of an inflammatory exudate on infection—just by changing pH.

Kilbourne Is it not a little late in the game? The inflammatory exudate comes well after.

Couch I would just like to make the point that the initial pH change with acute inflammation is to become slightly alkaline. If I remember correctly, Dr Smith has been talking about later stages, that would be with the polymorphonuclear leucocyte infiltration which is not characteristic of influenza; but maybe that is why we cannot find influenza virus when there is bacterial pneumonia, because it has been destroyed by that time.

Webster Do you have evidence that antibodies prevent the pH 5 conformational change? You alluded to it when you spoke.

Skehel No, we tried but I presume that anything that was bound came off at 5. We never prevented the pH 5 change in conformation *in vitro* by adding antibodies.

Chu I am interested in this carbohydrate business. As I understand it, the carbohydrate protects the antigenic site from combining with the antibody. Does the carbohydrate add anything new to antigenicity?

Skehel I suspect not. You would imagine it is seen as self by the host and, therefore, is not immunogenic. That is not the case for all carbohydrate side chains, in particular for one of them and the Australian people have tied that one down to a sulphated carbohydrate side chain near the membrane at 154 of HA2. The carbohydrate chains in HA1 are not immunogenic, I would imagine.

Chu Is it possible that the linking of the carbohydrate to the protein is part of the structure, or what?

Skehel Since the enzymes involved in the synthesis of the carbohydrate side chains are host enzymes, you would imagine that their structure is the same as the structure of the side chains on host glycoproteins. I do not know whether there could be modifications to that; there are certainly some, since sialic acid is removed from virus glycoprotein, and such modifications might on some occasions give rise to a new immunogen. I would say that is open, but I do not think there is any evidence for it.

Brownlee With reference to the carbohydrate, we are considering the possibility that there might be a monoclonal antibody that could see both the carbohydrate and some protein determinants. But the weight of the evidence at the moment suggests that carbohydrate is acting by this indirect role—that it is modulating or masking what would otherwise be a determinant. I hope you will allow me to go on, Mr Chairman, and ask what may be a naive question, but it relates to the discussion. What is the significance of, say, the monoclonal variants you find in neuraminidase? This is really a question for Laver. As I understand it the antibodies to neuraminidase are not thought of as neutralizing *in vivo*; rather we think of them as acting at a later stage than the initial infection. You do not describe these monoclonal antibodies as neutralizing antibodies, do you?

Laver I think Dr Webster believes they do neutralize.

Webster They neutralize, as Kilbourne found, on the way out of the cell. I think the selection occurs by inhibiting virus release. The monoclonal antibodies to NA do not prevent the virus from getting into the cell.

Kilbourne I think we have a semantic problem here which we really ought to pause and address. Geoffrey Schild is talking about polio virus neutralization and the point that David Tyrrell was making earlier was that neutralization has a very specific meaning in virology. Neutralization usually implies specifically inhibition of the initial event in terms of attachment of the virus. I think there is no doubt that other antibodies—neuraminidase antibody included—can affect virus replication but in multicycle replication you have various effects, either aggregation or pinning the virus to the cell surfaces as it comes out of the cell, aggregating the virus particles directly. The biologic end point is one of the inhibition of virus-replication. But I think it is very important to pinpoint that we are talking of neutralization specifically at the stage of initial viral attachment. I would like to adhere to the conventional definition.

John, I had a point for you in reference to the carbohydrate matter again. There have been recognized in the past some protease-susceptible variants, some of which we have studied and they have been interesting variants in the sense that the two NWS variants that we described also had slight antigenic differences one from the other. Do you suppose they might be carbohydrate variants in the sense of, being susceptible of insusceptible? Are their arginines shielded from trypsin or what?

Skehel Again, it is a possibility. The function of carbohydrate side-chains on surface proteins is not known. It is one of the possibilities that people always mention, that they protect the amino acid residues which would otherwise be susceptible to proteolysis. So you might imagine that if you do get such things which are susceptible to proteolysis they may have lost a carbohydrate side chain.

Kilbourne We will ask you to look at them.

Schild I think that as usual Webster will have the answer. Frequency of selection of antigenic variants for neuraminidase with monoclonal antibodies is similar to that of haemagglutinin, is that right? Like 10^{-3}–10^{-4}?

Webster Yes, the same range as with the haemagglutinin—approximately 10^{-5}.

Fiers So far the question about this shielding by the carbohydrate groups has been discussed in black and white terms. I do not know how it is in influenza, but in a number of other glycoproteins you really have a certain probability that the protein slips through without accepting the carbohydrate. In other words, I would expect that also in influenza, you would always have a certain percentage of viral particles which are not glycosylated in a particular site. So I wonder how good your backgrounds really are and whether it is not the case that, even for a particular region, which should be masked, a minority of the population does not have that region exposed and, therefore, can give rise to a certain low titre antibody.

Skehel It depends what figure you put on a minority. One assay is an immune-precipitation and the other is a haemagglutination-inhibition reaction. I would say the backgrounds in both cases were reasonably high, at the level of 5·0% but whether you put a minority at that level I do not know. In terms of micro-heterogeneity of carbohydrate chains I would agree with what you say. In terms of absolute lack of chains, I am not sure that those cases are very well documented.

Fiers Microheterogeneity is due to differences in secondary superadditions and is a different matter. But there is also evidence that for each particular site a fraction of the population exists at a level of perhaps 1·0 to 5·0%, which has not accepted a glycosyl group at all.

Skehel I do not know those studies. I do not know whether similar information exists for influenza.

Klenk We have looked very carefully and in great detail at the carbohydrate structures and also at the distribution of the carbohydrate on the fowl plague virus haemagglutinin. Although we have no direct evidence for this, we cannot exclude the possibility that a small percentage of the attachment sites do not contain carbohydrate. However, it is remarkable that, on the fowl plague virus haemagglutinin and on other haemagglutinins, specific potential attachment sites never contain carbohydrates. So there are certainly factors which determine whether a given carbohydrate site is glycosylated or whether it is not glycosylated.

Fiers That is still a different aspect; some protective target sites exist which are not accessible for glycosylation.

Skehel Right, yes.

Brownlee In vivo a small amount of non-glycosylation would not matter if, indeed, the carbohydrate was masking the ability of antibody to recognize a given region. So that, even if such a small amount existed according to this hypothesis, it may not interfere with the ability of the virus to survive.

Mahy I just wanted to return once more to clarify something that I thought I heard John Skehel say on the question of neutralization of infectivity. Are we now fairly certain, or do you have evidence, John, that virion RNA transcriptase activity is not being inhibited by combination with neutralizing antibody?

Skehel There is a report that certain monoclonal antibodies against fowl plague virus are able to inhibit transcriptase activity, and the suggestion comes from that, that such inhibition may be involved in neutralization of infectivity. The reason for my comment is that using the same monoclones, which turned out to be ours anyway, we tried to repeat those experiments and we could not. So that is the reason for my scepticism. But, of course, it is just one against one I would say in the moment.

Mahy You do not have a view on the question as to whether virus plus neutralizing antibody goes into cells? You have not done experiments in that area?

Skehel No. I think it is remarkably difficult to do uptake experiments with viruses, largely because of the difference between particle number and infectious particle number. So you do not really know whether what you see in terms of microscopy is the actual particle responsible for the infection.

Klenk I have a question for Dr Skehel, and this also relates to Dr Webster's talk this morning. You find that an amino acid exchange in position 226 determines the receptor-binding with respect to a 2, 3-versus 2, 6-bound neuraminic acid. Now Webster finds that this also determines enterotropism, if I understand correctly, with an additional amino acid exchange in position 228. To go one step further, one should then assume that in the epithelium of the digestive tract only one type of neuraminic acid should be accessible to the haemagglutinin. Is that correct? Has that been shown?

Webster No, it has not been looked at yet.

Klenk But you assume it is a possibility.

Both Does anybody know how many molecules of antibody it takes to neutralize a virus?.

Webster I go back to my days with Stephen Fazekas, who found that a small number of antibodies is required. I will not say "one" but a small number.

Both How many molecules of haemagglutinin on the surface of the virus?

Webster Approximately 500 molecules.

Both I am trying to get a feeling for whether we are dealing with a situation where there are a few antibody molecules and lots of haemagglutinin on the surface. The question is: if that is the case, if antibody binds one haemagglutinin on one side of the virus, why cannot a molecule on the other side be used to attach the virus to the cell?

Skehel It seems to me that in the artificial situations that we use to generate the mutants it might be different. If you have just got a cell with an FC receptor which is in the business of eating anything with a single antibody or more than one antibody attached to it, that is neutralization, and that may be the main basis for saying that a small number of antibody molecules is required. It seems to me that in the *in vitro* situation, as with the monoclone selection situation, you probably need considerably more. You probably need to swamp it.

Chu Dr Skehel, you talked about the mutants induced with horse serum. I think that in 1957, after the isolation of H2N2, these viruses have been very sensitive to horse serum. Some of them are; some of the isolates are not. In the early days, those which are sensitive to horse serum are usually more avid. Of course, that parallelism may not include it much longer. With H2N2 you can find horse serum resistance in the sensitive ones but they do not run parallel with avidity to antibody. Still, you do find viruses very often; some are very heavy and some are very resistant. I wonder whether your explanation comes closer to the molecular basis of the change to the inhibitor as well as the avidity to antibody.

Skehel It seems to me, from the work that people are doing on antigenic changes in receptor-binding mutants, that it might help to sort out what is meant by avidity. The avidity that you talk about is scored in the haemagglutination-inhibition test, which is a competition reaction, so you have got an affinity of antibody for haemagglutinin and an affinity of haemagglutinin for receptor to consider, and I imagine that a complex of that is what is usually referred to as avidity. It is interesting that some of these binding mutants score also as antigenic mutants, and that might be in some way related to what is observed with natural strains, in addition to differences in specificity of binding.

Kilbourne I should like the record to show that the comment about inhibitors by Dr Chu was a comment by one of the world's pioneers in the study of influenza virus inhibitors.

Scholtissek Do you know whether there is a correlation between the easiness of cleaving off the neuraminidase from the virus and the size of the stalk? You know that neuraminidases have different molecular weights. Some have insertions, or deletions depending how you look at the problem, and others do not have this. Is there any correlation between the size of the stalk and the cleavability of the neuraminidase?

Kilbourne Is this to be answered by Dr Webster or Dr Laver?

Laver As neither of us know the answer, it does not matter! I have no idea.

Structure, Genetics and Role of Non-glycosylated Proteins

C. SCHOLTISSEK

Institut für Virologie, Justus-Liebig-Universität Giessen, Giessen, Germany

INTRODUCTION

The genes of many influenza A and B strains have been sequenced (for reviews see Scholtissek, 1983; and McCauley and Mahy, 1983). For the PR8 strain the sequence of all eight RNA segments, and, therefore, we hope, the primary structure of the corresponding gene products are known (Allen et al., 1980; Baez et al., 1980; Fields and Winter, 1982; Fields et al., 1981; Van Rompuy et al., 1981; 1982; Winter and Fields, 1980; 1981; 1982; Winter et al., 1981a,b). To our knowledge six out of eight RNA segments of influenza A and B viruses code for non-glycosylated viral proteins: the three P-proteins encoded by the three largest RNA segments, the nucleoprotein (NP) encoded by RNA segment 5, the membrane (M) protein (RNA segment 7), and the non-structural (NS) proteins, two of them are encoded by RNA segment 8. The first four proteins together with virion (v) RNA form the RNA polymerase complex synthesizing viral mRNA.

Each virus particle consists of about 15 molecules of each of the three

"The Molecular Virology and Epidemiology of Influenza" (Eds Sir Charles Stuart-Harris and Professor C.W. Potter). Academic Press, London, New York and Orlando, 1984.

P-proteins, of about 1000 molecules of the NP, and of about 2500 molecules of the M-protein (Inglis *et al.*, 1976). The synthesis of the P-proteins, the NP and one of the NS (NS1)-protein starts relatively early in the infectious cycle, while the other viral proteins are produced relatively late. The viral protein synthesis is regulated mainly by the availability of their corresponding mRNAs (Hay *et al.*, 1977; for a review see Skehel and Hay, 1978; Inglis and Mahy, 1979).

THE THREE P-PROTEINS

The three P-proteins are involved in the synthesis of three different kinds of virus-specific RNAs. The first step after adsorption and penetration is the synthesis of viral mRNA by the incoming RNA polymerase complex. For this step protein synthesis is not required. After primary transcription and translation a second type of viral complementary (c) RNA is produced, the so-called replicative cRNA, which—in contrast to the mRNA—is not modified, and which functions presumably as template for vRNA synthesis (Skehel and Hay, 1978).

By two-dimensional polyacrylamide gel electrophoresis the three P-proteins can be separated. Two are basic proteins (PB1 and PB2), and one is an acidic protein (PA) (Horisberger, 1980). According to the open reading frames of the sequenced RNA segments the PB1 protein of PR8 consists of 757 amino acids, the PB2-protein of 759, and the PA protein of 716 amino acids (Fields and Winter, 1982; Winter and Fields, 1982). The function of the different P-proteins in the various steps of the synthesis of viral mRNA has been elucidated mainly by R. M. Krug and his colleagues. This synthesis can be dissected into at least three steps as outlined in Fig. 1. (1) The polymerase complex first binds to a fully methylated cap structure of cellular high molecular weight heterogeneous nuclear (hn) RNA. Using a specific endonucleotytic activity of the influenza polymerase complex, an oligonucleotide of 10–13 bases is cleaved off from the 5-end. At the 3′-end this oligonucleotide has a G or, preferentially, an A. (2) This starter molecule, which has no complementary base sequence to the vRNA, starts the synthesis of the viral mRNA by incorporation of G complementary to the penultimate C of the vRNA (= initiation step). (3) Thereafter elongation continues in a normal fashion (for a review see Krug, 1981). At the 3′-terminus the viral mRNAs are polyadenylated. Sixteen nucleotides complementary to the 5′-end of the vRNA are lacking (for a review see Skehel and Hay, 1978; Robertson *et al.*, 1981).

If viral cores as enzyme source and a cellular mRNA with a labelled cap are mixed in an *in vitro* system omitting NTPs, following UV irradiation and

Cleavage

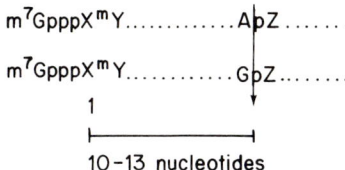

Initiation

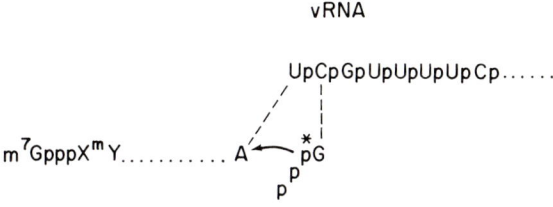

Elongation

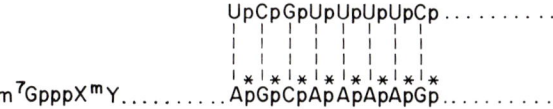

Fig. 1 Three steps in the priming of influenza viral mRNA synthesis by capped host RNA. Taken from Krug (1981).

RNase treatment, radioactivity is cross-linked only to the PB2-protein. Thus, the PB2 protein is the cap-recognizing protein (Ulmanen et al., 1981; Blaas et al., 1982a,b; Penn et al., 1982). If to the same system with nonlabelled cellular mRNA radioactive GTP is added, following UV irradiation and RNase treatment, radioactivity is recovered only with the PB1-protein, indicating that this protein is involved in chain initiation (Ulmanen et al., 1981). However, if in addition to radioactive GTP also ATP and CTP are added, omitting UTP (U would be incorporated not before position 13) following UV irradiation and RNase treatment, radioactivity is found bound only to the PA-protein, indicating that this protein is involved in chain elongation (Krug, 1982). As a further approach, ts mutants with defects in the genes coding for the various P-proteins have been investigated. The results obtained with these mutants are in full agreement with the findings described above (Nichol et al., 1981; Horisberger, 1982; Ulmanen *et al.*, 1983). For example, *ts* 1 and *ts* 6 mutants of the WSN strain, which have a *ts* defect in the PB2-gene, were found to be unable to cleave the cap-containing mRNA substrate at the non-permissive temperature. In this case it is not yet known whether the mutants at 40°C did not recognize the cap, which is a prerequisite for any further steps, or whether they have a *ts* defect in their endonucleotytic activity (Ulmanen *et al.*, 1983).

THE NUCLEOPROTEIN

As a rule, RNA segment 5 codes in most influenza A strains for the basic, arginine-rich nucleoprotein (NP). The NP of the PR8 and A/NT/60/68 strains consists of 498 amino acids as deduced from the base sequence of RNA segment 5 (Van Rompuy *et al.*, 1981; 1982; Winter and Fields, 1981; Huddleston and Brownlee, 1982). It is the major constituent of the nucleocapsid, which according to electron micrographs has a helical left-handed configuration (Compans *et al.*, 1972; Murti *et al.*, 1980; Heggeness *et al.*, 1982). The vRNA embedded into this structure is accessible to ribonuclease (Schäfer and Wecker, 1958; Duesberg, 1969) and it can be replaced by polyvinyl sulphate (Pons *et al.*, 1969). *In vitro* studies have shown that NP forms complexes very rapidly using vRNA or cRNA with equal affinity (Scholtissek and Becht, 1971). This might explain why after disrupting infected cells, vRNA as well as cRNA was found in nucleocapsid structures (Pons, 1971; 1975; Krug, 1972). The NP is one of the group-specific antigens, by which the three types of influenza virus, i.e. A, B and C, are classified.

A complex of the three P-proteins and vRNA, which does not contain NP, can accomplish viral mRNA synthesis *in vitro*, indicating that the NP is not required for the production of mRNA (Kawakami and Ishihama, 1983). However, there exist several mutants with a *ts* lesion in the NP gene which at the non-permissive temperature are unable to synthesize vRNA (Palese, 1977; Scholtissek, 1978). The precise role of the nucleoprotein and the various P-proteins in the synthesis of the replicative cRNA (poly A^-) and vRNA, for which no *in vitro* system is available yet, is not known.

At least one mutant of fowl plague virus (FPV, H7N1) with a *ts* defect in the NP gene (*ts* 19) synthesizes all types of viral RNA and proteins; however, no infectious particles are formed at the non-permissive temperature. This indicates that the NP also plays a role in virus assembly (Scholtissek and Bowles, 1975).

The NP is one of the two known phosphoproteins of influenza virus (Privalsky and Penhoet, 1977, 1978, 1981; Petri and Dimmock, 1981;

Almond and Felsenreich, 1982). Privalsky and Penhoet (1981) have shown, that the NP of the A/NWS/33 (H1N1) strain grown in MDCK cells contains only one tryptic phosphopeptide. We have analysed NPs of different influenza strains, which were grown in chick embryo or MDCK-cells in the presence of ^{32}P-orthophosphate, by tryptic fingerprinting (Kistner et al., manuscript in preparation). As shown in Fig. 2, the fingerprints of the human A/PR/8/34 (H1N1) and A/Hong Kong/1/68 (H3N2) strains, which are highly related in their NP genes (Scholtissek et al., 1978; Van Rompuy et al., 1981, 1982; Winter and Fields, 1981; Huddleston and Brownlee, 1982), look completely different. In the NP of the Hong Kong strain only one major phosphopeptide was found, which is in agreement with the finding by Privalsky and Penhoet (1981) on the NWS strain. In the NP of PR8 we found six phosphopeptides, one migrating to the position corresponding to that of the Hong Kong virus. The fingerprint of FPV (H7N1) is similar but not identical to that of PR8, while the fingerprint of virus N (H10N7) (not shown here) resembles rather that of the Hong Kong virus. If one and the same virus, e.g. PR8, is labelled in two different host cells like MDCK or primary chick embryo cells, the phosphorylation patterns of the NP look significantly different (Fig. 2). Thus, the phosphorylation pattern is not only strain-specific, but depends also on the host cell. Recently we have speculated on the involvement of host factor(s) in influenza virus replication to explain changes of host range, organ tropism and pathogenicity by reassortment (Scholtissek, 1979). According to our results, specific host phosphokinases could fulfil all the requirements expected for such an involvement.

The NP after its synthesis migrates to the cell nucleus, where it first accumulates (presumably as nucleocapsid) as shown by fluorescent antibodies. Later in the infectious cycle it can be demonstrated also in the cytoplasm (Breitenfeld and Schäfer, 1957). In abortively infected cells (Franklin and Breitenfeld, 1959) or after treatment with p-fluorophenylalanine (Zimmermann and Schäfer, 1960) or under von Magnus conditions (Rott and Scholtissek, 1963) the NP does not leave the nucleus.

THE MEMBRANE PROTEIN

The M-protein is located beneath the viral lipid bilayer. According to the sequence of the largest open reading frame of RNA segment 7 and the size of the corresponding mRNA, the M-protein of three different influenza A subtypes consists of 252 amino acids, and that of the B/Lee/40 strain of 248 amino acids (Winter and Fields, 1980; Allen et al., 1980; Lamb and Lai, 1981; McCauley et al., 1982; Briedis et al., 1982). There are several regions

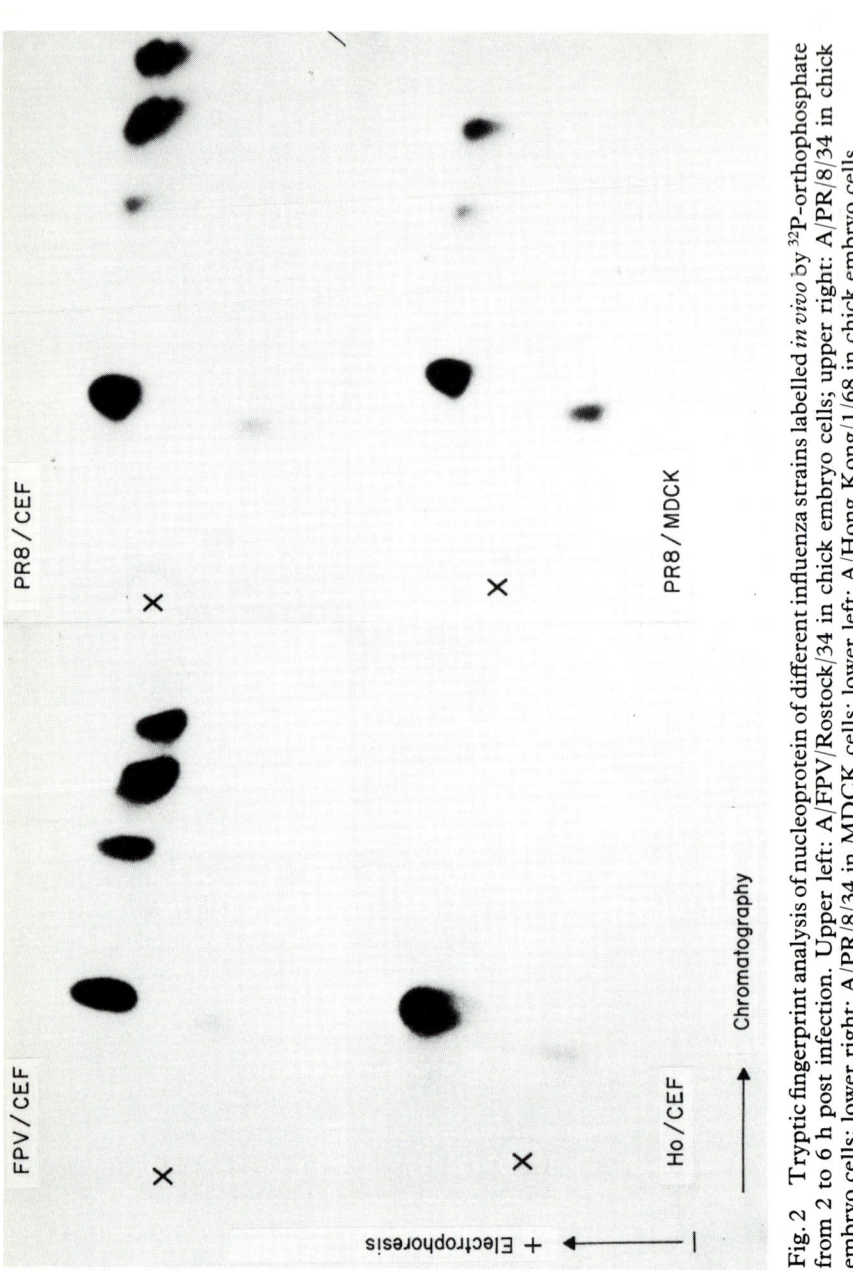

Fig. 2 Tryptic fingerprint analysis of nucleoprotein of different influenza strains labelled *in vivo* by ^{32}P-orthophosphate from 2 to 6 h post infection. Upper left: A/FPV/Rostock/34 in chick embryo cells; upper right: A/PR/8/34 in chick embryo cells; lower right: A/PR/8/34 in MDCK cells; lower left: A/Hong Kong/1/68 in chick embryo cells.

of 10 or more hydrophobic amino acids. It is possible to construct a three-dimensional structure of the M-protein with a highly hydrophobic domain, which might be embedded in the lipid membrane, and a more hydrophilic domain interacting possibly with the nucleocapsid. There is circumstantial genetic evidence that the M-protein might interact also with the C-terminus of the haemagglutinin (HA), which penetrates the lipid bilayer. During studies on the rescue of *ts* mutants of fowl plague virus the genes coding for HA- and M-protein segregated in no case where human, swine, or equine influenza A strains were investigated. Only with genetically highly related avian strains like virus N or A/turkey/England/63 (H7N3) was segregation observed with a relatively high frequency (Scholtissek *et al.*, 1976; Rott *et al.*, 1979).

The M-protein is synthesized relatively late in the infectious cycle, and it seems to become rate-limiting for virus maturation. There is a specific underproduction of M-protein in abortively infected cells, which is thought to be responsible for the lack of production of virus particles in these cells (Bosch *et al.*, 1978; Valcavi *et al.*, 1978; Lohmeyer *et al.*, 1979).

NON-STRUCTURAL PROTEINS

Non-structural (NS) proteins are virus-specific proteins, which are found in infected cells, but which are not constituents of virus particles. RNA segment 8 of influenza A and B viruses code for two of such NS-proteins via two different mRNAs, one of which is generated by splicing (Lamb and Choppin, 1979; Inglis *et al.*, 1979; Briedis *et al.*, 1981; Lamb and Lai, 1980; Briedis and Lamb, 1982). NS1 and NS2 of the influenza A viruses studied have 10 amino acids at their N-terminus in common, the sequence of the other amino acids is different. NS1 is found relatively early in the infectious cycle, while NS2 appears relatively late (Lamb *et al.*, 1978). Studies with monospecific antibodies have revealed that NS1 accumulates early in infection in cell nuclei or nucleoli, depending on the influenza strain under investigation (Dimmock, 1969; Young *et al.*, 1983). Late in the infectious cycle it can be visualized by electron microscopy as paracrystalline inclusions in the cytoplasm (Morrongiello and Dales, 1977; Shaw and Compans, 1978). The NS1-proteins of some influenza A virus strains are phosphoproteins, while those of other strains do not carry a phosphate group (Privalsky and Penhoet, 1978, 1981; Petri *et al.*, 1982).

Very little is known concerning the function of these NS-proteins. *Ts* mutants with a defect in RNA segment 8 were found either to be unable to synthesize sufficient vRNA and NS2- and M-protein at the non-permissive temperature (Wolstenholme *et al.*, 1980), or to have a defect in regulation by synthesizing very little HA- and M-protein (Koennecke et al., 1981). There is circumstantial evidence that the NS-protein(s) cooperate with the RNA polymerase complex. (1) During reassortment between FPV and virus N, RNA segments 2, coding for the PB1 protein, and 8 did not segregate readily, presumably because the RNA segments 8 of FPV and virus N are genetically relatively distantly related. With strains with genetically highly related segment 8, segregation occurs frequently (Scholtissek et al., 1976). (2) Certain ts mutants with defects in RNA segment 8 can be phenotypically suppressed by replacement of genes coding for the one or the other protein of the polymerase complex (Scholtissek and Spring, 1982).

From RNA segment 7 of influenza A viruses up to three different mRNAs are transcribed, two of them generated by splicing. From one of these spliced mRNAs another non-structural protein (M2) is translated, which contains 96 amino acids (Lamb et al., 1981; Inglis and Brown, 1981). RNA segment 7 of an influenza B virus also has two different open reading frames, one of which could code via a spliced mRNA for a corresponding M2-non-structural protein (Briedis et al., 1982). The function of M2 is completely obscure.

In other RNA segments there are also consensus donor and acceptor sites for splicing. However, corresponding mRNAs or proteins have not been identified so far; hence, the exact number of non-structural proteins is not yet known.

CONCLUSION

Influenza A, B, and C virus particles contain five non-glycosylated proteins. The structure and localization within the viral particle or within the infected cell, the synthesis after infection and the functions are fairly well known for most of these viral proteins. They are surrounded by a lipid bilayer and therefore—as far as this has been studied—do not react with specific antibodies unless the particles are disrupted. Since influenza viruses cannot be neutralized with antibodies directed against the internal type-specific proteins, the corresponding genes are not under selective pressure from the immune system of the host. This may be one of the reasons why they are relatively conserved as compared with the genes coding for the subtype-specific surface glycoproteins.

There are additional viral proteins in infected cells, which are not incorporated into viral particles during maturation and therefore are called non-structural proteins. The exact number of them is not known. We are just beginning to understand the function of two of these NS-proteins, those which are coded by RNA segment 8 of the influenza A virus.

In terms of genetic relatedness of RNA segment 8, avian influenza A viruses can be divided into two groups. Within each group the NS-gene is highly conserved. This is independent of the bird species (Scholtissek *et al.*, 1976; Scholtissek and von Hoyningen-Huene, 1980). Since there is no selective pressure from the immune system of the host against the gene products of RNA segment 8, the question arises, what were the driving forces responsible for this divergent development.

In contrast to most of the other RNA-containing viruses, influenza viruses need a nuclear phase for their replication. It has been claimed that the peculiar synthesis of viral mRNA, in which cellular hnRNA is involved (see Fig. 1), would necessitate this nuclear phase (Krug, 1981). This also would explain the sensitivity of influenza virus multiplication toward actinomycin D (Barry *et al.*, 1962) and α-amanitin (Rott and Scholtissek, 1970). However, in an *in vitro* system, most cellular mRNAs can act as primers for the synthesis of influenza virus mRNA. Since cellular mRNAs are available in the cytoplasm of the host there must be another yet unknown reason for the nucleocapsid to accumulate in the cell nucleus. Once in the nucleus, the viral RNA polymerase will of course find only host hnRNA, which normally is transported rapidly to the cytoplasm after splicing. Thus, if its regeneration is inhibited by actinomycin D or α-amanitin, influenza virus mRNA synthesis also ceases. The only known step in influenza virus multiplication, for which the cell nucleus would be necessary is splicing leading to the different species of mRNA as found for RNA segments 7 and 8. However, the real driving force, and the mechanism by which the nucleocapsids accumulate in the cell nucleus, is not known.

REFERENCES

Allen, H., McCauley, J. W., Waterfield, M. and Gething, M.-J. (1980). Influenza Virus RNA segment 7 has the coding capacity for two polypeptides. *Virology* **107**, 548–551.

Almond, J. W. and Felsenreich, V. (1982). Phosphorylation of the nucleoprotein of an avian influenza virus. *J. Gen. Virol.* **60**, 295–305.

Baez, M., Taussig, R., Zazra, J. J., Young, J. F., Palese, P., Reisfeld, A. and Skalka, A. M. (1980). Complete nucleotide sequence of the influenza A/PR/8/34 virus NS gene and comparison with the NS genes of the A/Udorn/72 and A/FPV/Rostock/34 strains. *Nucl. Acids Res.* **8**, 5845–5858.

Barry, R. D., Ives, D. R. and Cruickshank, J. G. (1962). Participation of deoxyribonucleic acid in the multiplication of influenza virus. *Nature* (Lond.) **194**, 1139–1140.

Blaas, D., Patzelt, E. and Kuechler, E. (1982a). Identification of the cap binding protein of influenza virus. *Nucl. Acids Res.* **10**, 4803–4812.

Blaas, D., Patzelt, E. and Kuechler, E. (1982b). Cap-recognizing protein of influenza virus. *Virology* **116**, 339–348.

Bosch, F. X., Hay, A. and Skehel, J. J. (1978). RNA and protein synthesis in a permissive and an abortive influenza virus infection. In "Negative Strand Viruses and the Host Cell" (Eds B. W. J. Mahy and R. D. Barry). Academic Press, London and New York, pp. 465–474.

Breitenfeld, P. M. and Schäfer, W. (1957). The formation of fowl plague virus antigens in infected cells, as studied with fluorescent antibodies. *Virology* **4**, 328–345.

Briedis, D. J. and Lamb, R. A. (1982). The influenza B virus genome. Sequences and structural organization of RNA segment 8 and the mRNAs coding for the NS1 and NS2 proteins. *J. Virol.* **42**, 186–193.

Briedis, D. J., Lamb, R. A. and Choppin, P. W. (1981). Influenza B virus RNA segment 8 codes for two nonstructural proteins. *Virology* **112**, 417–425.

Briedis, D. J., Lamb, R. A. and Choppin, P. W. (1982). Sequence of RNA segment 7 of the influenza B virus genome: Partial amino acid homology between the membrane proteins (M1) of influenza A and B viruses and conservation of a second open reading frame. *Virology* **116**, 581–588.

Compans, R. W., Content, J. and Duesberg, P. H. (1972). Structure of the ribonucleoprotein of influenza virus. *J. Virol.* **10**, 795–800.

Dimmock, N. J. (1969). New virus-specific antigens in cells infected with influenza virus. *Virology* **39**, 224–234.

Duesberg, P. H. (1969). Distinct subunits of the ribonucleoprotein of influenza virus. *J. Mol. Biol.* **42**, 485–499.

Fields, S. and Winter, G. (1982). Nucleotide sequence of influenza virus segments 1 and 3 reveal mosaic structure of a small viral RNA segment. *Cell* **28**, 303–313.

Fields, S., Winter, G. and Brownlee, G. G. (1981). Structure of the neuraminidase gene in human influenza virus A/PR/8/34. *Nature* (Lond.) **290**, 213–217.

Franklin, R. M. and Breitenfeld, P. M. (1959). The abortive infection of Earle's L-cells by fowl plague virus. *Virology* **8**, 293–307.

Hay, A. J., Lomniczi, B., Bellamy, A. R. and Skehel, J. J. (1977). Transcription of the influenza virus genome. *Virology* **83**, 337–355.

Heggeness, M. H., Smith, P. R., Ulmanen, I., Krug, R. M. and Choppin, P. W. (1982). Studies on the helical nucleocapsid of influenza virus. *Virology* **118**, 466–470.

Horisberger, M. A. (1980). The large P proteins of influenza A viruses are composed of one acidic and two basic polypeptides. *Virology* **107**, 302–305.

Horisberger, M. A. (1982). Identification of a catalytic activity of the large basic P polypeptide of influenza virus. *Virology* **120**, 279–286.

Huddleston, J. A. and Brownlee, G. G. (1982). The sequence of the nucleoprotein gene of human influenza A virus strain A/NT/60/68. *Nucl. Acids Res.* **10**, 1029–1038.

Inglis, S. C. and Brown, C. M. (1981). Spliced and unspliced RNAs encoded by virion RNA segment 7 of influenza virus. *Nucl. Acids. Res.* **9**, 2727–2740.

Inglis, S. C. and Mahy, B. W. J. (1979). Polypeptides specified by the influenza virus genome. 3. Control of synthesis in infected cells. *Virology* **95**, 154–164.

Inglis, S. C., Carroll, A. R., Lamb, R. A. and Mahy, B. W. J. (1976). Polypeptides specified by the influenza virus genome. 1. Evidence for eight distinct gene products specified by fowl plague virus. *Virology* **74**, 489–503.

Inglis, S. C., Barrett, T., Brown, C. M. and Almond, J. W. (1979). The smallest genome RNA segment of influenza virus contains two genes that may overlap. *Proc. Nat. Acad. Sci. USA* **76**, 3790–3794.

Kawakami, K. and Ishihama, H. (1983). RNA polymerase of influenza virus III. Isolation of RNA polymerase–RNA complexes from influenza virus PR8. *J. Biochem.* (Tokyo) **93**, 989–996.

Koennecke, I., Boschek, C. B. and Scholtissek, C. (1981). Isolation and properties of a temperature-sensitive mutant (ts 412) of an influenza A virus recombinant with a ts lesion in the gene coding for the nonstructural protein. *Virology* **110**, 16–25.

Krug, R. M. (1972). Cytoplasmic and nucleoplasmic viral RNAs in influenza virus-infected MDCK cells. *Virology* **50**, 103–113.

Krug, R. M. (1981). Priming of influenza viral RNA transcription by capped heterologous RNAs. *Curr. Top. Microbiol. Immunol.* **93**, 125–150.

Krug, R. M. (1982). The unique interaction of influenza viral RNA transcription with the host-cell transcriptional machinery. Data presented at the symposium on "The Origin of Pandemic Influenza Virus" held in Beijing, China, in November 10–12, 1982.

Lamb, R. A. and Choppin, P. W. (1979). Segment 8 of the influenza virus genome is unique in coding for two polypeptides. *Proc. Natl. Acad. Sci. USA.* **76**, 4908–4912.

Lamb, R. A. and Lai, C.-J. (1980). Sequence of interrupted and uninterrupted mRNAs and cloned DNA coding for the two overlapping nonstructural proteins of influenza virus. *Cell* **21**, 475–485.

Lamb, R. A. and Lai, C.-J. (1981). Conservation of the influenza virus membrane protein (M) amino acid sequence and an open reading frame of RNA segment 7 encoding a second protein (M2) in H1N1 and H3N2 strains. *Virology* **112**, 746–751.

Lamb, R. A., Etkind, P. R. and Choppin, P. W. (1978). Evidence for a ninth influenza virus polypeptide. *Virology* **91**, 60–78.

Lamb, R. A., Lai, C.-J. and Choppin, P. W. (1981). Sequences of mRNAs derived from genome RNA segment 7 of influenza virus: Colinear and interrupted mRNAs code for overlapping proteins. *Proc. Natl. Acad. Sci. USA.* **78**, 4170–4174.

Lohmeyer, J., Talens, L. T. and Klenk, H.-D. (1979). Biosynthesis of the influenza virus envelope in abortive infection. *J. Gen. Virol.* **42**, 73–88.

McCauley, J. W. and Mahy, B. W. J. (1983). Structure and function of the influenza virus genome. *Biochem. J.* **211**, 281–294.

McCauley, J. W., Mahy, B. W. J. and Inglis, S. C. (1982). Nucleotide sequence of fowl plague virus RNA segment 7. *J. Gen. Virol.* **58**, 211–215.

Morrongiello, M. P. and Dales, S. (1977). Characterization of cytoplasmic inclusions formed during influenza/WSN virus infection of chick embryo fibroblast cells. *Intervirol.* **8**, 281–293.

Murti, K. G., Bean, W. J. and Webster, R. G. (1980). Helical ribonucleoproteins of influenza virus: An electron microscopic analysis. *Virology* **104**, 224–229.

Nichol, S. T., Penn, C. R. and Mahy, B. W. J. (1981). Evidence for the involvement of influenza A (fowl plague Rostock) virus protein P2 in ApG and mRNA primed *in vitro* RNA synthesis. *J. Gen. Virol.* **57**, 407–413.

Palese, P. (1977). The genes of influenza virus. *Cell* **10**, 1–10.

Penn, C. R., Blaas, D., Kuechler, E. and Mahy, B. W. J. (1982). Identification of the cap-binding protein of two strains of influenza A/FPV. *J. Gen. Virol.* **62**, 177–180.

Petri, T. and Dimmock, N. J. (1981). Phosphorylation of influenza virus nucleoprotein *in vivo*. *J. Gen. Virol.* **57**, 185–190.

Petri, T., Patterson, S. and Dimmock, N. J. (1982). Polymorphism of the NS1 proteins of type A influenza virus. *J. Gen. Virol.* **61**, 217–231.

Pons, M. W. (1971). Isolation of influenza virus ribonucleoprotein from infected cells. Demonstration of the presence of negative-stranded RNA in viral RNP. *Virology* **46**, 149–160.

Pons, M. W. (1975). Influenza virus messenger ribonucleoprotein. *Virology* **67**, 209–218.

Pons, M. W., Schulze, I. T., Hirst, G. K. and Hauser, R. (1969). Isolation and characterization of the ribonucleoprotein of influenza virus. *Virology* **39**, 250–259.

Privalsky, M. L. and Penhoet, E. E. (1977). Phosphorylated protein component present in influenza virions. *J. Virol.* **24**, 401–405.

Privalsky, M. L. and Penhoet, E. E. (1978). Influenza virus proteins: identity, synthesis, and modification analyzed by two-dimensional gel electrophoresis. *Proc. Natl. Acad. Sci. USA* **75**, 3625–3629.

Privalsky, M. L. and Penhoet, E. E. (1981). The structure and synthesis of influenza virus phosphoproteins. *J. Biol. Chem.* **256**, 5368–5376.

Robertson, J. S., Schubert, M. and Lazzarini, R. A. (1981). Polyadenylation sites for influenza virus mRNA. *J. Virol.* **38**, 157–163.

Rott, R. and Scholtissek, C. (1963). Investigations about the formation of incomplete forms of fowl plague virus. *J. Gen. Microbiol.* **33**, 303–312.

Rott, R. and Scholtissek, C. (1970). Specific inhibition of influenza replication by α-amanitin. *Nature* (Lond.) **228**, 56.

Rott, R., Orlich, M. and Scholtissek, C. (1979). Correlation of pathogenicity and gene constellation of influenza viruses. III. Non-pathogenic recombinants derived from highly pathogenic parent strains. *J. Gen. Virol.* **44**, 471–477.

Schäfer, W. and Wecker, E. (1958). Über die Wirkung von Ribonuclease auf ^{32}P-markiertes "gebundenes Antigen" des Virus der Klassischen Geflügelpest. *Arch. Exptl. Vet. Med.* **12**, 418–422.

Scholtissek, C. (1978). The genome of the influenza virus. *Curr. Top. Microbiol. Immunol.* **80**, 139–169.

Scholtissek, C. (1979). Influenza virus genetics. *Adv. Genetics* **20**, 1–36.

Scholtissek, C. (1983). Genetic relatedness of influenza viruses (RNA and protein). In "Genetics of Influenza Viruses" (Eds P. Palese and D. W. Kingsbury). Springer Verlag, Berlin, pp. 99–126.

Scholtissek, C. and Becht, H. (1971). Binding of ribonucleic acids to the RNP-antigen protein of influenza viruses. *J. Gen. Virol.* **10**, 11–16.

Scholtissek, C. and Bowles, A. L. (1975). Isolation and characterization of temperature-sensitive mutants of fowl plague virus. *Virology* **67**, 576–587.

Scholtissek, C. and Spring, S. B. (1982). Extragenic suppression of temperature-sensitive mutations in RNA segment 8 by replacement of different RNA segments with those of other influenza A virus prototype strains. *Virology* **118**, 28–34.

Scholtissek, C. and von Hoyningen-Huene, V. (1980). Genetic relatedness of the gene which codes for the nonstructural (NS) protein of different influenza A strains. *Virology* **102**, 13–20.

Scholtissek, C., Harms, E., Rohde, W., Orlich, M. and Rott, R. (1976). Correlation between RNA fragments of fowl plague virus and their corresponding gene functions. *Virology* **74**, 332–344.

Scholtissek, C., Rohde, W., von Hoyningen, V. and Rott, R. (1978). On the origin of the human influenza virus subtypes H2N2 and H3N2. *Virology* **87**, 13–20.

Shaw, M. W. and Compans, R. W. (1978). Isolation and characterization of cytoplasmic inclusions from influenza A virus-infected cells. *J. Virol.* **25**, 608–615.

Skehel, J. J. and Hay, A. J. (1978). Influenza virus transcription. *J. Gen. Virol.* **39**, 1–8.

Ulmanen, I., Broni, B. A. and Krug, R. M. (1981). Role of two of the influenza virus core P proteins in recognizing cap 1 structures (m^{7}GpppNm) on RNAs and in initiating viral RNA transcription. *Proc. Natl. Acad. Sci. USA* **78**, 7355–7359.

Ulmanen, I., Broni, B. and Krug, R. M. (1983). Influenza virus temperature-sensitive cap (m^{7}GpppNm)-dependent endonuclease. *J. Virol.* **45**, 27–35.

Valcavi, P., Conti, G. and Schito, G. C. (1978). Molecular synthesis during abortive infection of KB cells by influenza virus. *In* "Negative Strand Viruses and the Host Cell" (Eds B. W. Mahy and R. D. Barry). Academic Press, London and New York, pp. 475–482.

Van Rompuy, L., Min Jou, W., Huylebroeck, D., Devos, R. and Fiers, W. (1981). Complete nucleotide sequence of the nucleoprotein gene from the human influenza strain A/PR/8/34 (HON1). *Eur. J. Biochem.* **116**, 347–353. Corrections: (1982). *Eur. J. Biochem.* **126**, 645.

Winter, G. and Fields, S. (1980). Cloning of influenza cDNA into M13: the sequence of the RNA segment encoding the A/PR/8/34 matrix protein. *Nucl. Acids Res.* **8**, 1965–1974.

Winter, G. and Fields, S. (1981). The structure of the gene encoding the nucleoprotein of human influenza virus A/PR/8/34. *Virology* **114**, 423–428.

Winter, G. and Fields, S. (1982). Nucleotide sequence of human influenza A/PR/8/34 segment 2. *Nucl. Acids Res.* **10**, 2135–2143.

Winter, G., Fields, S. and Brownlee, G. G. (1981a). Nucleotide sequence of the haemagglutinin gene of a human influenza virus H1 subtype. *Nature* (Lond.) **292**, 72–75.

Winter, G., Fields, S., Gait, M. J. and Brownlee, G. G. (1981b). The use of synthetic oligonucleotide primers in cloning and sequencing segment 8 of influenza virus (A/PR/8/34). *Nucl. Acids Res.* **9**, 237–245.

Wolstenholme, A. J., Barrett, T., Nichol, S. T. and Mahy, B. W. J. (1980). Influenza virus-specific RNA and protein synthesis in cells infected with temperature sensitive mutants defective in the genome segment encoding nonstructural proteins. *J. Virol.* **35**, 1–7.

Young, J. F., Desselberger, U., Graves, P., Palese, P., Schatzman, A. and Rosenberg, M. (1983). Cloning and expression of influenza virus genes. *In* "The Origin of Pandemic Influenza Virus" (Ed. W. G. Laver). Elsevier, Amsterdam, pp. 129–138.

Zimmermann, T. and Schäfer, W. (1960). Effect of p-fluoro-phenylalanine on fowl plague virus multiplication. *Virology* **11**, 676–698.

DISCUSSION

Kilbourne That is a masterful summary of a lot of information.

Skehel With regard to the location of transcriptase activity in the nucleus, it seems to me that just because you can feed an *in vitro* system with a capped messenger RNA and get that RNA to function as a primer it does not remove the requirement of the transcriptase complex to be in the nucleus in order to have an available cap to recognize. The question is, are caps free in the cytoplasm, are they recognizable in the cytoplasm, or are the capped messages in the cytoplasm present as protein complexes and cap recognition could be prevented? The nucleus might be the only place where a naked cap was available for recognition.

Scholtissek I agree with you, but we do not know whether free caps are available in the nucleus either. That is a question which is not solved. But since a capped messenger RNA can function in the *in vitro* system, it shows that this must not be the reason why influenza viruses need a nuclear phase. We certainly need a nuclear phase for splicing. That is clear.

Skehel If the only place in the cell where there are free caps is the nucleus then you need it for transcription.

Mahy One point which bears upon Skehel's comment, which I know only from a personal communication from Dr Kolakovsky, is that apparently in La Crosse virus infection there are also capped heterogeneous extensions on the messenger RNA and, so far as we know, La Crosse virus does not require the nucleus for its replication. The only difference, a very big difference to influenza with La Crosse virus, is that if you add a protein synthesis inhibitor all messenger RNA synthesis ceases. It suggests, possibly, that the capped structures are available to be spliced in the cytoplasm, at least in that system.

Fiers You are suggesting this possible association between the matrix protein and the carboxyl terminal and the haemagglutinin. Could you not also make the same argument for the neuraminidase or is it a category apart?

Scholtissek You are right. There is free segregation between the neuraminidase and the M-protein genes in the crosses we have done. The neuraminidase might not need the M-protein at its N-terminus during maturation. There is another difference between the haemagglutinin and neuraminidase which has not yet been mentioned. This is that haemagglutinin at the carboxyl terminal end has fatty acids bound covalently to the protein backbone, so that it is anchored much more firmly into the lipid bilayer than neuraminidase. You do not have fatty acids at the N-terminus of the neuraminidase.

Mahy Could I mention a recent piece of work which Charles Penn has done in my laboratory which bears upon the function of PB2 in relation to cap-containing structures? What he was able to show was that, using various cap analogue structures, at least in an *in vitro* system, there is modification of the PB2 protein itself which occurs on interaction with the cap structure. This can be shown because we have a *ts* mutant which is defective in this function. Although the cap structure is still used as a primer, stimulation of transcription does not occur. There is thus a stimulation function during the interaction of the cap structure with the polymerase, in addition to the use of the capped RNA as a primer (Penn and Mahy, 1984).

Murphy Does anyone have additional information on the role of the NS protein in replication that was not summarized by Dr Scholtissek?

Mahy No, we cannot really say any more than the fact that with the particular mutants which we have—we have two mutants we are working on extensively, both of which are now almost completely sequenced—we do not see any virion RNA synthesis in cells infected with these mutants at the non-permissive temperature. Unfortunately, one which has been sequenced has a mutation which lies in the overlapping reading frame between NS1 and NS2, so we cannot say which protein we are talking about. With the other one we have recently located a change just in the NS1 region, but we have not finished the sequence, so we do not know whether there might be another change in the NS2 region. It is very difficult when you have two proteins made from overlapping frames to be certain what is going on.

Skehel Could I ask if anyone knows any more about Horisberger's report of covalent attachment of the initiating nucleotide triphosphate to PB1 (Horisberger, 1982).

Kilbourne Deafening silence! Dr Scholtissek, did you mention the recent finding of Dr Lamb that he reported with reference to the non-structural protein coded by the neuraminidase gene of influenza B—I should say the RNA?

Scholtissek Dr Lamb talked about this at the negative strand virus meeting last week. This second protein which is synthesized from the RNA of the neuraminidase gene of influenza B virus is a glycoprotein. I did not mention this here. I was bound to talk only about non-glycosylated proteins. Indeed, he showed that there is presumably not a second messenger RNA but there is a second initiation site, and it is a glycoprotein.

Mahy Could I direct Dr Skehel's question back at him? I thought, in fact, that in his own laboratory recent work had shown an interaction between PB1 and initiation.

Skehel The question is whether there is a covalent linkage between the initiating nucleotide and PB1. The involvement of PB1 in initiation seems established. This was done by Mike Romanos. He did not look at covalent linkage, and the only report I know about is that from Horisberger.

Kilbourne This is a session on the molecular virology of influenza. Sir Christopher left us with an important question. I have not heard it addressed by any of the molecular virologists so far. Would anyone care to become wildly speculative at the end of this afternoon? Do we have any insight about what is now known about the molecular virology of the virus that would lead us to think about possible latency mechanisms? Certainly there is no reverse transcriptase that has been found for gene incorporation or incorporation of cDNA copies. Are there other reasonable or even unreasonable explanations that would address this very important and provocative question?

Brownlee The fact that there is no reverse transcriptase in the influenza RNA sequences might not prevent influenza-specific sequences from getting into the genome very, very rarely. There could be infection with a retrovirus at the same time as an influenza infection and the retrovirus could just grab any odd RNA that is there and perhaps incorporate into the genome. We know enough from the general molecular biology of—say globin genes, that very, very rarely in evolution funny things happened and the process pseudogenes are believed to be examples of the kind of thing I have just imagined for influenza genes. I would not exclude the possibility that influenza homologous segments would not be found at some stage in time in the mammalian genome.

Kilbourne That is a brave statement.

Both I think there is a situation where, with the availability of cloned genes we probably have some of the tools available to look for these kinds of sequences in a sensitive way. The question really comes down to: "Is there any clue at all that these sequences might exist in any kind of tissue?" I think it would be a brave person who would want to tackle a project like that with no guarantee of any results at the end of a lot of work. That is the situation we are in, I think.

Couch I do not really remember the specific details, but we submitted to Marcel Pons some time ago about 20 or 25 lung and tracheal/bronchial specimens as fresh as we could get them from autopsy for this purpose. My recollection is that his probe was for complementary RNA, and all of those specimens came up negative. I am unable to tell you the sensitivity or of the details of that particular evaluation, but I presume that is the kind of evaluation you were referring to.

Kilbourne Of course, a negative experiment is only a negative experiment.

Scholtissek I had a discussion—I do not remember exactly with whom—at the negative strand virus meeting. They had also established a system in which some of the virus genes were retained—not all of them—and they could passage these cells *in vitro*. This is some kind of establishment of such a persistently infected cell system.

We tried to do very similar things several years ago just by inactivating fowl plague virus, stepwise. We used Bayer A39, and we inactivated the virus to such a stage that no infectious virus was any longer produced. Then we infected cells with these preparations. Most of the cells survived, but they still synthesised nucleoprotein. At least they did not synthesize any more haemagglutinin and neuraminidase. We passaged these cells, and after about 10 passages they were just filled with nucleoprotein and then they died out. We have tried to repeat this several times. Of seven trials, I guess we were successful in about four.

Tyrrell It seems to me that it is important to get the epidemiology and the clinical side to give you a clear indication that in a certain population at a certain time there may be a latent virus. I think that what Dr Glezen has been saying suggests that the human may be the wrong place to look. If a virus actually does come and go again, there is no reason to suppose that it is lying latent in human beings.

I remember talking to Easterday some years ago. We had been talking about Shope's findings, to which Sir Christopher referred. He said that his Department had done a detailed study of the epidemiology of swine influenza in certain well-run herds in this area. They had formed the conclusion that the virus was persisting in the sows and that the virus disappeared and was not reintroduced from anywhere; nevertheless, when the piglets were born and had lost their maternal antibody, they were infected, and the only place that they could see for the virus was the sows. If that is correct and can be confirmed, then the right experiment to do is to use the best probe you can on a sow at a time when from the epidemiologist's data she is transmitting virus or likely to transmit virus to the piglets.

Kilbourne All that has to be put in the fresh context of what Webster told us this morning, that swine viruses can now replicate in turkeys. I think the old construction of it as only being a swine disease has to be re-examined in the light of the possible avian sources of virus.

Tyrrell But, on the other hand, in that epidemiological setting, it did appear it was the same virus all the time. I thought that what we heard earlier today suggested that there was a real difference between the American strains and the European ones, which gave evidence of a derivation from birds. Incidentally, I do not think that many of these farms where the pigs are kept have turkey flocks as well.

Webster I would like to make a comment along the same line. Martin Kaplan, who has been fascinated by this question for many years, went to Czechoslovakia with Blascovitch where they built special piggeries and went through all kinds of rigmarole to keep people out when they had influenza. They ran this experiment over an extended period and found that at intervals some of the pigs developed swine influenza. The mechanism of persistence is unknown but worth investigating.

Kilbourne Dr Dowdle, some years back you published evidence of serologic conversions as evidence of cryptic 'flu infections in the human population in the summertime. Is that not true? In other words, this is a credible alternative hypothesis to any true kind of biological latency; it is evident, as Dr Tyrrell was saying, for the continued circulation of viruses at times when we do not suspect them.

Dowdle We did publish such data but to be honest with you, I certainly would not stand here and say that it is evidence of continued virus transmission. It was simply an observation to raise the question. There was no virus isolation and one always wonders about serologic data.

Kilbourne I am astounded.

Mahy Could I just ask the clinicians one other point on this? There are those of us who have been privileged enough to hear Dr Hope-Simpson telling us about latency, and he bases many of his arguments on the possible influence of the sun-spot cycle on the eruption of new epidemics, and on the fact that simultaneously in several parts of the world very large distances apart the same strains of virus appear. I would have thought probably that this was not a very firm basis but I would be glad of any comment.

Kilbourne I do not want to terminate this session on molecular virology, but we have wandered far afield from it. As I see it, the purpose of this symposium is to keep going back and forth between the molecules and men.

REFERENCES

Penn, C. A. and Mahy, B. W. J. (1984). Capped mRNAs may stimulate the influenza virion polymerase by allosteric modulation. *Virus Research* **1**, (in press).

Horisberger, M. A. (1982). Identification of a catalytic activity of the large basic P polypeptide of influenza virus. *Virology* **120**, 279–286.

Immunological Reactions and Resistance to Infection with Influenza Virus

ROBERT B. COUCH, JULIUS A. KASEL,
HOWARD R. SIX, THOMAS R. CATE and
JOHN M. ZAHRADNIK

Influenza Research Center and the Department of Microbiology and Immunology, Baylor College of Medicine, Houston, Texas, USA

INTRODUCTION

Immunity to infection with influenza virus has been clearly demonstrated in studies involving challenge of human volunteers and observations of naturally occurring infections (Stuart-Harris and Schild, 1976). Serum antibody to the virus as measured by haemagglutination-inhibition (HI) or neutralization tests was the first described and most commonly used immune correlate of resistance to infection (Couch et al., 1969). Shortly thereafter, the presence of antibody to influenza virus was also identified in respiratory secretions following infection and it was reasoned that this antibody must mediate the resistance to infection (Couch et al., 1969). While evidence that such antibody can contribute to immunity has only been recently provided, (Couch et al., 1969; Couch et al., 1981; Clements et al.,

"The Molecular Virology and Epidemiology of Influenza" (Eds Sir Charles Stuart-Harris and Professor C.W. Potter). Academic Press, London, New York and Orlando, 1984.

1983) the relative significance of secretion and serum antibody as protective mechanisms against naturally occurring infection remains uncertain.

More recently, a variety of humoral and cell-mediated immune reactions that might play a role in resistance to influenza have been described. Considerable information is available on their importance in animal models and exploration in humans of these reactions is an area of active clinical research. Moreover, availability of more sensitive techniques for measuring immunoglobulin-specific classes of antibody to the virus has permitted a reconsideration of the relative significance of the predominant immunoglobulin (Ig) in secretions, IgA, and that in serum, IgG, in protection against infection.

In this report, consideration is given to the duration and specificity of immunity in man as derived from studies involving challenge of volunteers and observations of naturally occurring disease. The properties of the major immune reactions and how they relate to the information on immunity in man is then presented. Finally, a role for the various mediators in immunity to naturally occurring infection is proposed.

DURATION AND SPECIFICITY OF IMMUNITY

In the past 10 years, the potency of immunity to reinfection with homologous virus and existence of a considerable degree of heterotypic immunity to variants within a sub-type have been documented. In addition, data to support the long standing contention that infection with one sub-type induces little or no immunity to different sub-types was provided.

Homotypic and Heterotypic Immunity

In a series of studies we assessed the duration of homologous and heterologous immunity among type A (H3N2) influenza viruses in young adult volunteers. A group of individuals who had a prior documented infection with an A/Hong Kong/68 (H3N2)-like virus one to four years earlier were artificially rechallenged intranasally with A/Hong Kong virus (Couch, 1975). Surveillance detected a serologic response in only 15% of the group and no febrile influenzal illnesses were identified during the four-year period preceding virus challenge. The occurrence of a serologic response in only two of 35 volunteers and the absence of any illnesses demonstrated a potent homologous resistance for at least four years.

Another group of volunteers infected with A/England/72 (H3N2) virus two years earlier were challenged with homologous A/England-like or heterologous A/Port Chalmers/73 (H3N2)-like virus. No interim infections were detected in this group. As shown in Table I, infection was detected in one of seven volunteers challenged with A/England-like virus and this individual was not ill; none of the five challenged with A/Port Chalmers/73-like virus developed infection. The two illnesses in the rechallenged group were mild and not accompanied by evidence of influenza virus infection.

After the appearance of the A/Scotland/74 (H3N2) virus, volunteers who had experienced a documented infection with an earlier H3N2 variant were challenged with an A/Scotland-like virus. No interim infections had occurred in volunteers who had been infected with an A/Hong Kong-like virus four to seven years earlier or with an A/England or A/Port Chalmers-like virus one year earlier. As shown in Table II, infection was detected in a volunteer who had been infected with an A/Hong Kong-like virus seven years earlier and in two infected with an A/England-like virus one year earlier; no illnesses occurred among these rechallenged volunteers. The absence of infection and illness contrasts with the results of challenge of a newly selected group with no serum neutralizing antibody to the A/Scotland-like virus. Thus, a potent immunity against the challenge virus was shown to extend over a period of four to seven years and to span antigenic changes in the HA protein represented by three major variants of the H3N2 sub-type.

An assessment of the relation between infection and neutralizing antibody in serum or secretions showed that 96% of volunteers who resisted challenge in each of the studies possessed serum antibody to the challenge virus whereas only half had antibody in secretions. This suggested that,

TABLE I
Resistance of volunteers with prior influenza A/England virus infection to challenge with homologous or heterologous virus

Challenge virus	Group	No. vol.	Response to challenge			
			No. with virus isol.	No. with Ab rise	No. ill	No. with fever
A/Eng[a]	Prior A/Eng infection	7	1	0	1	0
	Control[b]	10	7	8	3	3
A/PC[c]	Prior A/Eng infection	5	0	0	1	0
	Control[b]	9	6	7	3	3

[a] Challenge dose was 1500 $TCID_{50}$. [b] Selected to be free of serum neutralizing antibody to challenge virus. [c] Challenge dose was 150 $TCID_{50}$.

TABLE II
Resistance of volunteers with prior influenza type A virus infection to challenge with heterologous virus[a]

Variant producing prior infection	No vol.	Years since infection	Response to challenge			
			No. with virus isol.	No. with Ab rise	No. ill	No. with fever
A/Hong Kong	6	4–7	1	1	0	0
A/England	6	1	0	2	0	0
A/Port Chalmers	3	1	0	0	0	0
Control[b]	13	—	9	10	3	2

[a] Challenge was with 3200 $TCID_{50}$ of A/Scotland virus. [b] Selected to be free of serum neutralizing antibody to challenge virus.

remotely after infection, immunity to reinfection relates best to the antibody in serum. In this regard, it is of interest that fewer and milder illnesses occurred among control volunteers in the two heterologous challenge studies than among controls for the homologous A/Hong Kong virus rechallenge. This partial immunity among the control volunteers administered either A/England, A/Port Chalmers, or A/Scotland virus correlated with the presence of neutralizing antibody to the heterotypic A/Hong Kong virus (data not shown). A similar heterotypic immunity to naturally occurring A/England infection was reported by Greenberg et al. (1974) among persons with A/Hong Kong serum antibody.

TABLE III
Relation of homologous and heterologous serum antibody to infection after natural exposure to influenza A/Victoria virus

Group	No. vol.	Infection after A/Vic exposure by Ab group			
		A/Scot Ab Only		A/Scot + A/Vic Ab	
		No.	No. infected	No.	No. infected
Prior A/Scot infection[a]	11	6	4	5	0
No A/Scot infection	8	8	3	—	—

[a] Produced by intranasal inoculation with 3200 $TCID_{50}$ of A/Scotland virus.

The individuals with the varying H3N2 virus experiences were later exposed to a naturally occurring influenza epidemic caused by A/Victoria/75 (H3N2)-like viruses. Heterotypic immunity was not apparent unless the individual had experienced infection in the A/Scotland challenge study a few months earlier and developed serum neutralizing antibody that cross-reacted with A/Victoria virus (Table III). Five of the seven volunteers infected with A/Victoria virus reported to clinic with an influenza-like illness, whereas none of the remaining volunteers reported during the epidemic period. These evaluations of sub-type immunity among volunteers in a closed population challenged with different H3N2 variants of type A influenza virus indicated a potent resistance to reinfection with heterologous H3N2 viruses that lasts for several years and spans antigenic changes exhibited by a number of variants.

Data on the duration of heterotypic immunity to reinfection with type A influenza viruses among persons in open communities was provided by Gill and Murphy (1976, 1977). During an A/England/72 (H3N2) epidemic, neither illness nor infection was detected among a relatively large group of persons with a confirmed A/Hong Kong/68 (H3N2) infection two to three years previously, although sub-clinical or mild illnesses may have been missed. Prior to a 1974 epidemic caused by A/Port Chalmers/73 (H3N2) virus, a more comprehensive evaluation of heterotypic immunity was undertaken. In that epidemic less than 3% of those with a prior A/Hong Kong or A/England infection experienced an infection with A/Port Chalmers whereas about 23% with no documented prior infection were infected; moreover, severe influenza was seen only in the latter group. In 1976, a similar evaluation performed during an A/Victoria/75 (H3N2) epidemic revealed infection in only 11% of a study group who experienced an earlier infection with H3N2 virus, whereas 27% of those lacking such a history experienced infection. In contrast to the A/Port Chalmers experience, when infection rates were similar regardless of the year of first infection, an increasing frequency of infection with time since first infection was noted; higher infection rates, 18%, were seen among persons previously infected with A/Hong Kong (1969 and 1970), than among those infected with A/England or A/Port Chalmers virus, 8% and 4% respectively. In addition, a high frequency of cases of severe influenza occurred among infected persons with no prior H3N2 infection (54%) whereas only 13% of reinfected persons were severely ill and these illnesses occurred among those infected with A/Hong Kong virus in 1969 or 1970, six and seven years earlier.

A similar occurrence of heterotypic immunity was reported by Wright et al. (1977) among a group of small children. Protection against a natural exposure to A/Port Chalmers virus occurred six months and two years after experiencing infection with unattenuated A/Hong Kong vaccine (six months) or natural infection with A/England virus (two years). More recently, Frank and Taber (1983) reported near complete resistance to reinfection with A (H3N2) virus among children with documented A (H3N2) virus infection three years earlier, whereas they had not found resistance to reinfection among another group of young children at an earlier time (Frank et al., 1979). Fox et al. (1982) also recently reported resistance to reinfection with A (H3N2) viruses among family members who had experienced an earlier infection but only if they had serum HI antibody titres $> 1:40$.

In summary, there seems little doubt that homotypic and heterotypic immunity develops after infection with a type A (H3N2) influenza virus, and that it is potent, lasts for several years, and spans several variants. The frequency of infection increases with time since the initial infection and the degree of antigenic variation, as does the likelihood of illness occurring and of it being severe.

Natural Homotypic Immunity after Prolonged Periods

Demonstration that homotypic immunity to reinfection with the same sub-type of type A virus may be prolonged was provided by the recent epidemiologic experience with the H1N1 influenza virus that reappeared in human populations in 1977. Despite a relatively certain exposure to persons infected with the H1N1 subtype, individuals born before 1952 (ensuring a high degree of probability of infection with closely related H1N1 viruses circulating between 1947 and 1957) have rarely been infected with the H1N1 variants circulating since 1977. Surveillance studies of influenza among persons in Houston, Texas presenting to health care facilities with febrile respiratory disease showed that 154 of 677 (23%) type A H3N2 isolates obtained during the 1977–8 epidemic, that was caused predominantly by A/Texas/1/77 (H3N2)-like virus, were from persons over age 35. However, during an epidemic a year later caused predominantly by A/Brazil/11/78 (H1N1) virus, only 2% of isolates were from this age group (Glezen et al., 1982). Similar evidence for immunity on reexposure of older persons to H1N1 viruses was provided by measurements of HI antibody in sera from Finnish residents (Pyhala, 1979). Among young persons, frequency of detection of antibody-positive sera between 1977 and 1978, the first year of recurrence of H1N1 virus, changed from 0% to 38% while the corresponding figures for older persons were relatively unchanged. Thus, it seems clear that a substantial degree of immunity to reinfection with variants of the H1N1 subtype can persist for more than 20 years.

In the recent report by Frank and Taber (1983) resistance to reinfection with H1N1 virus was as potent as that seen for H3N2 viruses. This contrasts with the findings of Fox *et al.* (1982) who did not find evidence of resistance to reinfection with H1N1 virus. Moreover, the same was true in his studies for reinfection with type B influenza virus. The basis for lack of demonstrable immunity to both types of influenza in these latter studies is unknown.

Since extensive infection and illness accompanies introductions of a new sub-type of type A influenza virus in human populations, immunity to type A viruses has been assumed to be limited to variants within a sub-type (Stuart-Harris and Schild, 1976). Evidence obtained in 1968, when the H3N2 (Hong Kong) sub-type appeared, suggested that immunity might extend to other sub-types. Hope-Simpson in England (1973) and Gill and Murphy in Australia (1976) reported that persons infected with an H2N2 virus during the year preceding occurrence of the first A/Hong Kong (H3N2) epidemic were immune to illness from this H3N2 virus on first exposure. That such immunity was probably a function of pre-existing antibody to the related N2 neuraminidases (NA) in both sub-types rather than antibody to the haemagglutinin (HA) is supported by recent information derived from longitudinal surveillance for influenza virus infections in a group of families in Houston, Texas. Both the H3N2 and H1N1 sub-type viruses circulated simultaneously in the Houston area in two different epidemic seasons of influenza (Frank *et al.*, 1983) so that persons were exposed to sub-types with distinct HA and NA proteins. In 1977–8, 40% of 238 persons were infected with a type A H3N2 virus, 11% with a type A H1N1 virus, and 4% with both sub-types; in 1980–1 the rates were 27%, 20%, and 5%, respectively. Assuming infection with each sub-type occurred independently of the other led to a predicted double infection frequency that was nearly identical to the actual frequency for the total group as well as for different age groups. This suggested that there was no significant cross-reactive immunity between sub-types when both surface antigens were distinctive. Moreover, both sub-types were isolated from six children and five were ill with both infections.

Present information available on the pathophysiology of influenza and of the duration and specificity of immunity to reinfection define a set of characteristics that immunological reaction-mediators must exhibit in order to be considered candidates for a significant role in prevention of infection with influenza viruses. They must exhibit sub-type specificity, exhibit reduced cross-reactivity to succeeding variants that appear during a type A sub-type era, be present for decades, and be active at the mucosal level. For participation in recovery from an established infection, an immune reaction-mediator must be active at the mucosal surface but need not exhibit the other

TABLE IV

Characteristics of the major candidate immunological reactions (mediators) for prevention of influenza virus infection

Characteristic	Anti-HA[a] Ab	Anti-NA[a] Ab	T-CTX[b]	T-DTH[b]	NK-CTX[c]	Activated macrophages	Interferon
Specificity	Sub-type/variant	Sub-type/variant	Type/sub-type	Type/sub-type	None	None	None
Develop early after infection	Yes	Yes	Yes	No[d]	Yes	Yes	Yes
Effect on infection	Prevent and decrease	Decrease	Decrease	None	None	Decrease	Decrease
Long term persistence (present before reinfection)	Yes	Yes	No	No	Yes	No	No
Effective at mucosal level	Yes	Yes	?Yes[e]	?	—	?Yes	Yes

[a] Antibody to the haemagglutinin (HA) and neuraminidase (NA) glycoproteins. [b] T-lymphocyte mediated cytotoxicity or delayed type hypersensitivity. [c] Natural killer cell cytotoxicity. [d] Development in the mouse is suppressed by infection and not by inactivated vaccine. [e] Are functional in the lung.

characteristics listed. A variety of cell-mediated and humoral-immune mechanisms have been proposed for affecting resistance to and recovery from an influenza virus infection; their major described characteristics are compared in Table IV.

CELL-MEDIATED IMMUNE REACTIONS

Recent developments of methods for assessing various aspects of the cell-mediated immune (CMI) response provided a basis for extensive evaluations of these responses and their relation to influenza. Although an extensive amount of data is available on responses in mice, minimal information is available thus far in man. Moreover, some reservations must be maintained regarding direct applicability of findings in mice because most humans have experienced several infections with influenza viruses, a circumstance not generally used in studies with mice.

Cell-mediated T cell Cytotoxic Reactions

The major CMI reactions or mediators that are candidates for a role in immunity to influenza virus infection are T-lymphocyte mediated cytotoxicity (T-CTX), T-lymphocyte mediated delayed type hypersensitivity (T-DTH), natural killer cell cytotoxicity (NK-CTX), macrophage antiviral effects, and interferon. Although the latter mediator is a humoral mediator of antiviral effects, it also acts as an immunomodulator for CMI (see later).

The development of T-CTX, its characteristics and role in influenza have received considerable attention recently. A summary of the major characteristics emerging from these studies is shown in Table V. Initial studies of T-cell cytotoxicity were performed in inbred mice and results showed that lysis of viral-infected cells by this mechanism exhibits specificity for cell surface antigens of the virus and the H-2K or D antigens of the major histocompatibility complex (Ada *et al.*, 1981). Both the effector and the target cells must possess compatible H-2K or D antigens. McMichael *et al.* (1977) using autologous and isologous infected lymphocytes as targets showed that T-cell cytotoxicity in humans also required that the target and cytotoxic cells must be syngeneic for the histocompatibility loci.

Other studies in mice have shown that T-cell cytotoxicity develops early after onset of influenza virus infection and reaches a peak level of activity before antibody is detectable; levels then return to baseline and are not detectable in the resting state (Ennis *et al.*, 1977). When adoptive transfer of

TABLE V
Summary of characteristics of T-lymphocyte cytotoxicity for influenza virus infected cells

---

Requires histocompatibility for expression.
Exhibits type specificity (also sub-type in mice).
Inducer potency varies; live > whole inactivated > sub-unit vaccine.
Level attained directly related to level of infection.
Prevention of infection prevents development.
Exhibits anamnestic responses.
Will decrease lung virus titres, lung consolidation, and mortality.
? T-CTX memory decreases with time.
? Inducer is immune interferon.

---

actively cytotoxic cells is employed in infected mice, a reduction in viral content of lungs and severity of pneumonia results (Yap and Ada, 1978). Although the T-cell cytotoxic reaction exhibits both type and sub-type specificity in mice, only type specificity has been seen, thus far, in humans (Ada et al., 1981; McMichael et al., 1977). Cytotoxic T-cells appear to recognize the HA and NA antigens; both the matrix (M) and nucleoprotein (NP) antigens are expressed on the surface of infected cells and, although reported as such, current evidence suggests that they do not appear to be target antigens (Askonas, 1980). The target antigen for the type-specific expression of cytotoxicity does not cross between type A and B viruses.

The level of T-CTX attained in mice is directly related to lung virus titers attained (Armerding and Liehl, 1981; Armerding et al., 1982). When the level of infection in the mouse is reduced by actively or passively acquired antibody, the level of T-CTX is similarly reduced. When infection of the mouse is prevented in the same manner, T-CTX does not develop (Armerding and Liehl, 1981; Armerding et al., 1982). When the level of infection in the mouse is reduced by actively or passively acquired antibody, the level of T-CTX is similarly reduced. When infection of the mouse is prevented in the same manner, T-CTX does not develop (Armerding and Liehl, 1981; Armerding et al., 1982). These findings in combination with the reductions in infection and disease with adoptive immunization argue strongly for a role of T-CTX in recovery from infection but not in prevention of infection.

Ennis et al. (1981a, 1982) described the dynamics of T-cell cytotoxic cells in the peripheral blood of volunteers infected with influenza virus or vaccinated with inactivated whole virus or sub-unit vaccine. Cells directly from peripheral blood were negative at seven days but exhibited T-cell cytotoxicity at 14 and 21 days; values had returned to baseline at 180 days. Cells stimulated *in vitro* for seven days with infected cells before use in cytotoxicity tests exhibited high levels of cytotoxicity; some activity was detected before exposure and there was a notable increase at seven days. By 180 days these values had also returned to baseline. Ennis *et al.* (1981a) saw little difference between infection and either of the vaccines, although McMichael *et al.* (1981) in humans and others with studies in mice (Webster and Askonas, 1980) suggested that sub-unit vaccines may be less efficient stimulators of T-CTX.

More recently, McMichael *et al.* (1983) has evaluated the relationship of T-CTX memory in volunteers to responses after challenge with an A/H1N1 virus. A relationship between T-CTX memory, as determined by *in vitro* stimulation tests before challenge and level of virus in nasal secretions three and four days after challenge, was observed. A similar relationship for serum HI antibody prompted an assessment of an effect of T-CTX among HI antibody-negative persons and an effect was noted. Because of the inability to separate the effects of T-CTX and HI antibody in the population studied, the possibility remains that the two mechanisms may work in concert or that antibody is dominant since the HI test is a relatively insensitive test for antibody (Six and Kasel, 1978). Nevertheless, the suggestion of a significant cellular effect at the nasal mucosal level is interesting. In this regard, Small (1982) was unable to find evidence of T-CTX at the mucosal level in the ferret model.

McMichael did not observe any relationship between symptom scores and T-CTX levels; this suggested to him that T-CTX aids in the clearance of virus and shortening of the duration of illness but does not appear in time to exert a beneficial effect on acute illness. Finally, a significant reduction in frequency of persons with T-CTX memory over a period of five years, suggesting a limited duration of effectiveness for this CMI reaction, was noted.

Other Studies Including Interferon

Mouse studies indicate that delayed type hypersensitivity (DTH) may be mediated by type and sub-type specific T lymphocytes (Ada *et al.*, 1981). Both type specific and sub-type specific cells are stimulated by infection and both are capable of mediating DTH and cytotoxicity (Ada *et al.*, 1981). In unprimed mice, inactivated vaccine may preferentially stimulate a population of lymphocytes capable of mediating sub-type specific DTH but not cytotoxicity (Ada *et al.*, 1981). When the latter cell population was adoptively transferred into mice, increases in lung infiltrates and mortality and absence of an effect on virus titres resulted; whereas, transfer of a population exhibiting cytotoxicity resulted in decrease in pneumonia mortality and lung virus titres (Yap and Ada, 1978). Characteristics of the cells involved in cutaneous DTH reactions in man have not been described, but Jennings et al. (1978) failed to find a relationship between serum anti-HA antibody titres and the extent of skin reactions.

Lung and peritoneal macrophages obtained from unprimed mice are able to inactivate influenza viruses (Rodgers and Mims, 1981). A contribution of macrophages to immunity in the unprimed host may exist but would be limited in effectiveness by a lack of access to the virus. Macrophages are present in the lung alveolus but not on the mucosal epithelial surface of the respiratory tract and this is the primary site of infection with influenza viruses. Moreover, they lack any specificity for virus and sub-type specificity of immunity is characteristic of influenza. Resting lymphocytes exhibit a similar ability to inactivate influenza viruses; however, this response is variable and lacks specificity (Hackemann et al., 1974). Moreover, lymphocytes are also uncommon in the normal mucosa.

Macrophages may become "activated" as a consequence of influenza virus infection and, in mice, are more effectively antiviral than in the resting state (Rodgers and Mims, 1981). Large numbers of them may gain access to virus and viral-infected cells at the mucosal surface as part of the inflammatory response to influenza virus infection. When functions of the macrophages are impaired, viral clearance in the mouse is delayed (Schulman, 1982). Macrophages "activated" by influenza virus and lymphocytes stimulated to undergo blastogenesis release interferon and other mediators into the surrounding medium; interferon could render uninfected cells resistant to infection with newly synthesized virus from infected cells.

In human studies, Cate et al. (unpublished observations) and Lazar et al. (1980) have shown that interferon released by lymphocytes stimulated by inactivated virus exhibits properties of alpha interferon; however, Ennis and Meager (1981) reported that lymphocytes stimulated by autologously infected lymphocytes secreted gamma interferon. The latter type of interferon is weakly antiviral but is active as an immunomodulator. Since its development *in vitro* in the presence of virus-infected stimulator lymphocytes was similar for all type A virus sub-types, Ennis suggested that immune interferon might mediate development of the type-specific T-CTX. Support for this suggestion was recently provided by Burlington et al. (1983), who reported that suppression of *in vitro* generation of T-CTX for influenza virus occurred in the presence of anti-gamma interferon antibody. A more detailed explanation of the mechanism of development, the role of interleukin 2, and the basis for type specificity is required before this explanation for generation of T-CTX can be accepted.

In addition to direct antiviral effects, interferon is also known to enhance the activity of natural killer (NK) cells, a cytotoxic mechanism that is not virus-specific. Ennis et al. (1981b) showed that volunteers infected with a type A virus developed increased NK activity early after inoculation and the activity was still elevated on day six. The level of cytotoxicity correlated with production of interferon and clinical severity of the illness. Since illness has been shown to reflect the intensity of infection, the level of NK activity must reflect the level of interferon which, in turn, reflects the intensity of infection. This suggests a role for NK-CTX and interferon in control of virus infection. However, Wells et al. (1983) was unable to relate differences in lung virus titres among mice to NK-CTX activity exhibited by adoptively transferred cells. Similarly, Leung and Ada (1981) failed to detect differences in responses to influenza virus challenge between inbred mice of a strain that lacked NK-CTX activity and those of a strain that possessed this activity. Finally, virus infection proceeds at a high level in the nude mouse despite high levels of NK-CTX (Wells et al., 1981). These combined findings suggest participation of NK-CTX in influenza is minimal and of little significance.

Thus, our present understanding of the various CMI reaction-mediators in influenza support a role for these defence reactions in recovery from influenza. The various characteristics described, however, do not support a role for CMI in resistance to infection although, on occasion, a rapid onset of a response might abort an infection so that it would be scored at the clinical level as no infection.

ANTIBODY

Antibody to influenza viruses develops after infection to at least four of the virion proteins, the HA, NA, M protein, and NP. Anti-M and anti-NP exhibit type-specificity primarily (Stuart-Harris and Schild, 1976). Passive treatment of mice with specific antibody to these latter two proteins before virus challenge failed to provide protection (Virelizier et al., 1976), and prior presence of NP antibody in humans is not associated with protection against influenza. Thus, antibody with these specificities does not appear to mediate resistance to infection. Antibody to both the HA and the NA proteins have been associated with prevention or modification of infection in both animals and man.

Anti-NA Antibody

Antibody specific for the NA reduces the quantity of newly synthesized virus from infected cells thereby limiting spread of infection (Stuart-Harris and Schild, 1976). Anti-NA develops in serum and respiratory secretions after infection although available data indicate that at least one priming infection is required before it is easily detected (Kasel, unpublished observations). The appearance and duration of anti-NA in nasal secretions is similar to that described for anti-HA but it generally appears at lower frequency and persists poorly (Hruskova et al., 1976). Its presence in serum before challenge is associated with reduced occurrence and severity of illnesses accompanying infection (Couch et al., 1974); it may prevent infection at the clinical level if present in high titre (Couch et al., 1974).

Anti-HA Antibody

Anti-HA antibody exhibits the characteristics required of a mediator for explaining the described patterns of naturally occurring immunity to influenza and it remains the major candidate for mediating resistance to infection. Serum antibody with this specificity is primarily IgG whereas a prominent antibody in secretions, particularly of the upper respiratory tract, is dimeric (11 S) IgA.

The most complete data on the kinetics of the anti-HA antibody response to primary infection has been provided by Murphy et al. (1982) using an enzyme-linked immunoadsorbent assay (Elisa) for the quantitation of class-specific antibodies to the HA sub-unit among persons challenged with live attenuated virus vaccines (H1N1 and H3N2). IgM, IgA, and IgG antibodies appeared simultaneously within two weeks after inoculation of virus. IgM and IgA antibody levels peaked at two weeks and then began to decline whereas IgG antibody, which was first detectable during the same period, continued to increase in titre until a maximal level was reached at four to seven weeks. Of the three class-specific antibody responses, IgM and IgG antibody occurred in all persons but an IgA antibody response was less frequent (50%). In nasal secretions, the time and rate of measurable antibodies paralleled the systemic response; although the frequencies of IgM and IgG anti-HA antibody were lower, the IgA antibody response frequency was nearly 100%.

Information relating to humoral immune responses in the lower respiratory tract of humans to infection with influenza virus is virtually non-existent. Zahradnik et al. (1983) examined the compartmental distribution of immunoglobulin-specific anti-HA responses in a small number of individuals exposed to an experimental intranasal challenge with a low dose of a live attenuated H1N1 virus vaccine. An analysis of bronchial lavage fluids showed that the most frequent antibody response was of the IgG isotype and it was mainly limited to persons with pre-existing serum antibody.

Duration of serum anti-HA antibody as determined by the HI test has been assessed after vaccination and infection. For both kinds of exposure to type A and B viruses there is an initial fall in mean titres over the first six months after achieving peak titres; titres then remain stable for at least two to three years without a further antigenic stimulus (Cate et al., 1977; and L. H. Taber, unpublished data). The level of fall can vary between two and ten-fold with the degree of fall being generally proportional to the peak titres. That serum anti-HA antibody may persist for long periods of time is indicated by the finding of H1N1 antibody in 80% of older persons during the 1976 swine immunization campaign, despite the fact that they should not have encountered a related antigen for at least 20 years, and the finding of antibody to the H3 HA in 1968 among persons alive before 1892 (Knight and Kasel, 1973). In a similar analysis for recently introduced H1N1 viruses, Cate (unpublished data) found that about 70% of elderly persons possessed serum neutralizing antibody to the A/Brazil/11/78 (H1N1) virus prior to its reappearance in human populations in 1977 although most had low titres. Serum antibody to the NA protein also persists for many years.

Antibody to the HA protein is less likely to persist in detectable concentrations in nasal secretions. In primed adults about 60% of persons have detectable neutralizing anti-HA antibody early after infection but only about 30% will have detectable antibody at 12 months; a progressive decline during a 12-month interval has been described (Waldman et al., 1970). In unprimed children administered live attenuated H1N1 and H3N2 virus vaccines nasal neutralizing antibody levels, after peaking between two and four weeks, declined significantly by nine weeks (Wright et al., 1982).

A great deal of evidence exists that the serum antibody response to influenza virus glycoproteins is sub-type specific. Both animal and human sera fail to exhibit cross-reactions between the HA or the NA antigen of the different sub-types (Stuart-Harris and Schild, 1976). This is probably also true for the secretory response.

Further insights into the specificity of the anti-HA antibody response have been provided mostly from investigations dealing with H3N2 viruses. The use of viral immunoadsorbants has permitted some discernment of the antibody population. Sera from individuals immunized with an inactivated virus vaccine containing the A/Port Chalmers/73 (H3N2) variant and who had been initially primed to A/Hong Kong/68 (H3N2) HA exhibited different patterns of response. While all vaccinees developed a cross-reacting antibody, a surprising finding was that 88% developed a response to a specific determinant(s) located on the A/Hong Kong/68 HA while only 30% developed antibody specific for the vaccine virus, A/Port Chalmers/73. Patterns of specificity similar to these have also been shown to occur for other H3N2 variants, A/England/72, A/Scotland/74, and A/Victoria/75, when these were used as vaccines for inducing anti-HA responses (Oxford et al., 1979). The finding that antibody to the strain-specific antigenic determinant(s) occurs in higher frequency among persons experiencing natural infection suggested that infection provided the broadest antibody response (Kasel et al., 1979). Overall, these various adsorption studies revealed that antibodies induced by exposures to influenza virus are mainly directed toward determinants shared by the different sub-type variants. This should be expected, since the HA molecule carries multiple determinants only a few of which are altered in different variants. Since the total antibody response reflects combined antibody specificities, a number of variant changes are required before little or no cross-reactivity is detectable for succeeding variants.

Anti-HA antibody may function in a variety of ways against influenza virus. These include neutralization for infection, opsonization for phagocyte destruction, complement-mediated lysis, aggregation of particles, and activation of antibody-dependent cellular cytotoxicity (ADCC). ADCC to influenza virus infected cells may be mediated by K lymphocytes from the non-T—non-B fraction, macrophages, and possibly neutrophils. Each of these cells contains receptors for the Fc portion of the Ig molecule of IgG but apparently not for IgA. Greenberg et al. (1975) showed that the level of ADCC activity correlated with the titre of serum anti-HA antibody. He also showed that antibody concentrations too small to be detected by neutralization but detectable by sensitive radioimmunoprecipitation (RIP) assays could mediate potent ADCC (Greenberg et al., 1977). Initial assessments of changes in ADCC activity after infection and vaccination revealed a rise early after antigen challenge with a fall by 30 days to a level commensurate with the titre of serum antibody (Greenberg et al., 1978b). After all antibody was removed from the system, the early rise remained and it was subsequently shown to represent an *in vitro* secretion of antibody by circulating B cells (Greenberg et al., 1979). ADCC also appears and increases early after infection and may play a role in recovery since Greenberg et al. (1978b) showed activity as early as day four after inoculation of neutralizing antibody-negative volunteers with a type A virus.

Anti-IgG and IgA in Secretions

There is little reason to doubt that antibody must be at the mucosal surface for optimal effect. Most attempts to discriminate between serum and local IgA antibody for a resistance to influenza virus infection have involved artificial intranasal challenge with large doses of *in vitro* propagated virus early, generally four to six weeks after an infection or vaccination. Definitive conclusions regarding the mechanism of natural immunity are not possible from such studies because influenza is presumed to be initiated most commonly by low doses of virulent virus contained in small airborne particles that deposit in both the upper and the lower respiratory tract and the interval between these natural rechallenges is months to years (Knight and Kasel, 1973). Noteworthy is the fact that, despite conditions in artificial challenges that would appear to favour nasal secretory antibody, only serum antibody has consistently related to protection (Couch et al., 1981). In the experiments summarized in Tables I to III, measurements of neutralizing antibody indicated a close parallel between detection of neutralizing antibody in serum and a demonstration of immunity; failure to detect cross-reacting antibody to the challenge virus in most persons did not occur until the A/Victoria/75 (H3N2) variant appeared. Moreover, in a separate study, Couch et al. (1979) showed that the level of serum antibody related best to protection whether the antibody was cross-reacting or strain-specific for the challenge virus.

The infrequent detection of nasal secretion neutralizing antibody after a remote infection suggested to us that this antibody was not primarily responsible for the immunity. Possible reasons for the inconsistency in demonstrating a major role for secretory IgA antibody include lack of a satisfactory collection and processing of secretions so that uniformity between individuals and collections is assured, and sensitivity of assays for antibody. It is of interest that, using a sensitive Elisa assay for quantitation of antibody, Murphy and colleagues have recently achieved some consistency in demonstrating a correlation between protection and secretory IgA antibody in volunteers challenged intranasally four to six weeks after infection with a live attenuated virus.

In a recent study of ours, Cate et al. (unpublished data) used sensitive radio immune precipitation (RIP) assays to compare neutralizing and IgG antibody in serum and IgG and IgA antibody in nasal secretions to resistance to an A (H1N1) influenza virus challenge. Volunteers had received a live attenuated vaccine, an inactivated vaccine, or placebo two months earlier. A summary of the findings are given in Table VI. Serum neutralizing antibody titres correlated with serum RIP IgG antibody titres, nasal secretion IgG antibody titres, and approached significance for a correlation with nasal secretion IgA antibody titres. When the results were examined for a correlation between antibody titre and severity of the infection and illness response, a significant inverse correlation with infection severity for all antibody assays ($P < 0.001$ for serum neutralization and RIP IgG; $P < 0.01$ for nasal secretion RIP IgG and IgA) were evident. Thus, the two antibodies in nasal secretions appeared of equal significance in resistance to this nasal challenge.

In a search for an independent effect of antibody in secretions, Cate examined the relation of days of virus shedding and titre of antibody in

TABLE VI
Response of volunteers to intranasal challenge with wild-type influenza A/USSR (H1N1) virus according to prechallenge serum and nasal secretion antibody titres

No. of Volunteers	Serum Antibody[a] Neutralizing	IgG[c]	Nasal Secretion Antibody[a] sIgA[d]	IgG[d]	Virus Shedding[b] % of Volrs.	Avg. days	Percent of Volrs. ill Total	Febrile
11	1·0 (<2)	104 (<50–386)	7·5 (<5–68)	4·3 (<5–34)	91	4·2	45	36
8	3·7 (3–6)	341 (150–780)	8·2 (<5–35)	5·5 (<5–51)	25	4·0	25	13
7	33·1 (8–128)	1154 (342–5045)	22·4 (<5–121)	18·5 (5–54)	0	—	0	—

[a] Antibody expressed as geometric mean titre (range). [b] All infected volunteers shed virus.
[c] Dilution of serum that precipitated 20% of radiolabelled HI-A/USSR with antiserum to IgG.
[d] Dilution of nasal wash that precipitated 10% of radiolabelled HI-A/USSR with antiserum to secretory component (sIgA) or to IgG, divided by the concentration (mg/dl) of the respective Ig in the specimen.

secretions among those volunteers with little or no serum neutralizing antibody. A significant inverse correlation with virus shedding was found for both RIP IgG and RIP IgA titres in secretions. In this analysis, no relation to serum RIP IgG was detected. Thus, these evaluations suggest that antibodies in both serum and nasal secretions aid in protection against influenza with the relative contributions of each related to antibody levels in both sites.

The lower respiratory tract contains a higher proportion of IgG than does the nasopharynx (Reynolds et al., 1978). Because most naturally occurring influenza is believed to be transmitted by small particle aerosols which would deposit in the lower respiratory tract and because antibodies in that location will have been acquired from an infection months or years earlier, we sought to compare anti-HA antibody concentrations in serum and in both upper and lower respiratory tract secretions remotely after an infection. Initial results using an Elisa method for separately quantitating IgA and IgG antibody (Murphy et al., 1981) to an H3 antigen are shown in Table VII. Subjects for this study were 25 students not previously given

TABLE VII
Distribution of concentrations of antibody to A/AICHI/68 (H3N2) influenza virus according to immunoglobulin class and body fluid

Body fluid	Ig class	No. with indicated μg/ml antibody						G/A mean (range)
		0·4–20	20–40	40–80	80–160	160–320	>320	
Serum	A	22	3					30·5 (1–250)
	G	1	5	2	7	9	1	

Body fluid	Ig class	No. with indicated μg/ml antibody						G/A mean (range)
		0–0·4	0·4–0·8	0·8–1·6	1·6–3·2	3·2–6·4	>6·4	
Nasal secretions	A	7	8	7	2		1	0·7 (0·1–2·7)
	G	16	5	2	1	1		
Bronchial lavage	A	13	6	4	1	1		3·6[a] (0·2–>15)
	G	7	6	4	2	5	1	

[a] Ratio for 24 specimens, one specimen did not contain IgA Ab.

vaccine. Lower respiratory secretions were collected by bronchial lavage with a fiberoptic bronchoscope and tested simultaneously with nasal secretions and serum for anti-HA to A/Aichi/68 (H3N2) influenza virus. This H3N2 variant had appeared over 10 years earlier and all students are presumed to have had at least one or two infections with this or a related H3N2 virus before specimens were collected. Results are expressed as μg/ml of IgA or IgG antibody as determined by reference to standard curves of O.D. readings for varying concentrations of purified IgA or IgG.

All serum specimens contained both measurable IgG and IgA antibody; concentrations of IgG antibody varied over a wide range but IgA antibody concentrations were low. The mean of IgG/IgA (G/A) antibody ratios for each student was 30·5 with a range of one to 250. This ratio contrasts to a G/A ratio of immunoglobulin concentrations in each serum of about four. Considerably lower antibody concentrations were detected in nasal and bronchial secretions than in serum. The distribution of concentrations for

IgA and IgG antibody in nasal secretions were similar but a slight excess of IgA antibody in most secretions resulted in a mean G/A ratio of 0·7. We presume that the IgA antibody measured is primarily 11 S. Assuming this is most likely to be true, then secretory IgA antibody will have been shown to persist for long periods of time in nasal secretions of most persons after infection with an influenza virus. Whether these concentrations of IgA or IgG antibody are sufficient to prevent initiation of infection in the nasopharynx has not yet been determined, although Clements et al. (1983) has indicated that low titres of remotely acquired IgA antibody are associated with protection against nasal challenge with attenuated influenza virus vaccines. Of interest are the distributions of antibody in bronchial wash fluids; higher concentrations of IgG antibody were detected in most specimens and the mean G/A ratio was 3·6.

The data in Table VII indicate that both IgA and IgG anti-HA antibody persist in both nasal and bronchial secretions. The greater proportion of IgG antibody in bronchial secretions is in keeping with the increasing proportion of IgG that is known to occur in secretions with increasing descent into the lower respiratory passages (Reynolds et al., 1978).

An integration of the information presented on immunoglobulins and antibody in respiratory secretions with available information on deposition sites of small particle aerosols and 50% human infectious doses for the

TABLE VIII
Relationship of location and Ig class of antibody to deposition site and infectivity estimates for a small particle aerosol containing a type A influenza virus

Respiratory level	Ratio IgG/IgA	Ratio IgG Ab/IgA Ab	% Deposition of inhaled 2μ particles[a]	Estimated inhalation dose required for infection at indicated site ($TCID_{50}$)
Nasopharynx	0·1[b]	0·7[b]	35	500[d]
Trachea and upper bronchi	0·6[b]	3·6[b]	±0	—
Lower bronchi and bronchioles	3[c]	—	12	3[e]
Alevolae	—	—	19	

[a] Data from Knight et al. (1970). [b] Data from this study. [c] Data from Reynolds et al. (1978). [d] Based on average of several HID_{50} for H3N2 viruses (Couch, 1973) and 35% deposition in nasopharynx. [e] Data summarized in Knight et al. (1970).

different sites is given in Table VIII. As noted, the G/A ratios for antibody in the two secretions exceeds the G/A ratios of Ig concentrations (determined in immunodiffusion plates with adjustment of values of IgA to reflect its dimeric structure (Greenberg et al., 1978a). The IgG/IgA ratio of 0·6 for bronchial secretions establishes that these washes were obtained from high in the tracheobronchial passages (Reynolds et al., 1978). Reynolds et al. (1978) has indicated that a high IgG/IgA ratio is found in secretions from more peripheral branchings of the bronchial passages (Table VIII).

Deposition sites for a 2μ particle aerosol are those provided by Landahl in Knight et al. (1970). The estimated HID_{50} for nasal drops represents an approximation from a number of determinations by Couch (1973) for A/Hong Kong/68-like viruses in serum neutralizing antibody-negative volunteers. The estimated HID_{50} by small particle aerosol of three $TCID_{50}$ was that reported for an H2N2 virus (Knight et al., 1970). As noted in the table, deposition of 35% of particles in the nasopharynx would indicate that an inhaled dose of about 500 $TCID_{50}$ is required for deposition of one HID_{50} at this site, considerably less virus need be contained in the aerosol in order to initiate infection in the lower respiratory passages. It seems likely that most infections are initiated by relatively dilute aerosols and that these infections are initiated in the lower respiratory tract (Knight and Kasel, 1973). IgG antibody would be the mediator of resistance to such a challenge. On the other hand, when acquisition is by a contact route or the virus dose inhaled is very large, then infection may be initiated in the nasopharynx; persisting IgA antibody may contribute to prevention of infection at that site.

Available data indicate that about 95% of IgA in nasal secretions and about 80% in bronchial lavage specimens is synthesized by B lymphocytes in the sub-mucosal tissues (Delacroix et al., 1982). Studies on nasal secretions by Butler et al. (1970) indicated that about 50% of the IgG in this secretion is derived from local synthesis and about 50% from serum. Optimal development of antibody in nasal secretions should, therefore, require local antigenic stimulation. In contrast to the findings for nasal secretions, studies of bronchial lavage fluids by Merrill et al. (1980) indicate that 100% of IgG in non-smokers is derived from serum whereas an average of 20% of IgG in smokers was synthesized locally.

Thus, a clear basis for the correlations between serum antibody and protection against influenza is provided by this current synthesis of available information. Furthermore, this proposal is supported by passive immunization data. Administration of antibody passively was shown very early to mediate protection in the animal model; more recently Puck et al. (1980) indicated that infants are protected from type A influenza by maternally-derived antibody.

The present information does not alter any existing concepts of optimal ways for immunization against influenza. A full complement of immunological reaction-mediators is best obtained by experiencing infection but immunization by means of inactivated vaccines can lead to significant levels of protection. The present information does suggest, however, that successful immunization requires a satisfactory serum antibody response.

SUMMARY

Immunity to infection with type A influenza viruses is sub-type specific since little or no resistance is conveyed to sub-types possessing immunologically distinct HA and NA proteins. Observations with H1N1 and H3N2 viruses indicate that homotypic resistance to subsequent infection and illness with the same virus is potent and of long duration. Within a sub-type, a prior antigenic experience with one variant may prevent or modify infection with another. The resulting degree of sub-type immunity depends on the extent of relatedness between variants.

The described immunological reactions that could influence the occurrence and course of influenza virus infection in man include the following: T-lymphocyte-mediated cytotoxic or DTH reactions; interferon, either through intracellular antiviral effects or stimulation of natural killer cytotoxic reactions; innate antiviral actions of macrophages and lymphocytes; and reactions involving antibodies to the HA and NA antigens in serum or respiratory secretions.

Assessments of the characteristics of the various mediators indicate that recovery from influenza virus infection must involve a variety of humoral and cell-mediated immune mechanisms; conclusions regarding the relative importance of each is not possible at the present time. Use of sensitive assays for IgA and IgG antibody in nasal secretions has suggested both classes of antibody play a role in resistance of volunteers to intranasal challenge with infectious virus.

Natural infection is considered to be acquired primarily by low doses of virus inhaled into the lower respiratory tract remotely after prior infection. A comparison of IgA and IgG antibody in bronchial lavage fluids remotely after an earlier infection indicated a predominance of IgG antibody. This finding in combination with the demonstrated prophylactic effect of passive antibody and the data indicating that most or all of IgG in the lower respiratory passages is derived from serum, suggests that serum IgG antibody is the primary mediator for prevention of naturally occurring influenza.

ACKNOWLEDGMENTS

The authors wish to thank Barbara Baxter for technical assistance and Linda Reckeweg for manuscript typing. Research presented in this manuscript was supported by the National Institute of Allergy and Infectious Diseases under contract no. NO1 AI 32685.

REFERENCES

Ada, G. L., Leung, K.-N. and Ertl, H. (1981). An analysis of effector T cell generation and function in mice exposed to influenza A or Sendai viruses. *Immunol. Rev.* **58**, 5–24.

Armerding, D. and Liehl, E. (1981). Induction of homotypic and heterotypic T-and B-cell immunity with influenza A virus in mice. *Cellular Immunol.* **60**, 119–135.

Armerding, D., Rossiter, H. and Liehl, E. (1982). Killer T cell responses to influenza A during a drift period: studies in mice. *Med. Microbiol. Immunol.* **170**, 255–264.

Askonas, B. A. (1980). Our immune defense against influenza. *Biochem. Soc. Trans.* **3**, 257–260.

Burlington, D. B., Djeu, J. Y., Langford, M., Wells, M. A. and Quinnan, G. V., Jr. (1983). Alpha and gamma interferons are required for the secondary *in vitro* generation of influenza A virus-specific cytotoxic T cells. *Abstracts of ICAAC, Am. Soc. of Microbiol.* 210.

Butler, W. T., Waldman, T. A., Rossen, R. D., Douglas, R. G., Jr. and Couch, R. B. (1970). Changes in IgA and IgG concentrations in nasal secretions prior to the appearance of antibody during viral respiratory infection in man. *J. Immunol.* **10**, 584–591.

Cate, T. R., Kasel, J. A., Couch, R. B., Six, H. R. and Knight, V. (1977). Clinical trials of bivalent influenza A/New Jersey/76-A/Victoria/75 vaccines in the elderly. *J. Infect. Dis.* **136** (Suppl.): S518–S525.

Clements, M. L., O'Donnell, S., Levine, M. M., Chanock, R. M. and Murphy, B. R. (1983). Dose response of A/Alaska/6/77 (H3N2) cold-adapted reassortant vaccine virus in adult volunteers: role of local antibody in resistance to infection with vaccine virus. *Infect. and Immun.* **40**, 1044–1051.

Couch, R. B. (1973). Summary of data in "Epidemiology of Influenza—Summary of Influenza Workshop IV". *J. Infect. Dis.* **128**, 361–386.

Couch, R. B. (1975). Assessment of immunity to influenza using artificial challenge of normal volunteers with influenza virus. *In* "International Symposium in Immunity to Infections of the Respiratory System in Man and Animals". London, 1974. *Develop. Biol. Standard.* **28**, 295–306. Karger, Bagel, 1975.

Couch, R. B., Douglas, R. G., Jr., Rossen, R. and Kasel, J. A. (1969). Role of secretory antibody in influenza. *In* "The Secretory Immunologic System" (Eds D. D. Dayton, D. A. Small, Jr., R. M. Chanock, H. E. Kaufman, T. Tomasi, Jr.), pp. 93–112. U.S. Government Printing Office, Washington, D.C.

Couch, R. B., Kasel, J. A., Gerin, J. L., Schulman, J. L. and Kilbourne, E. D. (1974). Induction of partial immunity to influenza by a neuraminidase-specific vaccine. *J. Infect. Dis.* **129**, 411–420.

Couch, R. B., Webster, R. G., Kasel, J. A. and Cate, T. R. (1979). Efficacy of purified influenza subunit vaccines and relation to the major antigenic determinants on the hemagglutinin molecule. *J. Infect. Dis.* **140**, 553–559.

Couch, R. B., Kasel, J. A., Six, H. R. and Cate, T. R. (1981). The basis for immunity to influenza in man. In "Genetic Variation Among Influenza Viruses" (Ed. D. P. Nayak) Vol. XXI, pp. 535–546. Academic Press, New York and London.

Delacroix, D. L., Dive, C., Ramband, J. C. and Vaerman, J. P. (1982). IgA subclasses in various secretions and in serum. *Immunol.* **47**, 383–385.

Ennis, F. A. and Meager, A. (1981). Immune interferon produced to high levels by antigenic stimulation of human lymphocytes with influenza virus. *J. Exp. Med.* **154**, 1279–1289.

Ennis, F. A., Martin, W. J., Verbonitz, M. W. (1977). Hemagglutinin-specific cytotoxic T-cell response during influenza infection. *J. Exp. Med.* **146**, 893–898.

Ennis, F. A., Rook, A. H., Hua, Q. Y., Schild, G. C., Riley, O., Pratt, R. and Potter, C. W. (1981a). HLA-restricted virus-specific cytotoxic T-lymphocyte responses to live and inactivated influenza vaccines. *Lancet* **ii**, 887–891.

Ennis, F. A., Meager, A., Beare, A. S., Hua, Q. Y., Riley, D., Schwarz, G., Schild, G. C. and Rook, A. H. (1981b). Interferon induction and increased natural killer-cell activity in influenza infections in man. *Lancet* **ii**, 891–893.

Ennis, F. A., Hua, Q. Y. and Schild, G. C. (1982). Antibody and cytotoxic T lymphocyte responses of humans to live and inactivated vaccines. *J. Gen. Virol.* **58**, 273–281.

Fox, J. P., Hall, C. E., Cooney, M. K. and Foy, H. M. (1982). Influenza virus infections in Seattle families, 1975–1979. I. Study design, methods and the occurrence of infections by time and age. *Am. Jour. Epidemiol.* **116**, 212–227.

Frank, A. L. and Taber, L. H. (1983). Variation in frequency of natural reinfection with influenza A viruses. *J. Med. Virol.* **12**, 17–23.

Frank, A. L., Taber, L. H., Glezen, W. P., Paredes, A. and Couch, R. B. (1979). Reinfection with influenza A (H3N2) virus in young children and their families. *J. Infect. Dis.* **140**, 829–836.

Frank, A. L., Taber, L. H. and Wells, J. M. (1983). Individuals infected with two subtypes of influenza A virus in the same season. *J. Infect. Dis.* **147**, 120–124.

Gill, P. W. and Murphy, A. M. (1976). Naturally acquired immunity to influenza type A. *Med. Jour. Aust.* **ii**, 329–333.

Gill, P. W. and Murphy, A. M. (1977). Naturally acquired immunity to influenza type A. A further prospective study. *Med. Jour. Aust.* **ii**, 761–765.

Glezen, W. P., Couch, R. B. and Six, H. R. (1982). The influenza herald wave. *Am. Jour. Epidemiol.* **116**, 589–598.

Greenberg, S. B., Couch, R. B. and Kasel, J. A. (1974). An outbreak of an influenza type A variant in a closed population: the effect of homologous and heterologous antibody in infection and illness. *Am. Jour. Epidemiol.* **100**, 209–215.

Greenberg, S. B., Criswell, B. S. and Couch, R. B. (1975). Lymphocyte-mediated cytotoxicity against influenza virus-infected cells: an *in vitro* method. *J. Immunol.* **115**, 601–603.

Greenberg, S. B., Criswell, B. S., Six, H. R. and Couch, R. B. (1977). Lymphocyte cytotoxicity to influenza virus-infected cells. II. Requirement for antibody and non-T lymphocytes. *J. Immunol.* **119**, 2100–2106.

Greenberg, S. B., Rossen, R. D., Six, H. R., Baxter, B. D. and Couch, R. B. (1978a). Determination of IgA concentrations in human nasal secretions using a serum IgA standard. *J. Clin. Microb.* **8**, 465–467.

Greenberg, S. B., Criswell, B. S., Six, H. R. and Couch, R. B. (1978b). Lymphocyte cytotoxicity to influenza virus-infected cells: response to vaccination and virus infection. *Infect. Immun.* **20**, 640–645.

Greenberg, S. B., Six, H. R., Drake, S. and Couch, R. B. (1979). Cell cytotoxicity due to specific influenza antibody production *in vitro* after recent influenza antigen stimulation. *Proc. Natl. Acad. Sci. USA* **76**, 4622–4626.

Hackemann, M. M. A., Denman, A. M. and Tyrrell, D. A. J. (1974). Inactivation of influenza virus by human lymphocytes. *Clin. Exp. Immunol.* **16**, 583–591.

Hope-Simpson, R. E. (1973). Summary of data in "Epidemiology of Influenza-Summary of Influenza Workshop IV" *J. Infect. Dis.* **128**, 361–386.

Hruskova, J., Syrucek, L., Tumova, B., Stumpa, A., Bruckova, M., Losova, M. and Berkovicova, V. (1976). Levels of immunoglobulins and antibodies to hemagglutinin and neuraminidase of influenza virus in nasal secretions after natural infection. *Acta Virol.* **20**, 126–134.

Jennings, R., Fenton, R. J., McEntegart, M. G. and Potter, C. W. (1978). A contribution of cellular immunity to protection against influenza in man. *Med. Microbiol. Immunol.* **166**, 51–62.

Kasel, J. A., Six, H. R., Couch, R. B., Greenberg, S. B. and Cate, T. R. (1979). Variant-specific antihemagglutinin serum response to Type A influenza natural infection and inactivated vaccines in adults. *Proc. Soc. Exp. Biol. and Med.* **161**, 519–521.

Knight, V. K., and Kasel, J. A. (1973). Influenza virus. *In* "Viral and Mycoplasmal Infections of the Respiratory Tract" (Ed. V. Knight) pp. 87–123. Lea and Febiger, Philadelphia.

Knight, V. K., Couch, R. B. and Landahl, H. D. (1970). Effect of lack of gravity on airborne infection during space flight. *J. Am. Med. Assoc.* **214**, 513–518.

Lazar, A., Okabe, N. and Wright, P. F. (1980). Humoral and cellular immune responses of seronegative children vaccinated with a cold-adapted influenza A/HK/123/77 (H1N1) recombinant virus. *Infect. Immun.* **27**, 862–866.

Leung, K. N. and Ada, G. L. (1981). Induction of natural killer cells during murine influenza virus infection. *Immunobiology* **160**, 352–366.

Merrill, W. W., Goodenberger, D., Strober, W., Matthay, R. A., Naegel, G. P. and Reynolds, H. Y. (1980). Free secretory component and other proteins in human lung lavage. *Am. Rev. Resp. Dis.* **122**, 156–160.

McMichael, A. J., Ting, A., Zweerink, H. J. and Askonas, B. A. (1977). HLA restriction of cell-mediated lysis of influenza virus-infected human cells. *Nature* **270**, 524–526.

McMichael, A. J., Gotch, F., Cullen, C., Askonas, B. and Webster, R. G. (1981). The human cytotoxic T cell response to influenza A vaccination. *Clin. Exp. Immunol.* **43**, 276–284.

McMichael, A. J., Gotch, F. M., Noble, G. R. and Beare, A.S. (1983). Cytotoxic T-cell immunity to influenza. *N. Engl. J. Med.* **309**, 13–17.

Murphy, B. R., Phelan, M. A., Nelson, D. L., Yarchoan, R., Tierney, E. L., Alling, D. W. and Chanock, R. M. (1981). Hemagglutinin-specific enzyme-linked immunosorbent assay for antibodies to influenza A and B viruses. *J. Clin. Microb.* **13**, 554–560.

Murphy, B. R., Nelson, D. L., Wright, P. F., Tierney, E. L., Phelan, M. A. and Chanock, R. M. (1982). Secretory and systemic immunological response in children infected with live attenuated influenza A virus vaccines. *Infect. Immun.* **36**, 1102–1108.

Oxford, J. S., Schild, G. C., Potter, C. W. and Jennings, R. (1979). The specificity of the anti-hemagglutinin antibody response induced in man by inactivated influenza vaccines and by natural infection. *J. Hyg.* (Camb.) **82**, 51–61.

Puck, J. M., Glezen, W. P., Frank, A. L. and Six, H. R. (1980). Protection of infants from infection with influenza A virus by transplacentally acquired antibody. *J. Infect. Dis.* **142**, 844–849.

Pyhala, R. (1979). H1N1 influenza and old people. *Fed. European Microbiol. Societies, Micro Letters* **6**, 175–176.

Reynolds, H. Y., Merrill, W. M., Amento, E. P. and Naegel, G. P. (1978). Immunoglobulin A in secretions from the lower respiratory tract. *In* "Secretory Immunity and Infection" (Eds J. R. McGhee, J. Mestecky and J. L. Babb) pp. 553–564. Plenum Press, New York.

Rodgers, B. C. and Mims, C. A. (1981). Interaction of influenza virus with mouse macrophages. *Infect. Immun.* **31**, 751–757.

Schulman, J. L. (1982). Summary of data in "Vaccination Against Influenza". *Immunology Today* **3**, 257–260.

Six, H. R. and Kasel, J. A. (1978). Radioimmunoprecipitation assay for quantitation of serum antibody to the hemagglutinin of type A influenza virus. *J. Clin. Microb.* **7**, 165–171.

Small, P. A. (1982). Summary of data in "Vaccination Against Influenza". *Immunology Today* **3**, 257–260.

Stuart-Harris, C. H. and Schild, G. C. (1976). "Influenza, the Viruses and the Disease." Edward Arnold, London.

Virelizier, J. L., Oxford, J. S. and Schild, G. C. (1976). The role of humoral immunity in host defense against influenza A infection in mice. *Postgrad. Med. J.* **52**, 332–337.

Waldman, R. H., Wood, S. H., Torres, E. J. and Small, P. A., Jr. (1970). Influenza antibody responses following aerosol administration of inactivated virus. *Am. J. Epidemiol.* **91**, 575–584.

Webster, R. G. and Askonas, B. A. (1980). Cross protection and cross reactive cytotoxic T cells induced by influenza virus vaccines in mice. *Eur. J. Immunol.* **10**, 396–401.

Wells, M. A., Albrecht, P. and Ennis, F. A. (1981). Recovery from a viral respiratory infection. I. Influenza pneumonia in normal and T-deficient mice. *J. Immunol.* **126**, 1036–1046.

Wells, M. A., Daniel, S., Djeu, J. Y., Kiley, S. C. and Ennis, F. A. (1983). Recovery from a viral respiratory tract infection. V. Specificity of protection by cytotoxic T lymphocytes. *J. Immunol.* **130**, 2908–2914.

Wright, P. F., Ross, K. B., Thompson, J. and Karzon, D. T. (1977). Influenza A infections in young children. *N. Engl. J. Med.* **296**, 829–834.

Wright, P. F., Okabe, N., McKee, K. T., Jr., Maassab, H. F. and Karzon, D. T. (1982). Cold-adapted recombinant influenza A virus vaccines in seronegative young children. *J. Infect. Dis.* **146**, 71–79.

Yap, K. L. and Ada, G. L. (1978). The recovery of mice from influenza virus infection. Adoptive transfer of immunity with immune T lymphocytes. *Scand. J. Immunol.* **7**, 389–397.

Zahradnik, J. M., Kasel, J. A., Martin, R. R., Six, H. R. and Cate, T. R. (1983). Immune responses in serum and respiratory secretions following vaccination with a live cold-recombinant (CR35) and inactivated A/USSR/77 (H1N1) influenza virus vaccine. *J. Med. Virol.* **11**, 277–285.

DISCUSSION

Dowdle Yesterday, Sir Christopher told us about some of the very early work on influenza viruses, the isolation of the virus and studies on pathogenesis; it was a natural step from there to devising methods for the control and prevention of influenza. I always find it amazing that the first influenza vaccine trials were held during the winter of 1935–6, two years after discovery of the virus. This first vaccine was produced in mouse lungs. Even at that early time it was felt there was a very close association between circulating antibody and protection against disease, although it was also noted at the time that indeed the correlates were not always perfect.

It was over 40 years ago that Dr Francis, Dr Fazekas and others pointed out that protection against disease was very likely to be associated with circulating antibody, but protection against infection itself was probably associated with antibodies found in the nasal secretions. That was a long time ago and so we might ask why we are talking about mechanisms of immunity this morning. First, it turned out it was not quite so simple and secondly, a great deal more has been learned and has been summarized in the review to which we have listened.

Schild I think one of the most intriguing natural experiments in the epidemiological context is the re-emergence of H1N1 in 1977 and the clear evidence from epidemiology that individuals who have been exposed some 20 years later, though they may be occasionally infected, do not get overt disease. So that some element of protection from disease is persisting following natural infection apparently for 20 years. Have you any comment on this in terms of your experimental work?

Couch We have no direct experimental challenge data that relate to this question; however, natural challenge has very clearly shown us that these persons exhibit partial and complete immunity. As indicated in my manuscript, we detected some serum antibody in most elderly persons. So a basis for the apparent partial or complete immunity exists. There is data to suggest, however, that H1N1 viruses are less virulent than H3N2 viruses. We found support for this with a low febrile illness rate among college students who were not alive before 1957. So, conclusions on illness occurrence after H1N1 among older persons must acknowledge that such an exposure to H3N2 or another influenza virus might not produce the same finding.

Schild I think the observations on older individuals, who are apparently protected from clinical disease associated with H1N1 virus, suggest that antibody to that virus is at very low levels or is sometimes undetectable. Is there a possibility that resistance may not necessarily be manifested by pre-existing antibody? It may be immunological memory or some other factor.

Couch We have recently used the Elisa method to test other age groups for antibody to A/USSR (H1N1) virus and find essentially all persons exposed to H1N1 viruses in the 1950s have antibodies. So there is data to support the proposal for a central role for serum IgG antibody in immunity. But I acknowledge that other mechanisms may be involved. Your comment on antibody memory raises a consideration of antibody-dependent cellular cytotoxicity (ADCC) which develops very early. Among primed persons, the rate at which ADCC develops and can be demonstrated is almost precisely that seen with T-cell cytotoxicity. The mediator for ADCC is a non-T, non-B lymphocyte but the mechanism is still cytotoxicity. So many possibilities exist that we simply cannot sort out the relative significance of mechanisms that could hasten recovery and prevent illness at present.

Fiers In the case of influenza B the nucleotide sequence data indicates that the drift occurs at a considerably slower rate. Is there any evidence that immunity in the human population persists for a longer time?

Couch I do not know how to best interpret the influenza B data. In volunteer studies there is no question that we can document the same kinds of resistance following vaccination or infection that we see for type A viruses. However, when individuals tried to look at naturally-occurring disease for immunity to B virus, they had much less success in detecting it. I am thinking mostly of the family studies which were reported by Fox where he indicated an inability to find any immunity at all to influenza B. Whether that results from the lack of precision in family studies or whether it is attributable to B virus is not clear. Influenza B exhibits all of the same kinds of immune mechanisms that we described for A and, while I do not think that we have adequate data, it is my own belief that we are dealing with the same type of immunity and of the same degree.

Fiers The fact that the virus itself changes at a slower rate means that one should be able by comparison to see when the resistance fades away, to what extent this is due to the time scale and how much is due to the change in the virus structure.

Couch Agreed. We have not done that.

Palese Based on sequencing data we know that there is about a 10% nucleotide change in the B virus haemagglutinins over a period of 30 years, whereas one sees a similar change in the H3 haemagglutinin genes over a period of only 10 years. I do not know if we should overinterpret those data, it appears that influenza B virus haemagglutinin genes change at a rate which is one-third of that found for influenza A (H3N2) virus haemagglutinins.

Murphy I want to respond to what Schild said about the possibility of immunological memory as it exists in the respiratory tract. Doctors Wright,

Karzon and I have recently been able to demonstrate local IgA memory for influenza haemagglutinin in the respiratory tract. At a time when the local HI antibody levels that had been induced by infection had gone down to an undetectable level we challenged individuals with an inactivated vaccine and were able to show an anamnestic response in the upper respiratory tract (Wright et al., 1983).

This is at least one of the reasons why it is difficult to measure and assess immunity to influenza viruses or the response to experimental challenge infections. This is so because one is usually attempting to assess a relatively dynamic system for measuring antibody levels in serum and nasal secretions. In the pre-challenge state you really have a capacity to respond at rates that differ from one individual to another. That is one reason why we were all plagued with the difficulty in the interpretation of the data of what is important in resistance.

Tyrrell I have a slight difference of outlook on one facet of this difficult subject, which is that when we do experimental infections with influenza virus we tend to use somewhat attenuated viruses; we give them in the upper respiratory tract; we have little clinical evidence of the lower areas being involved. Yet we find that the best correlate with resistance to infection is the presence of circulating antibody against haemagglutinin which probably means mainly IgG. In trying to understand what may be going on we have tried to visualize things at the cellular level; then, as you said we think maybe a small area of infection may develop but as there is plenty of antibody in the circulation this rapidly leaks from the plasma and prevents infection, so that nothing detectable takes place. You cannot find virus and there is no immune response. Therefore you say there is no infection. In fact, it is like having a small fire which is put out quickly. You may not know that there was one at all.

Couch I do not differ with what David Tyrrell said. I did not specifically state it, but a function of anti-haemagglutinin antibody is to prevent release of virus in the same way as does neuraminidase antibody; so, an aborted infection might occur. Also, we have shown that a very rapid and high quantity of IgG occurs in nasal secretions during the initial phases of inflammation and onset of respiratory symptoms. If you have substantial titres of antibodies in serum, this should be fairly effective for preventing the detection of infection. We do not have precise data that demonstrate this occurs, but we agree that this is one of the mechanisms by which antihaemagglutinin antibody can alter infection so that we end up scoring it as no infection at the clinical level.

Kilbourne I want to return to the H1N1 natural experiment with reference to the question of durability of homotypic immunity. This is, after all, a 1950 virus returning. Do you view this as then being a homotypic or a heterotypic challenge in the sense that something went on between 1950 and 1956?

Couch That question is more appropriate for the persons who spoke yesterday. The molecular biologists should be able to tell us whether it is exactly the same virus or not.

Kilbourne The question may be directed to those who sought out the antigenicity of the viruses such as Dowdle and Kendal—and perhaps myself. I do not know the answer as to how much antigenic variation actually did occur in that period, and how much the initial priming in that period was responsible.

It is an important question, and it is difficult to address also because of the fact that, as everyone has stated, the level of antibodies is so low and yet there is solid immunity.

Couch Although there is such evidence, I am not willing to say H1N1 viruses are less virulent than H3N2 although, as this group knows, a lot of people would like to say that. If we assume that it is not less virulent, then the H1N1 reoccurrence is not a heterotypic challenge of the kind that we saw with Victoria among persons with an earlier Hong Kong infection. So, if it is not a homotypic challenge, it is awfully close to it.

Dowdle We know a great deal and feel fairly comfortable with the information regarding H1N1 in protection, but what about the natural experiment that occurred with the H3 virus which seems to have circulated about the turn of the century? Here we had very high antibody titres in those of 60 and above. We did see some reduction in excess mortality, yet excess mortality was still occurring in that age group. Yet it does not occur now with H1N1.

Couch I tried to find at one time what happened to those individuals in the way of infection on re-exposure to H3 virus. I could not find any very good data. There was some soft data suggesting that a much lower infection frequency occurred in this group which would fit with the H1N1 data. Perhaps this is like the infant data in that some infection will fill the ecological niche to cause mortality.

Assaad The drift on H1N1 at the present-day is not necessarily the same drift as we had in 1950. However, the age-barrier is still the same. We really have no evidence—even with the latest ones which appeared in New Zealand or Chile—that there has been any disease in the age group that had the H1N1 30 years ago. Again, this is one of the areas where we need much more elucidation.

Couch Our concern is that we have been looking at a homotypic type of challenge with H1N1 virus and that future drift will be in a different direction from that seen earlier. A significant drift could then lead to the occurrence of significant H1N1 virus infection and disease among elderly patients.

Kendal My thoughts are regrettably rather qualitative and we really need some quantitative answers to the problems. Firstly, I am struck by the possible paradox between the existence of the doctrine of original antigenic sin which implies that people who previously were infected with viruses originally in the H1N1 sub-type, subsequently were susceptible to reinfection, otherwise the doctrine of original antigenic sin would never have been recognized. Yet we have the situation with the re-emergence of the H1N1 that says that protection within that sub-type is extremely strong and long-lasting, even now to viruses which have undergone a high degree of antigenic drift from the 1950 or 1977 strains.

Secondly, although the observations in terms of numbers are very small, nevertheless during the intensive efforts that were undertaken during the period of concern about swine 'flu re-emergence in 1976–7, which clearly shows a very high degree of antigenic difference from the H1N1 viruses that have circulated recently, appears only to have infected people of the same age group who are susceptible to the USSR or FW/50-like viruses.

This is qualitative data but the indications are that there may be a very strong degree of cross-protection against re-emergence of the H1N1 swine-like virus into older people at the present time, paralleling that with the USSR-like viruses and their derivatives. That was one of the reasons for the question I asked yesterday: do we know from the chemical structure of the haemagglutinin what it is that represents the shared antigenic determinants within the sub-type? It seems what we are lacking is knowledge about the epitopic specificity of antibodies in human sera, and also about the affinity or avidity of antibodies in human sera, which is relevant to answering the question about what antibody there is that is protective and where that antibody is.

Skehel Could I ask two questions? Is the specificity of the IgA antibodies the same as the IgG?

Couch That is a very germane question and I cannot answer it for you specifically. There is contradictory information in the literature on the specificity of IgA antibodies. There is information that says they are much less specific for A and B variants than are IgG antibodies and there is information published by Richman, that says that this may not be true, i.e. IgA antibodies have the same kinds of specificity as IgG antibodies.

Skehel The second question is in relation to the matter raised by Tyrrell and your answer to it. Is the mechanism of transfer of IgG into secretions dependent on injury or is the mechanism known?

Couch I do not think the IgG present during the resting state could possibly be a result of injury. When injury occurs there is a very clear outpouring of serum. The monitor for that is not IgG; it is albumin. This indicates something happens to the gradient during inflammation. I do not think anyone knows what the mechanism of transfer is in the base-line state. We tend to think of it as we think of transfer of immunoglobulins across the placenta—hence IgG. There is no significant transfer of IgA or IgM across either the placenta or the respiratory mucosa. That is the only reason for thinking that a similar kind of transport is involved.

Skehel That does not help me because I do not know what transfer across the placenta is!

Chu Reinfection in nature certainly looks to be very frequent, because with each variant—for instance, England/72 or Victoria or Texas—one started with a population with an antibody rate about 10% to 40% and at the end of the epidemic or period of that particular variant it goes to 80%, whether they are large epidemics or not. It looks as though reinfection occurs very frequently in nature.

The question I want to ask Dr Couch is whether he has any data to show whether there is any difference on the protection acquired from a single infection, in contrast to immunity acquired after repeated exposure to a succession of variants.

Couch I think that is a fairly complex question which, on the surface, might be considered fairly simple. We do not have specific data on the question but let me comment on the subject.

There are different ways to seek answers to that question. Consider first the infant. Does the first infection of an infant convey significant protection or is there a requirement for repeated infections before the infant gains immunity? The data is a bit contradictory. Most of us would like to believe the recent data by Frank in our family study, rather than the initial data he presented suggesting that an H3N2 infection in infants did not convey immunity to reinfection and illness. When Frank looked a second time, though the families had changed, he found very solid protection to reinfection with a closely related H3N2 or H1N1 variant. That is what I would like to believe occurs, though I have to concede that the data is a bit contradictory at the present time.

With older individuals, such as when the sub-type changed in 1968, one infection conveyed very substantial immunity. But then that is not a first infection; that may have been the tenth reinfection with a type A virus. Nevertheless, that reinfection with a new sub-type conveyed substantial immunity.

Finally, when one begins to dissect the problem further, suggestions again appear that immunity may be incomplete after a single infection. I was alluding to the Gill and Murphy data. They reported a 27% infection and illness rate with severe illnesses in half the persons when these were exposed to Victoria provided they had no medically-attended illness in earlier years. I cannot believe that Sydney, Australia has any less influenza than we have in Houston. Those people must have had an earlier H3N2 infection; I would have liked to see antibody tested against earlier variants. If you assume that an infection had occurred earlier, then they appeared fully susceptible to a second infection; whereas, those with a prior medically-attended illness were partially or completely immune. Then you would propose that the nature of the initial infection must influence the potency and duration of immunity. The more infection you have initially, the more immune response you get, the longer and more potent your protection.

So immunity, its duration, the likelihood of reinfection and the consequences of reinfection are complicated questions to which we do not have clear answers.

Murphy Responding to the question, how does IgG get across the mucosal barrier? We have looked at the specific activity of anti-haemagglutinin antibodies present in the serum and secretions to see what percentage of the anti-influenza antibodies present in the different isotypes are actively secreted into the upper respiratory tract. The study was done following first infection with an attenuated virus in infants and we found that about 20% of the IgG haemagglutination-antibody seems to be actively secreted (Wright et al., 1983). You can conclude that there is some transport mechanism that is actively secreting IgG. However, for IgA it is much higher: 80% to 90% of the individuals have a concentration of IgA anti-influenza antibody that is higher in the nasal wash than it is in the serum.

Couch The data on the lower respiratory tract suggests that IgG is synthesized locally in low quantities in smokers, presumably from cells included in the inflammatory response to smoke. There is no question about the nasal secretions. Good radio-label, specific-activity studies showed that a significant amount of IgG is synthesized locally in the upper respiratory tract.

Murphy This study measured antibody levels two weeks to one month after infection, with an attenuated virus at a time when there was no evidence of any kind of reaction.

Kilbourne It was true secretory antibody.

Murphy Yes. But secretory IgG.

Shortridge I would like to come back to the comment Dr Couch made about the apparent importance of airborne spread. This may be pre-empting Smith's talk later on, but one thing that struck me about the epidemiology of influenza is that whereas in temperate climates influenza always appears to occur commonly in the winter months, in the tropics—perhaps exemplified by Hong Kong, where we have the most data—influenza occurs all the year round at a fairly low level but tends to peak in the summer months. This raises a number of questions as to the mode of spread in the two different environments or geographical regions; implications arising from this include the emergence of pandemics, particularly in relation to the southern areas of our region. I wondered if you could make any comment in that respect?

Couch I do not know how the virus is transmitted in the tropics, but I would be glad to spend a sabbatical in Hong Kong studying the question!

Shortridge An excellent idea, all the data we have really comes from the temperate regions.

Couch You can correct me if it is wrong, but my understanding was that in most tropical areas influenza outbreaks occurred during the rainy season. I do not know what the rainy season is in Hong Kong but you are suggesting you do not have such outbreaks demonstrable. The belief is that people come indoors during winter and during the rainy season in the tropics. Then an opportunity to inhale the aerosol is optimal. But I am uncertain if you are suggesting that may not be true for Hong Kong.

Tyrrell My hypothesis is that the season of spread is when the weather sends you indoors and that varies from place to place, it may be raining, it may be stinking hot sun, or it may be stinking cold winter.

Couch You may be right. I think you must come into the household or classroom or institution; but that is also when the contact transmission is best as well.

REFERENCE

Wright, P. F., Murphy, B. R., Kervina, M., Lawrence, E. M., Phelan, M. A. and Karzon, D. T. (1983). Secretory immunological response after intranasal inactivated influenza A virus vaccinations. Evidence for immunoglobulin A memory. *Infect. Immun.* **40**, 1092–1095.

Cellular Immune Responses to Influenza Antigens—A Brief Review

G. C. SCHILD

National Institute for Biological Standards and Control,
London, UK

INTRODUCTION

The role of circulating and local antiviral antibodies in resistance to and recovery from infection by influenza virus has long been recognized, and has been reviewed in detail elsewhere (Potter and Oxford, 1979; Schulman, 1975; Couch, this vol. p. 119). It is clear however that there are limitations to the effectiveness of antibodies in protection against infection and disease. Neutralization of influenza virus is essentially brought about by antibody to haemagglutinin and is more or less specific for the virus sub-type stimulating the antibody. Antibody to neuraminidase (Schulman, 1975) does not commonly neutralize virus infectivity but modifies dissemination of virus infection in cell cultures or in the intact host, and likewise is essentially sub-type specific. Since in nature there is frequent antigenic "drift" and occasional antigenic "shift" in the surface antigens of prevalent influenza A viruses and since antibody in man also tends to be specific for the original sub-type experienced by the individual, circulating antibody offers less than complete protection against infection (Kilbourne, 1973; Hoskins *et al.*, 1979). The nature of cell-mediated immune responses to influenza

"The Molecular Virology and Epidemiology of Influenza" (Eds Sir Charles Stuart-Harris and Professor C.W. Potter). Academic Press, London, New York and Orlando, 1984.

antigens and their potential role in resistance to infection or recovery has been explored much more recently and to date much less completely. This article reviews briefly the present status of knowledge of cell mediated responses to influenza.

TYPES OF CELL-MEDIATED IMMUNITY (CMI)

During influenza virus infection of the mouse or man inflammation of the respiratory tract tissues occurs, which involves predominantly mononuclear cells. Thymus-derived lymphocytes (T cells) are known to be responsible for two different effector functions, delayed hypersensitivity (Td), and killer activity for virus-infected target cells (Tc) and two modulation functions either by "helping" B or T cell clonal expansion and maturation (Th) or by suppressing these events following antigenic stimulation (Ts) (Table I). It is hypothesized that distinct T cell sub-sets are responsible for each of these four functions. Two further classes of cells, natural killer cells, whose increase following infection appears to be non-specific, and antibody-dependent cytotoxic cells, are not further discussed here.

TABLE I
Cell responses to influenza antigens—current knowledge

Lymphoid cells designation	function	infection	inactivated virus	SA^a	Virus and antigen specificity
B	antibody	+	+	+	HA or NA sub-type and strain specific
T_c	Lysis of influenza infected cells	+	±	+	mainly react with all type A viruses[b]
T_d	DTH	+	+	NT	all type A viruses sub-type specific[c]
T_H	help T_c	+	+	NT	all type A viruses
T_H	help B	+	+	+	all type A viruses
T_s	suppress T_c	NT	+	NT	all type A viruses
T_s	suppress T_d	+	NT	NT	HA sub-type

NT not tested
+ indicates a response
− indicates there is no response
[a] induced by influenza surface antigen (SA) complexes (haemagglutinin and neuraminidase)
[b] a minor population of T_c are HA variant specific
[c] T_d data from Leung et al. (1980).

T CELLS WITH KILLER ACTIVITY (Tc) IN MICE

The role of Tc has received more attention that the activities of other T cells. The lysis of influenza virus infected cells by Tc does not involve either antibody or complement. The direct lytic activity of infected target cells by Tc is measured by the release of ^{51}Cr from labelled target cells when incubated with effector Tc cells. Such a direct test for Tc lysis is insensitive and generally low degrees of response are obtained even when the T cells are obtained from hosts which have been recently infected or immunized with influenza virus. Thus mature effector Tc are uncommon in peripheral blood and mainly memory Tc circulate. Tc memory activity may be measured by stimulating T cells from primed donors (e.g. from mouse spleen or peripheral human blood) *in vitro* by co-cultivating them with virus-infected lymphocyte cells for a few days before adding to the target cells (Fig. 1). The latter is a more sensitive test for Tc activity than the direct assay. An essential characteristic of Tc activity is its strong dependence on matching major histocompatability antigens of the effector and target cells (Fig. 2). This was first demonstrated in mice by Zinkernagel and Doherty (1974) using lymphocytic choriomeningitis virus, where both groups of cells must have H2 K or D markers (Blanden *et al.*, 1975), and later confirmed for influenza in man by McMichael (1978) where matching HLA A or B are required. Monoclonal antibodies to either HLA A or B inhibit virus type specific Tc activity (McMichael *et al.*, 1980).

In general Tc activity is not sub-type specific within, for example, type A influenza viruses. One sub-type of influenza A virus can sensitize the target

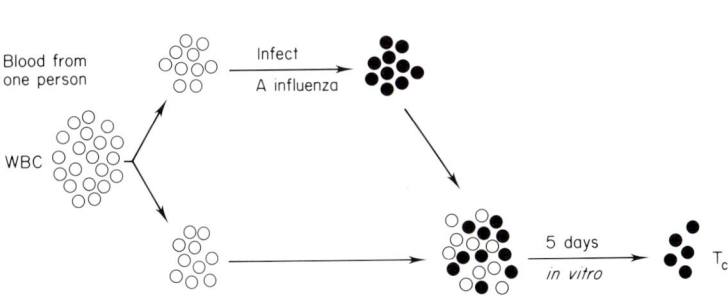

Fig. 1 Scheme for the generation of human Tc from peripheral white blood cells *in vitro*. Peripheral blood monocytes (PBM) are purified from blood, and a proportion of them are infected with influenza A virus to serve as stimulator cells. After washing the infected cells, they are added back to non-infected cells, and after several days (four to eight), Tc specific for influenza A virus are generated. Cytotoxicity is assayed on Cr-labelled A virus-infected syngeneic PBM. From Askonas *et al.* (1982).

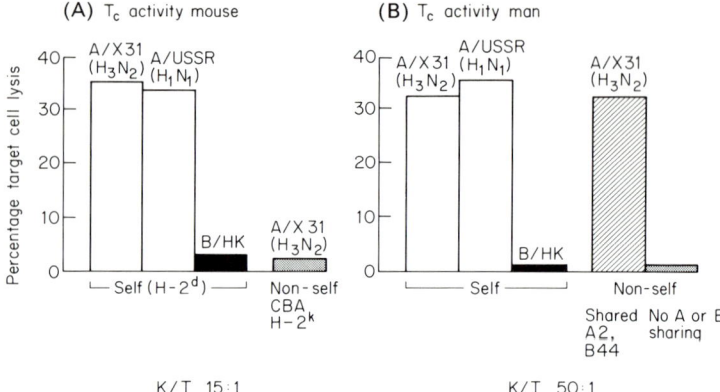

Fig. 2 Tc responses to influenza A virus in mouse and man: Virus specificity and H-2 or HLA restriction. (A) Donor BALB/c mice were primed by infection with A/X31 (H3N2) virus; two months later, spleen cells were cultured with A/X31-infected syngeneic lymphoblasts for five days. Cytotoxicity was assayed on ^{51}Cr labelled virus infected BALB/c or CBA (H-2) lymphoblasts infected with different influenza viruses as indicated. Target cell lysis is expressed as percentage of total ^{51}Cr released into the supernatant during a 3h assay. K/T = killer target cell ratio of 15:1. The influenza virus used for infection of the targets, A/X31 (H3N2) or A/USSR/77 (H1N1), is indicated above each bar. (B) Peripheral cells from one person (HLA A2 10, B18 44) were cultured for five days with syngeneic cells infected with A/USSR virus. Tc were assayed on ^{51}Cr labelled peripheral human cells infected with various influenza viruses as indicated. Self targets were from the same person. Two other targets were cells from other donors, one shared A2/B44, the other shared no histocompatibility antigens. K/T = killer target cell ratio of 50:1.

cell and a different strain can prime the Tc (Fig. 2). It is possible that there is recognition of a postulated common component of the viral haemagglutinin common to all strains of type A, in conjunction with the required histocompatibility antigen (Askonas et al., 1982), and some monoclonal antibodies to type A haemagglutinin inhibit the activity of Tc (Askonas and Webster, 1980). The broad specificity of Tc has been demonstrated in a single clone of cells and so is not due to a mixture of cells each with a different specificity (Lin and Askonas, 1980). Tc responses are, however, type specific and not shared between influenza viruses of type A and type B. Cells infected by type B virus are not affected by type A Tc and vice versa (Zweerink et al., 1977). In contrast to the above general finding of broad specificity of Tc activity within influenza viruses of virus type A, it has been possible to prepare a sub-set of Tc lymphocytes specific for a single haemagglutinin antigen sub-type (Effros et al., 1977).

Probably the most convincing evidence that haemagglutinin antigen has a role in Tc recognition and killing is provided by the finding (M. J. Gething,

T. J. Brachiale and J. F. Sambrook, unpublished data) that murine cells expressing only HA, following insertion of a rDNA vector, were specifically killed by Tc, although with low efficiency.

In mice, Tc is readily induced by infection with influenza virus, and the more prolific the virus growth, the better was the development of Tc memory (Cambridge et al., 1976). Tc response to inactivated influenza vaccines, and particularly to sub-unit vaccines was found to be low or absent (Webster and Askonas, 1980; Braciale and Yap, 1978). This may have important implications for attempts to induce Tc in humans by vaccination. However, a low positive Tc response to a purified vaccine containing haemagglutinin and neuraminidase antigens was found by Ennis (Ennis et al., 1977; Ennis, 1982; Ennis et al., 1982). McMichael et al. (1981) found Tc responses in six of eight volunteers given killed whole influenza virus A, but in only three of nine persons given sub-unit vaccine. The Tc memory response to inactivated whole virus was also reported. A definite rise in level of Tc was detected at day 28 rather than at day 7 and after a year the Tc level had fallen to baseline in four of the seven persons reporting for study.

The role of Tc in influenza immunity has been evaluated both in mouse models and in man by several investigations. A Tc clone (from BALB/c mice) selected in T-cell growth factor, on transfer into infected mice was shown to inhibit the replication of homologous or heterologous influenza A virus in the lungs of the host, thus limiting virus spread. The same Tc clone released immune interferon on contact only with its matched target cell (Askonas et al., 1982). Whether the protective effect of Tc is always dependent on interferon release needs further assessment (Virelizier et al., 1977; Tsukui, 1977; Ito et al., 1980).

Tc IN MAN

Available data indicate a close correspondence between the behaviour of Tc in the mouse and man, and support for the importance of Tc responses comes from studies in human volunteers. In one study (McMichael et al., 1983a) Tc memory was measured in volunteers before challenge with influenza. The results are illustrated in Fig. 3. Individuals with high Tc responses subsequently shed either low amounts of virus or no virus after intranasal inoculation with influenza A/Munich/78 (H1N1) virus. Volunteers with low levels of Tc immunity included all those who shed more than trace amounts of virus. This beneficial effect was observed in individuals with no detectable protective antibody in their serum. It implied that cross-reactive Tc could protect against influenza by contributing to early recovery. Ennis has shown that peripheral Tc were activated during

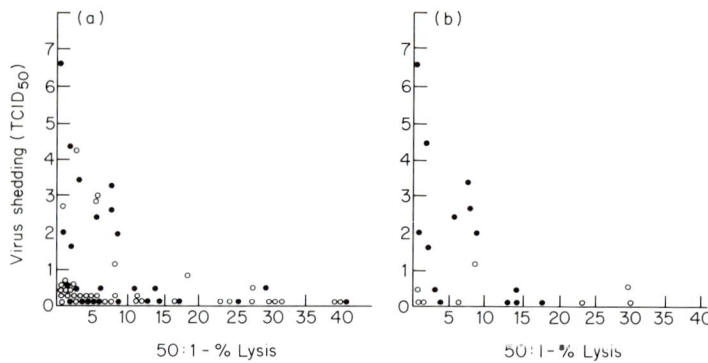

Fig. 3 The figure shows the relationship between cytotoxic (Tc) cell activity at the time of intranasal challenge of adult volunteers by live A/USSR/77 (H1N1) virus and the amount of virus shedding. For each volunteer degree of lysis of autologous target cells infected with A/USSR virus at an effector:target ratio of 50:1 is plotted against the amount of virus shed.

The left panel shows data for all 63 volunteers. The right panel shows data from 22 volunteers who lack antibody to A/USSR/77 haemagglutinin and neuraminidase (titres less than 1:10). Subjects born before 1957 are indicated by open circles and those born in or after 1957 by closed circles. From McMichael et al. (1983a, p. 15). Reproduced by kind permission of the authors and publisher of the New England Journal of Medicine.

infection *in vitro* after six to ten days but had decreased to baseline values by day 31 (Ennis *et al.*, 1981, 1982). He also reported a large vaccine trial where volunteers given live, whole inactivated or sub-unit influenza A vaccine showed a boost in their Tc memory. This increase was maximal at day 14 and declined to base levels by day 180 (Ennis *et al.*, 1981). Natural infection, on the other hand, appears to boost a more lasting response in Tc memory.

McMichael *et al.* (1983) have studied Tc activity and Tc memory in the peripheral blood lymphocytes of 189 volunteers aged 17–55 years over the six years 1977–82. Tc was measured as described above, using influenza viruses H3N2 and H1N1, and the cells were tested after *in vitro* culture for five to seven days. Controls were mismatched virus-infected cells, autologous cells infected with influenza B, and matched non-infected target cells. Using a killer cell:target cell ratio of 50:1 they confirmed histocompatibility restriction and influenza virus type-specificity. The study was carried out in Oxford, England where influenza isolations had been infrequent between 1977 and 1979. From 1977 to 1979 peripheral blood samples gave a generally high Tc response from most individuals; between 1980 and 1982 the level of response had declined and a confirmatory decline in values was found in serial blood samples from a number of individuals taken during the same years. One confirmed case of influenza during the period showed a four-fold rise in type A influenza virus specific Tc activity. McMichael et al. (1983b) concluded that Tc immunity declined when influenza A was scarce during the period 1977–82. Tc immunity appeared to rise following infection but to decline slowly thereafter, with a half-life of two to three years. This contrasts with the rise of Tc activity after vaccination with whole inactivated virus; in this situation the Tc response appears to last less than 12 months (Ennis et al., 1977, 1981; Ito et al., 1980).

SUMMARY

Immune responses stimulated by influenza infection include both humoral and cellular elements. Circulating and local antibodies are undoubtedly of importance in defence against influenza and protect against reinfection with the same variant. Antibodies in the humoral response are specific for individual variants arising in the population but permit influenza virus variants to escape immune control. Cell-mediated responses are far less discriminatory. The level of responsiveness of both B and T cells is regulated by helper and suppressor T cell subpopulations. Other sub-sets of T cells are responsible for T cell-mediated lysis of virus-infected cells and delayed hypersensitivity reactions. There is evidence that all of these types of responses occur in man and mouse after exposure to influenza infection. T cells predominantly recognize different features of the influenza virus, which is shared by all the different influenza A viruses but are specific for influenza viruses of types A and B. The molecules involved in T cell recognition remain elusive, but it appears that viral proteins, like other antigens, are seen by T cells in conjunction with products of the major histocompatibility locus (K and D end of H-2 or HLA and the I region). A summary of the types of cells involved in cell-mediated responses to influenza and their specificity are shown in Table I.

The cross-reactivity between the type A viruses of both types of T cell responses (Tc and Td) has implications for vaccination. Replicating virus is far more effective in generating Tc memory cells than killed virus preparations. Sub-unit vaccines appear to prime less efficiently for Tc responses than whole virus vaccines, but inactivated virus vaccines are still important for protection against a given influenza virus variant in people at risk during influenza epidemics.

REFERENCES

Askonas, B. A. and Webster, R. G. (1980). Monoclonal antibodies to the haemagglutinin and to H-2 inhibit the cross-reactive T-cell populations induced by influenza. Eur. J. Immunol. **10**, 151–156.

Askonas, B. A., McMichael, A. J. and Webster, R. G. (1982). The immune response to influenza viruses and the problem of protection against infection. *In* "Basic and Applied Influenza Research" (Ed. A. S. Beare). C.R.C. Press, pp. 166–173.

Blanden, R. V., Doherty, P. C., Dunlop, M. B. C., Gardner, I. D., Zinkernagel, R. M. and David, C. S. (1975). Genes required for cytotoxicity against virus infected target cells in K and D regions of H-2 complex. *Nature* (Lond.) **254**, 269–270.

Braciale, T. J. and Yap, K. L. (1978). Role of viral infectivity in the induction of influenza virus specific cytotoxic T-cells. *J. exp. Med.* **147**, 1236–1252.

Cambridge, G., Mackenzie, J. S. and Keast, D. (1976). Cell-mediated immunity to influenza. *Infect. Immun.* **13**, 36–43.

Effros, R. B., Doherty, P. C., Gerhard, W. and Bennink, J. (1977). Generation of both cross-reactive and virus-specific T-cell populations after immunization with serologically distinct influenza A viruses. *J. Exp. Med.* **145**, 557–568.

Ennis, F. A. (1982). Some newly recognized aspects of resistance against and recovery from influenza. *Arch. Virol.* **73**, 207–217.

Ennis, F. A., Martin, W. J. and Verbonitz, M. W. (1977). Cytotoxic T-lymphocytes induced in mice by inactivated influenza virus vaccine. *Nature* (Lond.) **269**, 418–419.

Ennis, F. A., Rook, A. A., Qi Yi-Hua, Schild, G. C., Riley, D., Pratt, R. and Potter, C. W. (1981). HLA restricted virus specific cytotoxic T lymphocyte responses to live and inactivated influenza vaccines. *Lancet* **ii**, 887–893.

Ennis, F. A., Qi Yi-Hua and Schild, G. C. (1982). Antibody and cytotoxic T lymphocyte responses of humans to live and inactivated influenza vaccines. *J. Gen. Virol.* **58**, 273–281.

Hoskins, T. W., Davies, J. R., Smith, A. J., Miller, C. L. and Allchin, A. (1979). Assessment of inactivated influenza A vaccine after three outbreaks of influenza A at Christ's Hospital. *Lancet* **i**, 33–35.

Ito, Y., Aoki, H., Kimura, Y., Takano, M., Maeno, K. and Shimokata, K. (1980). Generation and maintenance of immune interferon producing cells induced by allogeneic stimulation in mice *Infect. Immun.* **29**, 383–389.

Kilbourne, E. D. (1973). An explanation of the interpandemic antigen instability of influenza viruses. *J. Inf. Dis.* **128**, 668–670.

Lin, Y. L. and Askonas, B. A. (1980). Cross reactivity for different type A influenza viruses by a cloned T-killer cell line. *Nature* (Lond.), **288**, 164–165.

McMichael, A. J. (1978). HLA restriction of human cytotoxic T lymphocytes specific for influenza virus. *J. Exp. Med.* **148**, 1458–1467.

McMichael, A. J., Parham, P., Brodsky, F. M. and Pilch, J. R. (1980). Influenza virus specific cytotoxic T-lymphocytes recognize HLA molecules; blocking by monoclonal anti-HLA antibodies. *J. exp. Med.* **152**, 195S–203S.

McMichael, A. J., Gotch, F., Cullen, P., Askonas, B. A. and Webster, R. G. (1981). The human cytotoxic T-cell response to influenza A vaccination *Clin. Exp. Immunol.* **43**, 276–284.

McMichael, A. J., Gotch, F. M., Noble, G. R. and Beare, A. S. (1983a). Cytotoxic T-cell immunity to influenza. *N. Engl. J. Med.* **309**, 13–17.

McMichael, A. J., Gotch, F. M., Dongworth, D. M., Clark, A. and Potter, C. W. (1983b). Declining T-cell immunity to influenza 1977–82. *Lancet*, **ii**, 762–764.

Potter, C. W. and Oxford, J. S. (1979). Determinants of immunity to influenza infection in man. *Brit. Med. Bull.* **35**, 69–75.

Schulman, J. L. (1975). Immunology of influenza. *In* "The Influenza Viruses and Influenza" (Ed. E. D. Kilbourne) Academic Press, New York and London, pp. 373–392.

Tsukui, K. (1977). Influenza virus induced interferon production in mouse spleen cell cultures: T-cells as the main producer. *Cell Immunol.* **32**, 243–251.

Virelizier, J. L., Allison, A. C. and de Meyer, E. (1977). Production by mixed lymphocyte cultures of a type II interferon able to protect macrophages against virus infection. *Infect. Immun.* **17**, 282–285.

Webster, R. G. and Askonas, B. A. (1980). Cross protection and cross-reactive cytotoxic T-cells induced by influenza virus vaccines in mice. *Eur. J. Immunol.* **10**, 396–401.

Zinkernagel, R. M. and Doherty, P. C. (1974). Restrictions of *in vitro* T-cell mediated cytotoxicity in lymphocytic choriomeningitis within a syngeneic or semi-allogeneic system. *Nature* (Lond.) **248,** 701–702.

Zweerink, H. J., Courtneidge, S. A., Skehel, J. J., Crumpton, M. J. and Askonas, B. A. (1977). Cytotoxic T-cells kill influenza virus-infected cells but do not distinguish between serologically distinct type A viruses. *Nature* (Lond.) **267**, 354–356.

Evidence for Host Cell Selection of Antigenic Variants of Influenza A (H1N1) and B Virus: Antigenic Differences between the Haemagglutinins of Viruses Grown in Eggs and Mammalian Cells

G. C. SCHILD[a], J. S. OXFORD[a] and R. G. WEBSTER[b]

[a]Division of Viral Products, National Institute for Biological Standards and Control, London, [b]Division of Virology and Molecular Biology, St Jude Children's Hospital, Memphis, Tennessee, USA

The haemagglutinin (HA) antigens of influenza A and B viruses undergo frequent and progressive antigenic drift as a result of selection, under immunological pressure, of viruses possessing alterations in amino acid sequences at specific sites in the molecule (reviewed by Webster et al., 1982). We have recently reported (Schild et al., 1983) evidence for an additional selection mechanism for antigenic variants of influenza B virus that depends upon differing host cell tropisms of virus subpopulations. The cultivation of influenza B virus in eggs selects sub-populations which are antigenically

"The Molecular Virology and Epidemiology of Influenza" (Eds Sir Charles Stuart-Harris and Professor C.W. Potter). Academic Press, London, New York and Orlando, 1984.

distinct from virus grown from the same source but in mammalian cell cultures. From these studies it appeared likely that the observed co-variance between antigenic character of virus haemagglutinin and the cell substrate used for virus isolation and growth was that one or more of the antigenic sites of the HA molecule is indirectly associated with receptor binding specificity (for details of virus HA structure see Wiley et al., 1981; Krystal et al., 1982). We have now extended our findings to influenza A (H1N1) virus. Our findings may have implications for the understanding of the biology and antigenic variability of influenza virus. As antigenic characterization of influenza virus strains for epidemiological purposes and for the preparation of influenza vaccines (reviewed by Dowdle and Schild, 1975; Stuart-Harris and Schild, 1976) conventionally relies on the cultivation of virus in eggs, these observations may also have an important practical significance for the design and efficacy of influenza vaccines.

Tables I and II show the serological characteristics, as indicated by their reactions with anti-HA monoclonal antibodies, of influenza B and influenza A (H1N1) viruses isolated and passaged in eggs or cell cultures. The haemagglutination-inhibition (HI) reactions of eleven influenza B viruses representative of 27 strains, isolated and passaged in eggs or canine kidney cell cultures (MDCK) from specimens collected during a school outbreak of influenza in 1982 (Oxford et al., 1983) were investigated (Table I). The virus preparations were tested against monoclonal antibodies prepared against influenza B virus cultivated in eggs or MDCK cells (see footnote to Table I). Three patterns of serological reactivity were apparent. Monoclonal antibody 195 reacted to high titres with all the influenza B viruses tested. Monoclonal antibody 209 reacted with all the viruses that had been isolated and subsequently passaged in MDCK cultures but not with those that had been cultivated in eggs at any stage in their passage histories. Antibody 238 reacted only with viruses which had at least one passage in eggs and with none of the viruses that had been passaged in MDCK cultures alone. The mutual exclusivity of the reactions of antibodies 209 and 238 with the 27 virus preparations was striking.

Viruses having different passage histories in eggs or cell cultures would be expected to react differently with monoclonal antibodies if these were directed against antigens present as carbohydrate moieties derived from host-cell membrane and covalently linked to the haemagglutinin molecule (Harboe, 1963). However, this does not explain our findings. None of the monoclonal antibodies gave HI reactions which were entirely determined by the last culture system in which the test virus was grown. Moreover, the reactions were influenza B-specific and were not affected by absorbing the antibodies with homogenates of chorioallantoic membrane or MDCK cells.

Similar findings were obtained with influenza A (H1N1) viruses isolated during an outbreak in a residential school in 1983 (Table II). It is seen that

TABLE I
Haemagglutinin-inhibition reactions with monoclonal antibodies to haemagglutinin of influenza B viruses of different isolation and passage histories

Specimen No.	Isolation and passage history of B/England/82 viruses — Cell substrate for virus isolation[1] and passage[2]	Monoclonal antibodies to B/Oregon/5/80 virus					Monoclonal antibody to B/England/145/82
		124	146	162	195	238	209
145	M[1]–M[2]	<	<	<	25600	<	320
	M–M(×3)	<	<	<	12800	<	320
	M–A1	800	<	<	38400	9600	<
	M–A1(×3)	NT	<	<	12800	9600	<
	M–A1–M(×3)	NT	<	<	12800	9600	<
222	M–M	<	<	<	≥6400	<	160
	M–A1	<	1600	<	≥6400	6400	<
	Am–A1	<	3200	<	4800	6400	<
	Am–A1–M(×3)	<	1600	<	≥6400	6400	<
272	M–M	<	<	<	≥6400	<	40
	M–A1	50	400	<	6400	6400	<
	M–A1(×3)	<	400	NT	6400	6400	NT
	Am–A1	6400	NT	<	3200	4800	<
	Am–A1–M(×2)	NT	NT	NT	NT	12800	<
296	M–M	<	<	<	≥6400	<	NT
	M–A1	100	1600	100	6400	6400	NT
	M–A1–M(×3)	<	800	400	≥6400	≥6400	NT
203	M–M	<	<	<	≥6400	<	>1280
	M–A1	800	<	400	≥6400	≥6400	<
290	M–M	<	<	<	≥6400	<	>1280
	M–A1	<	3200	200	≥6400	≥6400	<
	M–A1–M(×3)	<	800	<	25600	≥6400	NT
183	M–M	<	<	<	≥6400	<	160
	M–A1	<	3200	<	6400	4800	<
188	M–M	<	<	<	≥6400	<	160
	M–A1	800	<	200	≥6400	6400	<
244	M–M	<	<	<	≥6400	<	640
	M–A1	100	>6400	<	≥12800	≥12800	<
278	M–M	<	<	<	≥6400	<	40
	M–A1	200	400	200	≥6400	≥6400	<
269	M–M	<	<	<	≥6400	<	>1280
	M–A1	1600	<	100	≥6400	≥6400	<
B/Oreg/5/80 egg-grown		6400	3200	3200	6400	4800	<

M indicates isolation or passage in MDCK cell cultures. A1 indicates passage in the allantoic cavity of embryonated eggs. Am indicates isolation in the amniotic cavity of embryonated eggs. ( ) indicates number of serial passages. < HI titres less than 1:50 or, for antibody 209, less than 1:10. NT not tested. Monoclonal antibodies (with the exception of 209) were prepared against purified, egg-grown B/Oregon/5/80 virus by standard techniques. Monoclonal antibody 209 was prepared by immunizing mice with virus cultivated in MDCK cells. Mice were immunized intraperitoneally with approximately 3000 HA units of purified influenza virus and approximately 21 weeks later boosted intravenously with purified virus. Spleens were removed four days later and spleen cells fused to SP2/OAg14 myeloma cells. Hybridomas secreting specific anti-HA antibodies were selected using HI and ELISA techniques and cloned in soft agar. Ascitic fluids were collected from mice injected intraperitoneally with 10^7 hybridoma cells. (For technical details see Kohler and Milstein, 1975; Lu Bao Ian et al., 1983.)

TABLE II
Haemagglutination inhibition reactions of anti-HA monoclonal antibodies with influenza A (H1N1) viruses of different isolation and passage histories

Specimen No.	Cell substrate[a] virus isolation and passage	A/Brazil/11/78[b] 2	A/Brazil/11/78[b] 29	A/England/333/80[b] 23	A/England/333/80[b] 61	A/England/333/80[b] 1	A/Baylor/1/83[b] 3	A/Baylor/1/83[b] 7	A/Eng/91/83[c] 384
920	M–M	3200	<	<	1600	1600	<	3200	2560
	M–A1	6400	1600	1600	3200	800	<	<	<
922	M–M	3200	<	<	1600	1600	<	6400	2560
	M–A1(×3)	6400	<	<	<	6400	>12800	1600	<
965	M–M	3200	<	<	1600	1600	<	6400	12800
	M–A1(×5)	3200	800	3200	3200	1600	<	<	<
81	M–M	3200	<	<	800	1600	<	3200	12800
	M–A1(×2)	3200	1600	1600	3200	1600	>12800	<	<
91	M–M	3200	<	<	1600	1600	<	3200	12800
	M–A1(×5)	3200	<	<	<	3200	>12800	<	<
157	M–M	3200	<	<	1600	1600	<	3200	NT
	M–A1(×5)	3200	<	<	<	3200	>12800	<	NT
162	M–M	3200	<	<	1600	1600	<	3200	NT
	M–A1(×2)	3200	3200	3200	3200	3200	<	<	NT
226	M–M	3200	<	<	1600	1600	<	6400	NT
	A1–A1	3200	<	<	<	6400	>12800	800	NT

[a] See footnote for Table I. [b] Monoclonal antibodies produced against egg-grown viruses. [c] Monoclonal antibody produced against MDCK-grown virus.

certain of the antibodies (1,2) reacted with all viruses irrespective of their passage histories, whilst others clearly differentiated between viruses isolated from the same specimen and grown in eggs or cell cultures. Antibodies 3, 23 and 29 reacted with viruses grown in eggs but not those passaged exclusively in cell cultures whilst antibody 7 and 384 reacted with virus which had been grown exclusively in cell cultures but mostly failed to react with virus passaged in eggs.

It is of interest that the antibodies which reacted exclusively with viruses passaged only in eggs were of narrow specificity, reacting only with a proportion of isolates, whilst the antibodies which reacted with MDCK-grown virus but not with egg-grown virus reacted with virus from all eight clinical specimens examined. A possible explanation for this observation is that the antigenic heterogeneity among the egg-grown viruses results from selection occurring as a result of their adaptation to growth in eggs, whilst such a selection does not occur on isolation of virus in MDCK cultures. This conclusion is supported by studies on plaque purification and gene sequence analysis of influenza virus (J. Robertson—unpublished data).

Further investigations (Schild et al., 1983) were carried out with plaque purified viruses derived from influenza B/England/145/82. Virus which had been isolated and further passaged twice on MDCK cultures, with an

TABLE III

Growth of plaque-purified clones of B/England/145/82 virus in MDCK cultures and fertile eggs and haemagglutinin-inhibition reactions of progeny virus with monoclonal antibodies and post-infection ferret sera

Substrate	Proportion of clones showing[a] growth of MDCK cultures and eggs No. plaques producing viral growth / No. tested	HI reactions of progeny virus with stated monoclonal antibodies: No. reacting / No. tested (range of titres)				HI reactions of progeny virus with post-infection ferret sera[b]					
		195	238	209			F1	F2	F3	F4	F5
MDCK cultures	$\frac{194}{200}$ (97%)	$\frac{190}{190}$ (2560–≥12800)	$\frac{0}{190}$ (all <100)	$\frac{112}{112}$ (40–640)		(a)	320^c	960	480	320	480
						(b)	160	640	320	120	320
Egg	$\frac{5}{200}$ (2.5%)	$\frac{5}{5}$ (9600–≥12800)	$\frac{5}{5}$ (all ≥12800)	$\frac{0}{5}$ (all ≤20)		(a)	40	120	80	30	120
						(b)	20	60	60	20	60

[a] Agar cores overlaying individual plaques in MDCK cultures were taken up with pasteur pipettes and the virus eluted into 0·3 ml volumes of PBS. To test growth in MDCK cells 0·15 ml of each eluate was inoculated into cultures grown in 12 well flat-bottomed tissue culture plates each well being 4·5 cm² in area containing 1·5 ml medium (MEM, 2% NaHCO3). The cultures were incubated 72 h at 36°C in an atmosphere of 5% CO_2. The medium was harvested and virus growth detected by haemagglutination assay with chick erythrocytes. To test growth in eggs 0·15 ml eluate was inoculated into the allantoic cavity of 10 day fertile eggs. Allantoic fluids were tested for haemagglutinin after 72 h incubation at 35°C. [b] Sera collected 14 days post-infection with B/England/145/82 virus. Ferrets F1, F2 and F5 were infected with virus isolated and grown in eggs, ferrets F3 and F4 were infected with virus isolated and grown in MDCK cell cultures. [c] Data is shown for the progeny of two plaques (a) and (b) picked from MDCK cultures and grown either in MDCK cells (upper half of table) or in eggs (lower half of table).

infectivity titre of $10^{7.7}$ pfu/ml in MDCK cells and $10^{3.5}$ EID/ml by the allantoic route in embryonated hens eggs, was seeded at high dilutions on MDCK monolayers. Two hundred well-separated plaques were harvested and eluted into small volumes of medium (see footnote to Table III).

The plaque eluates were inoculated undiluted into further MDCK cultures and also into the allantoic cavities of fertile eggs. A high proportion of the eluates successfully infected MDCK cells. In contrast, only five of the 200 plaque eluates tested produced growth in eggs. All 190 plaque-derived viruses harvested from MDCK cultures and the five plaque-derived viruses which grew in eggs reacted to high titres with the monoclonal antibody 195. Monoclonal antibody 238 reacted with each of the five viruses generated in eggs but failed to react with the 190 viruses prepared in MDCK cultures. The converse pattern of reactions was obtained with monoclonal antibody 209 which reacted with the MDCK harvests but failed to react with the egg harvests. The differing serological reactivities of the two groups of plaque-derived viruses with antibodies 238 and 209 were not simply a direct reflection of the last substrate in which the virus had been passaged. When the five viruses prepared in eggs were given a further passage in MDCK cultures, the HI reactions of the MDCK harvests were identical to those of the parental allantoic fluids, i.e. all reacted with antibody 238 and none reacted with antibody 209. Plaque isolation experiments were also carried out with B/England/145/82 virus initially isolated in MDCK cells and further passaged once in eggs. The infectivity titre of this virus was $10^{8.5}$ pfu/ml in MDCK cultures and $10^{9.7}$ EID$_{50}$/ml on allantoic inoculation in eggs. Twenty-four plaques were picked; the progeny of all plaques grew in the allantoic cavity and MDCK cultures. All harvests from eggs or MDCK cells reacted with monoclonal antibody 238 but not with antibody 209.

Clear antigenic differences between the influenza viruses described above which differed in their reactions with monoclonal antibodies were also detectable with polyclonal sera. For example, the influenza B virus preparations listed in Table I were tested with post-infection ferret sera to egg-grown B/England/145/82 and B/Singapore/222/79 viruses. The HI titres were between 2- and 40-fold higher (mean 10-fold higher) with viruses which had been passaged on MDCK cells only than with those that had been passaged at least once in eggs. The HI reactions of ferret sera with plaque purified B/England/145/82 viruses were also investigated (Table III). Viruses from the same two plaques were inoculated on MDCK cells and in eggs and the progeny tested with ferret sera. The HI titres against virus prepared in MDCK cultures were between 4- and 11-fold (mean 7-fold) higher than the titres against virus prepared in eggs.

Large differences were also observed in the frequency and the titre of HI antibody in the sera of unvaccinated children and young adults to influenza B viruses grown in eggs or MDCK cells from the same clinical specimen or from the same MDCK plaque or with corresponding pairs of influenza A

TABLE IV
Haemagglutination-inhibiting antibody in human sera to influenza A (H1N1) and influenza B viruses with different passage histories.

		Frequency and titre of HI antibody: % of sera with stated titres					
		Children[a]			Young adults[b]		
Virus origin and passage history		$\geqslant 10$	$\geqslant 40$	$\geqslant 160$	$\geqslant 10$	$\geqslant 40$	$\geqslant 160$
A/Eng/157/83	M–M	100	35	5	—	—	—
A/Eng/157/83	M–A1	34	6	1	—	—	—
A/Eng/91/83	M–M	—	—	—	61	38	10
A/Eng/91/83	M–A1	—	—	—	25	5	0
B/Eng/222/82	M–M	83	76	57	100	100	100
B/Eng/222/82	Am–A1	20	8	2	20	2	1
B/Eng/145/82	M–M	58	24	4	—	—	—
B/Eng/145/82	M–A1	7	3	1	—	—	—

[a] Sera collected in 1982 from 181 unvaccinated children aged 2–8 years attending hospital clinic for treatment or investigation. [b] Sera collected in October 1982 from 107 university students aged 18–22 years were treated with RDE before testing. — not done.

(H1N1) virus grown in MDCK cells or eggs (Table IV). Many sera showed high HI titres (≥ 1280) with viruses passaged exclusively on cell cultures and were negative (titre < 10) when tested with corresponding egg-grown virus.

In experiments to investigate any biological differences between the antigenically distinct sub-populations, the range of erythrocytes agglutinated by the viruses was compared. Erythrocytes may be used as a model for cell-receptor specificity for influenza virus (Burnet and Clarke, 1948). The preparations of B/England/145/82 and B/England/222/82 listed in Table I were tested with erythrocytes of chicken, turkey, man (group A, AB and O cells), rhesus monkey, guinea pig, sheep, rat and horse. The viruses, irrespective of passage history, agglutinated the cells of these species to similar titres with the exception of sheep, horse and rat erythrocytes. For cells from the latter three species, high agglutination titres were detected with virus which had been isolated or passaged in eggs but no agglutination was detected for virus passaged in MDCK cultures only.

In conclusion, our findings provide strong evidence that influenza A and B viruses isolated from clinical specimens and grown in MDCK cultures contain biologically and antigenically distinct sub-populations of virus. For influenza B virus a minor proportion of the MDCK-grown virus is capable of growth in the allantois of fertile eggs without prior adaptation, and possesses HA which is antigenically distinct from the majority of the virus which grows poorly or not at all in the allantoic cavity.

This novel "non-immune" selective pressure mechanism for generation of antigenic variants of influenza A (H1N1) viruses could have implications for the nature evolution of influenza viruses. A high frequency of occurrence of genetic and antigenic variants has been observed for RNA viruses (reviewed by Holland et al., 1982) including influenza (Palese and Young, 1982; Yewdell et al., 1979). Moreover, it has been well documented that point mutations in the gene coding for the HA molecule results in antigenic variants which are selected under immunological pressure in nature (reviewed by Webster et al., 1982; Yewdell et al., 1979) but host cell selection pressure provides an additional mechanism for antigenic selection. The verification of antigenic differences between the egg-grown and cell-grown influenza virus populations with polyclonal post-infection human sera in the present study suggests that the antigenic differences in the HA might be of epidemiological significance. The implications of these observations are not necessarily restricted to influenza viruses and similar.

ACKNOWLEDGMENTS

We would like to acknowledge the collaboration with J. C. de Jong, Rijks Instituut voor de Volksgezondheid with the studies on influenza B viruses. Alan Douglas, National Institute for Medical Research, Mill Hill, kindly provided monoclonal antibodies. Terry Corcoran, Bob Newman and Diana Major gave excellent technical assistance.

REFERENCES

Burnet, F. M. and Clarke, E. (1948). Walter and Eliza Hall Institute Monograph No. 4. Macmillan, Melbourne.
Dowdle, W. R. and Schild, G. C. (1975). In "The Influenza Viruses and Influenza" (Ed. E. D. Kilbourne) Academic Press, New York and London, pp. 243–268.
Harboe, A. (1963). The influenza virus haemagglutination-inhibition by antibody to host material. *Acta Path. Microbiol. Scand.* **57**, 317–330.
Holland, J., Spindler, K., Horodyski, F., Grabau, E., Nichol, S. and Uandepol, S. (1982). Rapid evolution of RNA genomes. *Science* **215**, 1577–1585.
Kohler, G. and Milstein, C. (1975) Continuous cultures of fused cells secreting antibody of predefined specificity. *Nature* (Lond.) **256**, 495–497.
Krystal, M., Elliott, R. M., Benz, E. W., Young, J. F. and Palese, P. (1982). Evolution of influenza A and B viruses: conservation of structural features in the haemagglutinin genes. *Proc. Natl Acad. Sci. (USA)* **79**, 4800–4804.
Leung, U.N., Ada, G.L. and McKenzie, I.F.C. (1980). *J. exp. Med.* **51**, 815–826.
Lu Bao, Ian, Webster, R. G., Brown, L. F. and Nerome, K. (1983). Heterogeneity of influenza B viruses. *Bull. WHO* **61**, 681–687.
Oxford, J. S., Hiyam Abbu, Corcoran, T., Webster, R. G., Smith, A. J., Grilli, E. A.

and Schild, G. C. (1983). Antigenic and biochemical analysis of field isolates of influenza B virus: evidence for intra- and inter-epidemic variation. *J. Gen. Virol.* **64**, 2367–2377.

Palese, P. and Young, J. F. (1982). Variation of influenza A, B and C viruses. *Science* **215**, 1468–1474.

Schild, G. C., Oxford, J. S., de Jong, J. C. and Webster, R. G. (1983). Evidence for host-cell selection of influenza virus antigenic variants. *Nature* (Lond.) **303**, 706–709.

Stuart-Harris, C. H. and Schild, G. C. (1976). *In* "Influenza—The Viruses and the Disease". Edward Arnold, London.

Webster, R. G., Laver, W. R., Air, G. M. and Schild, G. C. (1982). Molecular mechanisms of variation in influenza viruses. *Nature* (Lond.) **296**, 115–121.

Wiley, D. C., Wilson, I. A. and Skehel, J. J. (1981). Structural identification of the antibody-binding sites of Hong Kong influenza haemagglutinin and their involvement in antigenic variation. *Nature* (Lond.) **289**, 373–378.

Yewdell, J., Webster, R. G. and Gerhard, W. U. (1979). Antigenic variation in three distinct determinants of an influenza type A haemagglutinin molecule. *Nature* (Lond.) **279**, 246–248.

DISCUSSION

Couch There were a couple of matters I thought needed emphasizing: Dr Schild brought up both of them. One is the relationship between T cell cytotoxicity in the McMichael study and the occurrence of signs and symptoms. All of us have been interested in T cell cytotoxicity and the proposal that it is one of the major mechanisms for recovery. We found the McMichael data very disappointing because McMichael really suggested that T cell cytotoxicity does not develop fast enough to have a significant effect on the acute illness. So his proposal was that the role of T cell cytotoxicity would be limited to reducing the duration of illness; we would have liked for it to appear more significant than that and to have appeared early enough to have had an effect on the acute illness. I think we ought to hold reservations on conclusions but that is the proper interpretation of his data and is the interpretation he made.

The second matter was the disappearance of T cell memory with time. If a person returns to the baseline state with time and loses the anamnestic response which was described in mice, then there is another reason why T cell cytotoxicity may not have the kind of significance that most of us assumed it had for recovery.

I think we must hold reservations on conclusions, but this is clearly the first good complete study of T cell cytotoxicity in man. Perhaps further evaluations will clarify and amplify that result.

Skehel What evidence do you find most convincing that the virus component recognized by cytotoxic cells is the haemagglutinin?

Schild I do not think there is any complete evidence but there is work from animals which are immunized with purified haemagglutinin, which suggests that they get low levels of activity. That is probably the best evidence. But the level of activity was extremely low and in this case I think there was a question of specificity being narrow when compared with Tc responses following infection or immunization with whole virus.

Murphy I would like to make two comments. First, to answer Dr Skehel, Mary Jane Gething has presented some data at a meeting just recently held at Cold Spring Harbour. She has put the H2 haemagglutinin in a BPV vector and expressed it in a mouse cell line. She was able to use Dr Braciale's T cell clones to demonstrate that these T cell clones will specifically lyse the hetero-compatible cells expressing the integrated haemagglutinin on the surface. Clearly, cytotoxic T cells can recognize determinants on the haemagglutinin. This is the most convincing evidence to suggest that this can occur.

I also want to make a comment about McMichael's data. The weight of the data (Fig. 3 of Dr Schild's first paper) is based on only four individuals. He considers a significant response to be a response greater than 10%. There were four individuals on the slide that Schild presented who had a low level of virus present on days 3 and 4 after challenge and who had a high level of pre-challenge CTL. If you look at John Fox's data on antibody responses following natural infection with influenza viruses, 20% of individuals do not have HI or NI serum antibody responses following infection with influenza viruses.

One of the possible explanations for McMichael's four individuals are that these are individuals who were recently infected with the "Russian" H1N1 viruses during their first two or three years of circulation. These four individuals might just not have developed HI or NI serum response but they were immune to the H1N1 virus through an influenza-specific nasal wash antibody response. Also, if you look at this data, it is not statistically significant when you exclude individuals born prior to 1957. The data is suggestive but not statistically significant. I think the interpretations of that study need some reservations.

Couch We were interested in the same matter that Brian refers to. We used McMichael's data and set up a matching-out table for cytotoxicity versus antibody. If your cytotoxicity is less than 10% or greater than 10%, and antibody less than 10 or greater than 10, and you relate these to detection of little or no virus, the P values are greater than 0·10 for the antibody-positive group. This indicates no relationship of virus shedding with cytotoxicity among antibody-positive persons; this is what McMichael stated. Therefore, he had to look at those who are antibody-negative; then the P value for a relationship to cytotoxicity is 0·02. If you do the analysis for no virus shedding, then it loses significance.

If you evaluate antibody among those who are cytotoxic-negative, you have also a P value of 0·02 suggesting an independent effect of antibody.

The point to make on this is that you cannot, with the available data, draw the conclusion that one or the other of these mechanisms is paramount; there is data to indicate that both are contributing to the virus-shedding result. The matter that concerns us, as you might guess from the kind of data we presented in our manuscript, is that the HI test is crude for this kind of evaluation; more sensitive tests for antibody would help us feel confident a significant role for T cell cytotoxicity had been proven.

Murphy The point I was making was that of the seven individuals that were on Couch's slide, three were greater than 27 years of age and thus could have had prior but remote experience with H1N1 virus. Only four of those seven individuals would have been of the age at which they would never have had an infection. I just wanted to raise the possibility of these four having been recently infected with H1N1 virus and thus just fell into the spectrum of individuals who do not develop an HI or NI response after infection.

Mahy I wanted to clarify a technical point. I heard Dr de Jong last week presenting some of this data, and he was very insistent that in order to select virus from the population it was necessary to use monkey kidney cells and that these cells should be no further than a tertiary pass. In your data you referred mainly to MDCK cells. Is there any importance in the type of cell which you use in this initial selection?

Schild We have done little or no work with monkey kidney cells yet, so I really cannot give you any help in that respect. All our work has been done on MDCK.

Palese I thought your slides showed that you had baboon kidney cells.

Schild That is right. That was for H3N2 viruses. We know that in the case of isolating H3N2 viruses on eggs or baboon cells we can see differences between the matched-up pairs of viruses with monoclonal antibodies, but we have not investigated the phenomenon in these cells in any depth.

Kilbourne I should like to make a general comment on Dr Schild's very interesting findings with the B variants (Schild *et al.*, 1983). Of course, genetic antigeneity of viruses is not unsuspected and has been manifest many times in the past, particularly with 'flu, going all the way back to Alec Isaac's work in which you get the rapid attenuation of something in the egg as the virus comes from the human respiratory tract into the chick embryo. There have also been hints of dimorphism or perhaps polymorphism for many other characteristics of the virus that came out. Dr Schild has properly emphasized the practical importance of these findings, but I think the theoretical importance of the findings is enormous, particularly the point about the fact that selection by non-immunologic means can result in antigenic variations, which is something, of course, we discovered with the swine mutants a few years back. More specifically, we can find that if we look for the evolution of a large plaque mutant in MDCK cells with this line mutant we can predict that we then show on the basis of Both's sequencing of such an isolate that it is converted from one mutant form to another and simultaneously has changes of sub-type.

Klenk There is evidence that monkey kidney cells and MDCK cells differ in their proteolytic activating capacity and this may perhaps explain these differences in the behaviour of MDCK cells or monkey cells in the studies you mentioned. Do you need trypsin for the passages in MDCK cells?

Schild Yes, we were aware that proteolytic activity may be of importance in this respect. The influenza B viruses grow happily in these cells without adding trypsin but we did culture some of the viruses with trypsin and looked at the antigenic character, and the trypsin made no difference to the observations of reaction or not with monoclonal antibody.

REFERENCES

McMichael, A. J., Gotch, F. M., Noble, G. R. and Beare, P. A. S. (1983). Cytotoxic T-cell immunity to influenza. *New Engl. J. Med.* **309**, 13–17.

Schild, G. C., Oxford, J. S., de Jong, J. C. and Webster, R. G. (1983). Evidence for host-cell selection of influenza virus antigenic variants. *Nature* (Lond.) **303**, 706–709.

Pathogenesis of Influenza Virus Infection in Ferrets, a Model for Human Influenza

H. SMITH and C. SWEET

Department of Microbiology,
University of Birmingham,
Birmingham, UK

INTRODUCTION

Human influenza is predominantly an upper respiratory tract (URT) infection with some lung involvement but pneumonia or viraemia are rare (Douglas, 1975). Typical signs and symptoms are nasal discharge, cough, fever, headache, myalgia, malaise, anorexia, depression and occasionally neurological and gastro-intestinal disturbances (Stuart-Harris, 1965; Douglas, 1975). It is seldom lethal unless complicated by bacterial infection (Douglas, 1975).

Influenza in the ferret is a good model for human influenza since the patterns of infection are similar. After intranasal instillation of virus, infection is predominantly in the URT and nasal discharge, fever, listlessness and anorexia occur (Smith et al., 1933; Stuart-Harris, 1965). There is some lung involvement but both viraemia and pneumonia are rare

"The Molecular Virology and Epidemiology of Influenza" (Eds Sir Charles Stuart-Harris and Professor C.W. Potter). Academic Press, London, New York and Orlando, 1984.

and, as with humans, the infection is not usually lethal (Stuart-Harris, 1965). Differences in virulence between virus isolates from human influenza and between recombinant clones derived from such isolates, as assessed in ferrets, generally agree with those observed in volunteers (Toms et al., 1976; Davenport et al., 1977; Fenton et al., 1977; Campbell et al., 1979; Matsuyama et al., 1980).

We have therefore studied the pathogenicity of influenza virus in the ferret using the classical approach to the subject—a comparison of the behaviour of virulent and attenuated strains. Ferrets were inoculated by the intranasal route and, of the various criteria for assessing virulence (Sweet and Smith, 1980), we used 50% infectious dose (ID_{50}), the level and persistence of URT infection, the height and duration of fever and the level of lung infection. For the recombinant influenza virus system A/Puerto Rico/8/34–A/England/939/69 (H3N2), clones 7a and 64c were established as virulent strains and clone 64d and the parent PR8 as attenuated strains (Toms et al., 1976, 1977; Matsuyama et al., 1980). All four strains had similar ID_{50}s but differed in other parameters. Using these strains, we have investigated: (1) the viral and host factors influencing URT infection; (2) the origin of fever and other systemic effects of influenza; (3) the viral and host factors involved in infection of the lower respiratory tract (LRT); and (4) the enhanced susceptibility of the LRT of neonates to influenza virus infection.

UPPER RESPIRATORY TRACT INFECTION

Experiments began with the virulent clone 7a and the attenuated clone 64d (Toms et al., 1976, 1977). Following intranasal inoculation, titres of virus in nasal washings indicated that the clones replicated similarly in the nasal mucosa over the first 17–21h. Then, titres of clone 64d levelled out just below 10^5 50% egg bit infectious doses ($EBID_{50}$) ml^{-1} and began to fall rapidly 29–33h post-inoculation. In contrast, titres of clone 7a continued to rise to just below 10^6 $EBID_{50}$ ml^{-1} at 29h and, after a plateau of about 8h, declined. Thus, for clone 7a, the maximum titre was about 10-fold greater than that for clone 64d and the decline, although as rapid as for 64d, was about 8h later. A febrile response occurred in ferrets at about the same time for both viruses (25–29h after inoculation) but the pyrexia was more severe and prolonged for clone 7a than for clone 64d. A nasal inflammatory response, 90% polymorphonuclear cells (PMN) and 10% mononuclear (MN) phagocytes, also occurred at about the same time as the pyrexia and was similar in timing and extent for both viruses. The onset of pyrexia and the inflammatory response corresponded with the beginning of the decline in titres of clone 64d, but both were approaching maximum before the beginning of the decline of clone 7a. This more rapid association of the responses with decline of clone 64d was seen in mathematical correlations made between the rises of pyrexia and numbers of inflammatory cells and subsequent falls in virus titres (Toms *et al.*, 1977). In addition both clones induced interferon, the level of which in nasal washes was generally higher for clone 7a than for clone 64d. The onset and rise of interferon production occurred at the same time for both clones, were coincident with the rise in pyrexia and inflammatory cells and were, like them, associated with the decline in virus titres (Husseini *et al.*, 1981). Finally, non-specific inhibitors of influenza virus were induced in nasal secretions by both clones (Husseini *et al.*, 1981).

In less extensive experiments, URT infections with strain PR8 and clone 64c showed general patterns of virus, pyrexia and inflammatory response similar to those for clones 7a and 64d (Matsuyama *et al.*, 1980). The titres of PR8 in nasal washes were at least as high as those for 7a and their subsequent decline was not as rapid; fever was, however, as low as that for clone 64d and the inflammatory response was not only slightly delayed but 3- to 6-fold less than for the other strains. Initially, titres of clone 64c were somewhat lower than those for clone 7a but they declined more slowly; the febrile and the inflammatory responses were as high as for clone 7a. Levels of interferon and non-specific inhibitors were not monitored for infections with PR8 or clone 64c and it is possible that the relatively low inflammatory response to PR8 was reflected in reduced interferon production.

The Similar Action of Phagocytes, Interferon and Non-specific Inhibitors on Clones 7a and 64d

In tests *in vitro*, clones 64d and 7a were similarly adsorbed to, and rapidly destroyed by, nasal phagocytes from infected ferrets and peritoneal phagocytes from uninfected ferrets, both comprising about 90% PMN and 10% MN cells (Sweet *et al.*, 1977). Also, both clones were similarly sensitive to the action of interferon whether induced either by clone 7a or clone 64d (Husseini *et al.*, 1981). They were also similarly affected by non-specific inhibitors that were induced in nasal washes (Husseini *et al.*, 1981). Thus, phagocytes, interferon and non-specific inhibitors were probably responsible for the rapid decline of both clones in the URT on the second and third day after inoculation, but they were not responsible for the earlier decline of clone 64d. The interactions *in vitro* of clone 64c and PR8 with inflammatory phagocytes, interferon and non-specific inhibitors were not investigated but there is no reason to believe they would have behaved differently from clones 7a and 64d. Nevertheless, the reduced inflammatory response to PR8 observed *in vivo* (Matsuyama *et al.*, 1980) may have allowed the high initial nasal virus titre of PR8 and its relatively slow decline over the next two days, especially if there had been a correspondingly low interferon production (Matsuyama *et al.*, 1980). With regard to clone 64c, the nasal inflammatory response was as rapid and as high as those for clones 7a and 64d and so the slow decline in its nasal titres (Matsuyama *et al.*, 1980) must be attributed to other factors (see below).

The Differential Effect of Pyrexial Temperatures on the Replication of Virulent and Attenuated Strains in Nasal Turbinate Tissue

In uninfected ferrets, the temperature of the nasal mucosa is several degrees below core temperature (about 39°C) (Belshe *et al.*, 1978). In infected ferrets, however, during the 2nd and 3rd day after inoculation, the temperature of nasal epithelium will probably be similar to that of the rest of the body because inflammation and congestion will cause local heating in addition to the generalized pyrexia (Sweet *et al.*, 1978a). Hence, the temperature of the mucosa will be 34–36°C at the beginning of infection but will rise through the 2nd day to about 40°C for clone 64d and PR8 and to 41°C for clones 7a and 64c (Toms *et al.*, 1977; Matsuyama *et al.*, 1980). The effect of these different temperatures on virus replication was studied in organ cultures of ferret nasal turbinates to mimic the situation *in vivo*. At 34°C, clones 7a and 64d produced similar yields up to 19h after inoculation but thereafter until 27h, the yields of clone 7a were significantly higher (Sweet *et al.*, 1978b), a pattern similar to that occurring during the first day *in vivo* (Toms *et al.*, 1977). More importantly, the yield of clone 64d was 100-fold reduced at 40°C compared with that at 37°C, whereas that of clone 7a was almost unaffected (Sweet *et al.*, 1978a). Similarly, the yield of strain PR8 at 40°C was 10-fold lower than that at 37°C, whereas the yield of clone 64c, although somewhat lower than those of the other strains at 37°C, was not further reduced at 40°C (Matsuyama *et al.*, 1980). At 41°C, the yields of clone 64d and PR8 were reduced even more but these reductions are not relevant to the situations *in vivo* where the core maxima were not greater than 40·3°C following infection with these strains (Toms *et al.*, 1977; Matsuyama *et al.*, 1980). The yield of clone 7a was drastically reduced at 41°C (Sweet *et al.*, 1978a), a temperature reached *in vivo* later on the second day (Toms *et al.*, 1977), and therefore probably contributing to the subsequent rapid decline of virus titres. The yield of clone 64c was reduced at 41°C but not as much as that of clone 7a and this probably accounts for the less rapid decline of clone 64c in nasal washes after the fever reached its maximum of 41°C (Matsuyama *et al.*, 1980).

The Increase in Nasal Virus Titres *in vivo* when Fever was Suppressed

Ferrets inoculated with clones 64d and 7a were either shaven or treated with sodium salicylate, which had no apparent effect on the inflammatory response. In some ferrets (responders), the fever seen in untreated ferrets was reduced; in others (non-responders) it was not. Significantly more virus was shed in the nasal washes and its level decreased less rapidly in the ferrets whose fever was reduced compared with the situation in untreated ferrets and in non-responding ferrets (Husseini *et al.*, 1982). Furthermore, the effect was more apparent for infections with the attenuated clone 64d than those of the virulent clone 7a (Husseini *et al.*, 1982). Hence, a significant factor in the virulence of influenza virus in ferrets is an ability to replicate at pyrexial temperatures and a similar correlation between virulence and ability to replicate at pyrexial temperatures has been shown for recent isolates of H1N1 and H3N2 viruses in human volunteers (Chu *et al.*, 1982).

ORIGIN OF FEVER AND CONSTITUTIONAL EFFECTS

The respiratory effects of influenza almost certainly result from mucosal damage and inflammatory changes consequent upon virus replication in the URT and LRT (Fenner *et al.*, 1974; Sweet and Smith, 1980). The origin of the constitutional effects, fever, headache, myalgia, anorexia, malaise and depression has been less clear (Fenner *et al.*, 1974). It appears, however, that these effects may follow release of endogenous pyrogen from MN phagocytes in the respiratory tract after interaction with influenza virus during the inflammatory response which occurs during infection (Sweet *et al.*, 1979).

Work with clone 7a in the ferret provided evidence for the local origin of endogenous pyrogen. Firstly, insufficient infective virus or viral antigen escaped from the URT into the blood-stream over a period sufficiently long to produce, by virus interaction with phagocytes in the blood or reticuloendothelial system, the prolonged fever suffered after intranasal infection. Thus, ten half-hourly intravenous injections of 10^8 $EBID_{50}$ of clone 7a into ferrets were needed to produce a fever of short duration (3–8h) and, after one such injection, influenza virus antigen was detected in the spleen by immunofluorescence. In contrast, intranasal infection resulted in a 24h fever and the total virus content of the nasal mucosa was less than 10^8 $EBID_{50}$

before the onset of fever and only reached $10^{8.5}$ EBID$_{50}$ for 4h during the fever. Furthermore, just before or during the fever produced in ferrets by intranasal infection, influenza virus antigen could not be detected by immunofluorescence in their spleens. Secondly, the local origin of endogenous pyrogen in the URT during infection was indicated by the fact that the onset of fever coincided with the onset of inflammation in the URT (Toms *et al.*, 1977; Matsuyama *et al.*, 1980). Thirdly, immunofluorescence showed that the phagocytes of the inflammatory exudate contained influenza virus antigen. Fourthly, these infected phagocytes released a rapidly acting, heat-labile pyrogen on incubation *in vitro*; and a similar pyrogen was released from ferret peripheral blood leucocytes *in vitro* after interaction with influenza virus (Sweet *et al.*, 1979).

Work with human volunteers provided the connection between release of endogenous pyrogen and production of the constitutional effects of influenza, since the latter, including fever, were seen after intravenous inoculation of human endogenous pyrogen (Cranston *et al.*, 1971; Sweet *et al.*, 1979). Similar effects were produced in volunteers by inoculating large doses of interferon (Scott *et al.*, 1981; Gutterman *et al.*, 1982) which is also induced in the URT of ferrets and man by influenza virus (Husseini *et al.*, 1981; Jao *et al.*, 1965). Whether the amount of interferon induced in infection is sufficient to contribute to the unpleasant effects is not known.

The differences between strains in ability to evoke fever in the ferret model might relate to the variations in severity of constitutional effects noted in different human epidemics (Sweet and Smith, 1980). These differences could result from variation of: (1) the amount of virus in the URT; (2) the number of MN phagocytes in the URT; (3) the capacity of the virus strains to release pyrogen from phagocytes; and (4) a combination of these factors. Thus, the relatively low fevers produced by clone 64d and PR8 might be explained by the low content of the former in nasal washings and the relatively small inflammatory response induced by the latter. This may relate to the fact that the surface antigens (H1N1) of PR8 are different from those (H3N2) of the other strains (Toms *et al.*, 1977; Matsuyama *et al.*, 1980). Clone 64c may have a greater capacity than the other strains to release endogenous pyrogen, since it induced as severe a pyrexia as clone 7a despite its lower titre in the nasal tract (Matsuyama *et al.*, 1980).

LOWER RESPIRATORY TRACT INFECTION

Preliminary monitoring of virus in homogenates of the whole lungs of intranasally inoculated ferrets showed bigger differences in infection between the virulent and attenuated strains than existed in the URT. Thus, clones 7a and 64c produced high titres, 10^5–10^7 50% egg infectious doses (EID_{50}), in the homogenates whereas PR8 and clone 64d either produced low titres or failed to infect the lungs (Toms et al., 1976; Matsuyama et al., 1980).

Distribution of Infection

In subsequent work (Sweet et al., 1981; Husseini et al., 1983; Sweet et al., 1983), the distribution of infection was assessed daily and quantitatively by three methods: (1) titre of infectious virus in tissue homogenates; (2) degree of histological damage; and (3) location of virus-infected cells as detected by immunofluorescence. Trachea and external bronchi were examined in addition to the four lung lobes: the latter were divided into three zones with differing proportions of airway to alveolar tissue; the hilar, containing large bronchi, bronchioles and some alveolar tissue; the intermediate, containing small bronchi, bronchioles and more alveolar tissue; and the outer, containing predominantly alveolar tissue, some bronchioles but rarely bronchi. When examining the infectious virus in three ferrets for each strain, i.e. in three bronchi and 12 lung lobes, the pattern of virus distribution was illustrated best on the third day after inoculation. When the number of bronchi and lung lobes with relatively high titres, for example $> 10^6$ and $> 10^3$ EID_{50} respectively, was assessed two points emerged. Firstly, the attenuated strain PR8 and clone 64d produced much less infection than the virulent clones 7a and 64c. Secondly, clone 7a appeared to infect external bronchi less well and lung lobes better than clone 64c. However, the striking result was that for lung lobes infected with all virus strains, the hilar zone usually contained more virus than the intermediate zone and the outer zone contained the least. This was the first indication that lung infection was in airway epithelium and not in alveolar tissue. These results were supported by the survey of tissue damage which was assessed by projecting numerous sections onto a grid system and calculating the percentage of the total number of points counted that showed inflammation. Overall the damage was minimal. It was greater, however, in the bronchi, where epithelium and mucous glands were affected, than in the parenchyma of the lung where any damage that occurred was around the bronchioles and not in the alveoli. Strain differences were similar to those shown by monitoring infectious virus. The two attenuated strains produced less damage than clones 7a and 64c. Of the virulent viruses, clone 7a damaged bronchi less but lung parenchyma more than 64c. Finally, for infection with clone 7a the distribution of virus antigen in the three lung zones, assessed semi-quantitatively by immunofluorescence, confirmed that the infection was virtually absent from the alveoli and confined to airway epithelium, where it was predominantly bronchial rather than bronchiolar (Husseini *et al.*, 1983). The progressive pattern of immunofluorescence found in the trachea, bronchi and three lung zones on days 1–4 after inoculation indicated a descending infection (Husseini *et al.*, 1983).

Two important facts arose from the studies of distribution of infection within the LRT. Firstly, infection of the alveoli was virtually absent, even for virulent viruses, and this agrees with the rarity of alveolar pneumonia in human influenza. Secondly, LRT infection involved predominantly bronchial epithelium even within the lung; hence it is in comparisons of relative capacities to attack the lining of the bronchi that explanations might be found for the large differences in severity of LRT infection shown by virulent and attenuated strains.

Reasons for the Lack of Alveolar Infection

One possible explanation is that virus never reaches this region but this is unlikely. Some small infected droplets, able to reach the alveoli, would be formed by air rushing through and over the original nasal inoculum and the heavily infected URT during the first two days after inoculation (Sweet and Smith, 1980).

Assuming that virus reached the alveoli, are alveolar cells capable of supporting replication *in vivo*? Almost certainly, since infected organ cultures of the outer zone of the lung from which all visible airways had been removed produced yields of clone 7a as high as similarly infected cultures of bronchus, trachea and the hilar and intermediate zones of the lung. Also, immunofluorescence showed that alveolar cells were infected on the periphery of the pieces of outer zone tissue (Husseini *et al.*, 1983). Clearly, lack of alveolar infection *in vivo* must be due to factors which prevent virus attack on alveolar cells. However, lack of spread of infection from any alveolar cells that do become infected could contribute; the organ culture experiments showed that little virus was released from the infected alveolar cells of the outer zone compared with the release from organ cultures containing airway tissue (Husseini *et al.*, 1983).

Although, as shown for URT infection, interferon and inflammatory PMN phagocytes would be induced at, and reduce, any focus of infection in the alveoli, the predominant host defence present before infected foci developed would be alveolar macrophages. Tests *in vitro* (Bird *et al.*, 1983) showed that ferret lung macrophages adsorbed and destroyed the virulent clones 7a and 64c to the same extent as the attenuated strains not only at the normal ferret temperature, 39°C, but also at the pyrexial temperatures, 40–41°C, which occur *in vivo* on days 2 and 3 after inoculation when lung infection begins (Toms et al., 1977; Matsuyama et al., 1980). Thus, at 39, 40 and 41°C about 80% of each of the four strains adsorbed to the macrophages in 1h and to controls of heat-killed macrophages and ferret red blood cells. However, in contrast to the controls where treatment with neuraminidase followed by freezing and thawing released all the adsorbed virus for each of the four strains, only about one-third of that adsorbed (and probably ingested) by the active macrophages was recovered.

In summary, the lack of alveolar infection appears to be due to destruction by lung macrophages of any virus which reaches the alveoli, coupled with the lack of release, and therefore of spread, of virus from any alveolar cells that do become infected. Also, the antiviral action of induced interferon and PMN phagocytes would reduce infection at isolated loci.

Differential Infection of Bronchial Tissue

To investigate the second point raised by the distribution of infection in the LRT, organ cultures of bronchial rings derived from extra- and intra-pulmonary tissue were infected with each of the four strains at normal and fever temperatures. Similar amounts of all four strains were required to initiate infection (Sweet et al., 1984). Strain PR8 replicated poorly, its yield after 24h was almost 100-fold less than those of clones 7a and 64c at 39°C, with similar differences at 40°C, the temperature of pyrexia induced by PR8. This behaviour of strain PR8 is: (1) in striking contrast to the high yields obtained for PR8 in organ cultures of nasal turbinate tissue and of the intermediate zone of the lung, where alveolar cells were probably infected (Matsuyama et al., 1980); and (2) in accord with the behaviour of PR8 in vivo, where it lacked capacity to infect the LRT despite a high ability to infect the URT. The yields of the other attenuated strain, clone 64d, were greater than those of PR8 but significantly lower than those of the virulent strains at 39°C and 40°C. Again, a difference in replication in bronchial tissue compared with that in nasal turbinate and alveolar tissue was apparent. In the latter tissues the yield of clone 64d at 40°C was significantly reduced from that at 39°C (Sweet et al., 1978a; Matsuyama et al., 1980), whereas this was not so for the bronchial organ cultures (Sweet et al., 1984). The lower yield of clone 64d in bronchial tissue compared with those of the virulent strains explains to some extent its behaviour in the LRT in vivo but an additional factor also operates. In contrast to PR8 and the virulent clones, clone 64d produced a relatively low URT infection which was of short duration because of the influence of pyrexia (Toms et al., 1977; Sweet et al., 1978a). Thus, low seeding of the lung from the URT by clone 64d may compound its somewhat low ability to replicate in bronchial tissue. The superior ability of clones 7a and 64c to attack the LRT was reflected in a high ability to replicate in bronchial organ cultures; their 24h yields at 39°C were similar and not reduced at 40°C. The seemingly superior ability of clone 64c to attack bronchial tissue *in vivo* might be associated with the fact that at 41°C, the pyrexial temperature produced by clones 7a and 64c, although its yield in bronchial organ cultures was reduced, it was still 10-fold higher than that of clone 7a. However, there is no satisfactory explanation for the apparently superior ability of clone 7a over 64c to infect the lung lobes since bronchial tissue is the predominant tissue infected, although extra- and intra-pulmonary bronchial tissue may differ in some way in relation to replication of these two clones.

Clearly replication in bronchial organ cultures reflects to a considerable extent the position *in vivo* and the reasons for the differing abilities of strains to attack this tissue should be sought.

INCREASED SUSCEPTIBILITY OF THE LOWER RESPIRATORY TRACT IN NEONATAL FERRETS

In contrast to adult ferrets, infection of one-day-old ferrets with clone 7a was invariably fatal even with an inoculum 100 000-fold less than that used for adults (Collie *et al.*, 1980). All neonates showed severe involvement of the URT and some died apparently from obstruction of airways and with pathology akin to that seen in human sudden infant death syndrome or "cot death" (Collie *et al.*, 1980). A greater proportion of the neonates, however, appeared to have died from uncomplicated influenzal pneumonia (Collie *et al.*, 1980) and this indicated a much greater susceptibility of the LRT of neonatal ferrets compared with that of adult animals. The previous sections indicate this greater susceptibility might result from: (1) a greater susceptibility of alveolar and/or airway epithelial cells compared with corresponding adult cells; (2) a greater proportion of airway, i.e. ciliated, epithelium relative to alveolar tissue; (3) less mature macrophages; or (4) a combination of these three factors. Two of the three possibilities have been investigated so far and appear to play some role.

Comparisons were made between LRT infection with clone 7a in one-day-old (newborn) and fifteen-day-old (suckling) ferrets, the latter having been shown to be almost as resistant to the lethal effects of influenza as adult animals (Coates *et al.*, 1984a). In newborn ferrets, there was a rapid, severe and progressive infection of lung tissue with infection of alveolar cells as well as those of bronchial and bronchiolar epithelium, as assessed by monitoring virus infectivity and by immunofluorescence (Coates *et al.*, 1984a). In suckling ferrets, as previously shown for adult animals, the lung infection was less severe, less persistent and confined to the epithelium of bronchi with a smaller bronchiolar involvement and even less alveolar cell infection (Coates et al., 1984a). Thus, on day three after intranasal inoculation, about 100-fold more virus was found in homogenates of the combined intermediate and outer zones of the lung of newborn animals compared with those of suckling animals. At eight days after inoculation, these high levels of virus were maintained in the lungs of newborn animals whereas those of the suckling animals were reduced approximately 10-fold and eliminated by day 9. Correspondingly, in this area of the lung on day 3 about 20% of the bronchioles observed in sections from newborn ferrets contained virus antigen in their epithelium compared with 3% for the suckling animals. Also, many fluorescing alveolar cells were seen in the sections from newborn animals while few fluoresced in tissues from suckling animals.

Similar differences were seen in infected organ cultures of the combined intermediate and outer zones of the lungs of newborn and suckling animals (Coates et al., 1984a). The total virus yield at 24h from the tissue of newborn animals was 10–100-fold more than that from the tissue of suckling animals, and far more bronchioles and alveolar cells were seen to be infected in these organ cultures compared with those from the suckling animal tissue. Clearly, one factor in the increased severity of LRT infection in neonates is an increased susceptibility of alveolar and airway epithelial tissue to infection by influenza virus.

In human lung the proportion of airway tissue to alveolar tissue is greater in the neonate than in the adult (Doershuk et al., 1975). A similar situation in ferret neonates to that in human babies could be a significant factor in their increased susceptibility to infection, since airway tissue appears more prone to virus attack than alveolar tissue. Quantitative assessment of the proportion of ciliated and alveolar tissue in serial sections taken at intervals through the mid-lobe of the lungs of newborn, suckling and adult ferrets showed the proportion of the putatively more susceptible tissue, 0·12, 0·06 and 0·03 respectively, was greater in the younger animals (Coates et al., 1984b).

The final factor possibly operating in the increased susceptibility of the neonatal LRT, namely the immaturity of alveolar macrophages, has not yet been assessed. Also, the persistence of neonatal LRT infection to 8–9 days compared with the more transient situation in suckling and adult ferrets (Coates et al., 1984a) suggests a less well-developed immune system in neonates.

SUMMARY

The pathogenicity of influenza virus in the ferret has been studied as a model for human influenza using the classical approach of comparing the behaviour of virulent (clones 7a and 64c) and attenuated (PR8 and clone 64d) strains of the A/Puerto Rico/8/34–A/England/939/69 (H3N2) recombinant system.

The difference between the strains in producing URT infection is determined by differential ability to replicate in nasal turbinate tissue at pyrexial temperatures set against a background of a high capacity of inflammatory phagocytes, interferon production and non-specific inhibitors to reduce infection on the second day after inoculation, which is similar for all strains except PR8, where infection appears to benefit from a reduced inflammatory response.

Fever in ferrets follows from local release of endogenous pyrogen by virus-phagocyte interaction in the URT. Since in humans, injection of endogenous pyrogen produces not only fever but all of the constitutional effects of influenza, the local origin of these effects is indicated. The strain differences in producing fever noted in ferrets might relate to differences in severity of constitutional effects in different human epidemics. These differences might be explained by variations in amounts of virus and phagocytes in the URT and possibly by differing capacities of strains to induce endogenous pyrogen.

Infection of the LRT of ferrets is characterized by two principal features: a relative lack of alveolar involvement, which agrees with the rarity of influenzal pneumonia in human influenza, and infection predominantly confined to bronchial tissue. The lack of alveolar involvement is not due to lack of access of virus or insusceptibility of alveolar cells. The important factors appear to be a powerful defence provided by alveolar macrophages and a lack of release of virus from any alveolar cells which may become infected. The differences in severity of infection produced in the LRT by the different strains were largely but not wholly reflected in their abilities to infect organ cultures of bronchial tissue.

In contrast to adults, neonatal ferrets were killed by influenza virus as a result of an increased severity of LRT infection. This resulted from a greater susceptibility of their alveolar cells and airway epithelial cells to infection by influenza virus compared with adult tissue and possibly to a larger proportion of airway to alveolar tissue. Immaturity of the alveolar macrophages and a less developed immune system also probably contribute but have not yet been investigated.

REFERENCES

Belshe, R. B., Richardson, L. S., Prevar, D. A., Camargo, E. and Chanock, R. M. (1978). Growth and genetic stability of 4 temperature-sensitive (ts) mutants of respiratory syncytial (RS) virus in newborn ferrets. *Archiv. Virol.* **58**, 313–321.

Bird, R. A., Sweet, C., Husseini, R. H. and Smith, H. (1983). The similar interaction of ferret alveolar macrophages with influenza virus strains of differing virulence at normal and pyrexial temperatures. *J. Gen. Virol.* **64**, 1807–1810.

Campbell, D., Sweet, C. and Smith, H. (1979). Comparisons of virulence of influenza virus recombinants in ferrets in relation to their behaviour in man and their genetic constitution. *J. Gen. Virol.* **44**, 37–44.

Chu, C.-M., Tian, S.-F., Ren, G.-F., Zhang, Y.-M., Zhang, L.-X. and Liu, G.-Q. (1982). Occurrence of temperature-sensitive influenza A viruses in nature. *J. Virol.* **41**, 353–359.

Coates, D. M., Husseini, R. H., Collie, M. H., Sweet, C. and Smith, H. (1984a). The role of cellular susceptibility in the declining severity of respiratory influenza of ferrets with age. *Brit. J. Exp. Pathol.* **65**, 29–39.

Coates, D. M., Husseini, R. H., Rushton, D.I., Collie, M. H., Sweet, C. and Smith, H. (1984b). The role of lung development in age-related susceptibility of ferrets to influenza virus. *Brit. J. Exp. Pathol.* (in press).

Collie, M. H., Rushton, D. I., Sweet, C. and Smith, H. (1980). Studies of influenza virus infection in newborn ferrets. *J. Med. Microbiol.* **13**, 561–571.

Cranston, W. I., Rawlins, M. D., Luff, R. H. and Duff, G. W. (1971). Relevance of experimental observations to pyrexia in clinical situations. *In* "Pyrogen and Fever" (Eds G. E. W. Wolstenholme and J. Birch), A Ciba Foundation Symposium, Churchill Livingstone, London, pp. 155–164.

Davenport, F. M., Hennessy, A. V., Maassab, H. F., Minuse, E., Clark, L. C., Abrams, G. D. and Mitchell, J. R. (1977). Pilot studies on recombinant cold-adapted live type A and B influenza virus vaccines. *J. Infect. Dis.* **136**, 17–25.

Doershuk, C. F., Fisher, B. J. and Matthews, W. (1975). Pulmonary physiology of the young child. *In* "Pulmonary Physiology of the Fetus, Newborn and Child" (Ed. E. M. Scarpelli). Lea and Fibiger, Philadelphia, p. 166.

Douglas, R. G. (1975). Influenza in man. *In* "The Influenza Viruses and Influenza" (Ed. R. D. Kilbourne). Academic Press, London and New York, pp. 395–481.

Fenner, F., McAuslan, B. R., Mims, C. A., Sambrook, J. and White, D. O. (1974). "The Biology of Animal Viruses". Academic Press, London and New York.

Fenton, R. J., Jennings, R. and Potter, C. W. (1977). Differential response of ferrets to infection with virulent and avirulent influenza viruses: a possible marker of attenuation. *Archiv. Virol.* **55**, 56–66.

Gutterman, J. U., Fine, S., Quesada, J., Horning, S. J., Levine, J. F., Alexaniana, R., Bernhardt, L., Kramer, M., Spiegl, H., Colburn, W., Trown, P., Merigan, T. and Dziewanowski, Z. (1982). Recombinant leukocyte A interferon: pharmokinetics, single-dose tolerance, and biologic effects in cancer patients. *Annls. Int. Med.* **96**, 549–556.

Husseini, R. H., Sweet, C., Collie, M. H. and Smith, H. (1981). The relation of interferon and nonspecific inhibitors to virus levels in nasal washes of ferrets infected with influenza viruses of differing virulence. *Brit. J. Exp. Pathol.* **62**, 87–93.

Husseini, R. H., Sweet, C., Collie, M. H. and Smith, H. (1982). Elevation of nasal viral levels by suppression of fever in ferrets infected with influenza viruses of differing virulence. *J. Infect. Dis.* **145**, 520–524.

Husseini, R. H., Sweet, C., Bird, R. A., Collie, M. H. and Smith, H. (1983). Distribution of viral antigen within the lower respiratory tract of ferrets infected with a virulent influenza virus: production and release of virus from corresponding organ cultures. *J. Gen. Virol.* **64**, 589–598.

Jao, R., Wheelock, E. and Jackson, G. (1965). Interferon study in volunteers infected with Asian influenza. *J. Clin. Invest.* **44**, 1062–1068.

Matsuyama, T., Sweet, C., Collie, M. H. and Smith, H. (1980). Aspects of virulence in ferrets exhibited by influenza virus recombinants of known genetic constitution. *J. Infect. Dis.* **141**, 351–361.

Scott, G. M., Secher, D. S., Flowers, D., Bate, J., Cantell, K. and Tyrrell, D. A. J. (1981). Toxicity of interferon. *Brit. Med. J.* **282**, 1345–1348.

Smith, W., Andrewes, C. H. and Laidlaw, P. P. (1933). A virus obtained from influenza patients. *Lancet* **ii**, 66–68.

Stuart-Harris, C. H. (1965). "Influenza and Other Virus Infections of the Respiratory Tract". Edward Arnold, London.

Sweet, C. and Smith, H. (1980). Pathogenicity of influenza virus. *Microbiol. Revs.* **44**, 303–330.

Sweet, C., Bird, R. A., Toms, G. L., Woodward, C. G. and Smith, H. (1977). Thermal stability and interaction with ferret inflammatory exudates of two clones of influenza virus of differing virulence for both ferrets and man. *Brit. J. Exp. Pathol.* **58**, 635–643.

Sweet, C., Cavanagh, D., Collie, M. H. and Smith, H. (1978a). Sensitivity to pyrexial temperatures: a factor contributing to virulence differences between two clones of influenza virus. *Brit. J. Exp. Pathol.* **59**, 373–380.

Sweet, C., Cavanagh, D., Collie, M. H. and Smith, H. (1978b). Yields of a virulent and an attenuated clone of influenza virus from organ cultures of ferret nasal tissue: divergence with time of incubation. *FEMS Microbiol. Letts.* **4**, 191–194.

Sweet, C., Bird, R. A., Cavanagh, D., Toms, G. L., Collie, M. H. and Smith, H. (1979). The local origin of the febrile response induced in ferrets during respiratory infection with a virulent influenza virus. *Brit. J. Exp. Pathol.* **60**, 300–308.

Sweet, C., McCartney, J. C., Bird, R. A., Cavanagh, D., Collie, M. H., Husseini, R. H. and Smith, H. (1981). Differential distribution of virus and histological damage in the lower respiratory tract of ferrets infected with influenza viruses of differing virulence. *J. Gen. Virol.* **54**, 103–114.

Sweet, C., Bird, R. A., Husseini, R. H., Gem, J. and Smith, H. (1984). Differential replication of attenuated and virulent influenza viruses in organ cultures of ferret bronchial epithelium. *Archiv Virol.* **80**.

Toms, G. L., Bird, R. A., Kingsman, S. M., Sweet, C. and Smith, H. (1976). The behaviour in ferrets of two closely related clones of influenza virus of differing virulence for man. *Brit. J. Exp. Pathol.* **57**, 37–48.

Toms, G. L., Davies, J. A., Woodward, C. G., Sweet, C. and Smith, H. (1977). The relation of pyrexia and nasal inflammatory response to virus levels in nasal washings of ferrets infected with influenza viruses of differing virulence. *Brit. J. Exp. Pathol.* **58**, 444–458.

DISCUSSION

Palese Have you been able to correlate the virulence of your strains 64d, 7a and 64c with particular genes of the PR8, recombination system?

H. Smith No, together with Skehel who did the molecular biology, we reached the same conclusions as the Giessen group, namely, a constellation of genes was required, not any particular gene.

Palese What were the gene constellations?

H. Smith The haemagglutinin of the virulent parent appeared important, but with the limited number of recombinants examined no pattern emerged. In another recombinant system there were two pairs of strains that showed differences in behaviour in the lower respiratory tract despite an identical gene constellation. Later Skehel found subtle differences in the haemagglutinins of one pair by the use of monoclonal antibodies. Hence, there can be very subtle differences between strains which relate to the degree of lower respiratory tract infection.

Maassab As far as PR8 is concerned, how many passages in eggs have been undergone before you use it in ferrets?

H. Smith It must have been many. Originally we obtained the strain from Paul Beare. If it was passaged many times, it would probably become more virulent.

Maassab That is what I am trying to say, if you go back to mice once and then make a pool, and then go back to ferret, it might kill the ferret. The pattern of pathogenesis is completely different.

H. Smith I agree, and it would be interesting to see if that correlated with an increase in ability to infect the lower respiratory tract.

Maassab I have another question dealing with alveolar macrophages on which I have been instructed by a graduate student of mine to ask. We were able to have a productive infection of alveolar macrophages from ferrets using human influenza virus. The literature available nowadays says that because influenza in humans would not produce a productive infection in alveolar macrophages, so the results we have had in the last six months using two human viruses, H2N2 and another, an '83 strain, show that we were able to achieve productive infection in ferret alveolar macrophages grown *in vitro* and to produce about two logs of virus within eight to 15 hours post-infection. The criterion we had to use, as you are probably aware, is that we could not use any serum when infecting, because any animal serum, even in 0.1% fraction, could restrict growth of the virus, so the literature at least as far as the alveolar macrophages or the peritoneal macrophages are concerned used serum to grow viruses. Serum-free media was devised and it is enriched, and that has been able to support growth of the virus. You have cytolysis and you have an increase in antigen at the same time, so both infectious virus, FA production and cell lysis go along together.

We are fairly confident that it is a productive infection because if you take the rabbit alveolar macrophages and use the same two viruses under the same conditions, there was no productive infection; all you get is internalization of the virus and then in about one hour afterwards it all comes out and there is no evidence of increased fluorescence and minimal cytopathology. So the alveolar macrophages of ferret do lend themselves to some of these studies that we are talking about.

H. Smith We have not kept infected macrophages for a long time to see if there was a productive infection; our interest, of course, has been on how much of the virus was destroyed in the first hour or first two hours. We did not use human serum in our work; all materials came from the ferret.

Maassab The idea is that you cannot use any serum to maintain the macrophages with infection, and the composition of the media used throughout the infection has to be formulated, so you have all kinds of chemical additives without serum and that would give positive results; that will go along with the lack of results available in the literature dealing with macrophages and especially the mouse macrophage.

Tyrrell May I make three quick points. Firstly, about the question of PR8. It is my understanding that Paul Beare used the PR8 which had been used for the original production of the recombinants and it came from Mill Hill. It certainly had been passed frequently in eggs there. We are all aware that there are many different PR8s, and to try and make this whole study valid, it is important to use the PR8 which had been used when the recombinant experiments were done. There is one other point in this connection. I think you would agree it is still generally true that the pathogenicity of those strains and recombinants for ferrets reflects what happens in man. The human experiments are far less precise than the ferret ones, but it does suggest that some of the observations you have, may have rather more generality than just applying to the ferrets—at least generality in the direction of what goes on in human disease.

Secondly, I have a comment on your organ culture experiments, with peripheral lung; even alveolus contains many different sorts of cells and the fact that virus is not shed is a very interesting and possibly rather important point. I am reminded of some experiments which I did some years ago in which we cultured human type II pneumocytes and found that virus would replicate in there partly, but infection could not be passed to other cultures. Maybe some other cells perhaps type one pneumocytes which would be permanent in larger numbers may be behaving in a different way, so there is more subtlety there.

Finally, if I can speculate—and I believe we are supposed to speculate here—I wonder whether some really quite small and subtle change could have made the 1918–9 virus particularly pathogenic for man by enabling it to invade alveolar cells, because looking at some of the old sections of lungs—which Sir Charles used to tell me about—it appeared that the alveolus was very much involved by the virus which was going around at that time.

Dowdle Maybe Dr Smith would like to speculate on the H1N1.

H. Smith Our work with ferrets show that in the lower respiratory tract there can be subtle differences between strains and differences with behaviour in the upper respiratory tract. For example, PR8 produces a severe upper respiratory infection *in vivo* and in organ culture grows extremely well in nasal turbinates. In contrast it does not grow in bronchial organ cultures, which fits with the lack of lower respiratory infection *in vivo*. In addition clone 64d, the attenuated strain, shows a very drastic cutoff of its replication at 40° compared with 37° and 39° in nasal turbinates, whereas in bronchial organ cultures the replication is not cut off at this temperature obtained during pyrexia *in vivo*.

To answer the question directly H1N1 and H3N2 strains may vary in their ability to infect the lower respiratory tract and may be affected differently by different antibodies. I do not know whether that is true; but our work with ferrets suggests that there can be much variability in the behaviour of strains in the lower respiratory tract that may not be seen in upper respiratory infection. It is good to have heard from Bob Couch earlier that more attention is being paid to monitoring lower respiratory infection in man.

Dowdle Thank you. That ought to start something! As a matter of fact, it just so happens that Dr Kilbourne has had his hand up for quite a while, so it is a very appropriate moment.

Kilbourne I have a question and a comment, a comment first of all on Tyrrell's comment. He will recall that in 1957 Hans Hers and Mulder demonstrated evidence on the basis of immunofluorescence of alveolar implantation of the virus in that epidemic. That was not 1918. My interest in that is that that may be a very common reinforcing event for Couch's generalization about a small amount of aerosol.

Couch That was a factor indicated on the slide.

Kilbourne OK. It is important to bring that out. Also, the site of implantation is not always reflected by the site of later pathology. The specific question relates to how the virus was administered.

H. Smith Intranasally.

Kilbourne By that method you would not necessarily infect alveolar cells. In other words, the restriction may not be on tissue tropism but on the method of infection.

H. Smith It is possible that virus does not reach the alveoli but when there is a heavily-infected nasal tract and air rushing through it, it is probable that some small droplets will be formed and reach the alveoli. Nevertheless, we cannot be sure of this point of the story.

Kilbourne There is one further comment before I have a rebuttal on what I just raised. In terms of the neonatal susceptibility of ferrets, I think one must dissect that out from the general increased susceptibility of the young mammal to influenza virus as shown by Wagner many years ago where he gave NWS not only intra-cerebrally but intraperitoneally and found that there was much greater susceptibility than that of even slightly older animals.

H. Smith There are many factors that might operate and, almost certainly immature macrophages will be one. Another would be immaturity of the immune system. In the neonates, virus persists at a high level for eight days but not in the adult where the immune system coped with the infection. We think however, that an important factor is an increased inherent susceptibility of bronchiolar tissue and alveolar cells. The obvious way to try to investigate this is to obtain suspensions of these cells and conduct more specific studies than ever occur in organ culture.

Mahy Have you ever seen any evidence of viraemia in the ferret model?

H. Smith You would find from experiments summarized in the written article that virus escape from the infected respiratory tract is insufficient to produce a fever by systemic reaction with macrophages or to be detected in the spleen by fluorescent antibody. Hence, viraemia, if it occurs, is at a very low level.

Mahy Endogenous pyrogen is released, in your view, from macrophages locally and then into the blood stream?

H. Smith Yes, the evidence for this is summarized in the written article.

Klenk I wonder if you have any data concerning the effect of bacterial super-infection on the course of influenza infection?

H. Smith Yes, in experiments on neonates with PR8 bacterial superinfection we produced lethal effects which could be prevented by treatment with antibiotics. The virulent strain 7a killed antibiotic-treated neonates in the absence of bacterial superinfection.

O'Grady Could I ask two questions? I do not know how easy it is to handle these very small creatures, but is it not likely that the access of the inoculum to the lower respiratory tract is very much greater in them than in adults and that might account for some of the difference in the involvement of the lower tract?

The other is in relation to the alveolar cells. Were you able to look at the alveolar cells in the new-born animals and see whether there was any difference as compared with the adult animals, in relation to failure of the virus to get out again which might account for the greater involvement of the alveoli?

H. Smith To answer the first question, we do not know but I am almost certain that you are right. It would be difficult to obtain a precise answer without using radiolabelled aerosols.

With regard to release from alveolar cells of the neonate, certainly in the organ culture experiments there was a greater release of virus from neonatal lung than from adult lung. When we obtain these cells in suspension for experiments we should be able to give a more definite answer. But the indications are yes, the cells produced more virus and release more.

Tyrrell Can I go on from what Dr Klenk was saying about the interaction with bacteria because there is now quite a lot of information to show that both macrophages and polymorphonuclear leucocytes behave differently if they are taken from influenza-infected animals. Their chemotaxis is reduced, for instance. This can also be demonstrated to occur when cells are exposed to virus *in vitro*. There is some hint also that the whole animal may be more susceptible to bacterial infections if it has received a "virulent" recombinant. Considering this is the meeting where we are supposed to cross-fertilize ideas, I think it could be very important in relation to how dangerous the virus is, and virtually nothing is known about even the individual genes within the virus which are important, let alone the more detailed studies of which type of haemagglutinin or whatever. This would be open to investigation. I hope it will be one day.

Percival Coming back to the potentiation of pathogenicity by a virus infection, in this case influenza, most clinicians feel and say that staphylococcal pneumonia is more likely during an influenza epidemic, and there have been articles suggesting that meningococcal infections in children are more common following influenza. This has not really been touched on in the meeting so far. I wondered really how good is this type of evidence, and in particular the epidemiological evidence. Dr Glezen told me yesterday that he did not have any such evidence.

Conversely, could we ask if there is evidence of the reverse of bacterial interference, for instance parainfluenza virus infections making influenza infections less likely.

Tyrrell I should really get Sir Charles to comment on this because he knows all about staphylococcal pneumonia. I saw my first case of staphylococcal pneumonia on the ward and he said, "That will be an influenzal case" and the epidemic flourished from then on!

Stuart-Harris That was almost the last of the staphylococcal cases we had in Sheffield. We have not seen staphylococcus pneumonia to any extent in the last few years. I do not know why this should be, except that on the whole the staphylococcus seems to have changed its pathogenicity.

Tyrrell There is no question but that there is a frequent association. Professor Kilbourne saw this in New York City. It occurred in the great pandemic. There were certain outbreaks in which staphylococci were the main bacteria but when you ask exactly why it occurs no-one can give you a very good answer. Certainly staphylococcal pneumonia in adults is almost indicative of an influenza virus infection.

Dowdle But it does vary considerably from year to year.

Tyrrell And from place to place in any year.

H. Smith Dr Jakab in the USA has done some work with volunteers and mice indicating that after infection with influenza virus staphylococci and other bacteria adhere to the nasopharyngeal cells better than for controls. There is also work along these lines by others.

Kilbourne It apparently needs to be reiterated that most of the mortality from influenza is bacterial. With that simple statement I will pass. But whether it is staphylococcal, pneumococcal, Group A streptococcal or *Haemophilus influenzae*, this is a notorious association.

Dowdle In a study we carried out in Atlanta over several years relating to the 1968 epidemic, we looked at the risk factors associated with hospitalization during influenza epidemics. It would appear that the risk factors from pneumococcal disease were very much the same as any other year; it was simply that you had more of them.

Scholtissek I am not a bacteriologist, but is it not possible that such bacteria are involved here which provide some proteases which could cleave the HA of the virus, so that the virus could spread better?.

H. Smith It is possible. I do not know. There is plenty of evidence that viruses exacerbate bacterial infections but I do not have this evidence.

The Role of the Haemagglutinin as a Determinant for the Pathogenicity of Avian Influenza Viruses

HANS-DIETER KLENK, W. GARTEN, F. X. BOSCH
and R. ROTT

Institut für Virologie der Justus-Liebig-Universität Giessen,
Giessen, Germany

INTRODUCTION

Influenza A viruses have been isolated from a large variety of domestic and feral birds (for references see Hinshaw and Webster, 1982). While the clinical manifestations of influenza virus infection in mammals are virtually always a result of localized infection of the respiratory tract epithelium, the clinical disease in birds infected with highly pathogenic avian influenza viruses is commonly associated with systemic infection and death. The majority of avian influenza viruses, however, induce asymptomatic infection which is restricted to local sites in mucous membranes frequently in the gut and the respiratory tract. Avian influenza viruses occur with at least 13 different haemagglutinin sub-types and in many haemagglutinin-neuraminidase combinations (Hinshaw et al., 1981). In addition to variability of the genes coding for haemagglutinin and neuraminidase in one sub-type,

"The Molecular Virology and Epidemiology of Influenza" (Eds Sir Charles Stuart-Harris and Professor C.W. Potter). Academic Press, London, New York and Orlando, 1984.

there are also considerable differences in base sequence homologies or oligonucleotide fingerprints of the other genes (for references see Scholtissek, 1983). This suggests that avian influenza viruses arise in nature in a continuous process of segmented gene reassortment. Furthermore, these viruses show differences in their pathogenicity for chicken. Highly pathogenic virus strains exist among the H7 and H5 sub-types. So far as is known, virus strains of all the other sub-types are non-pathogenic (Easterday, 1975). Therefore, for studies on pathogenicity of influenza viruses the avian system offers the advantages that a variety of naturally occurring different virus strains can be used in their natural host. Furthermore, this virus–host system enables us also to analyse the contribution of the individual virus genes to pathogenicity. Genetic studies have usually been concerned with the analysis of virus recombinants obtained *in vitro*. Isolation of pathogenic recombinants has turned out to be a relatively infrequent event, even when both parents were pathogenic viruses. This has led to the concept that pathogenicity depends on an optimal gene constellation (for review see Rott *et al.*, 1983). It is reasonable to assume, however, that any field strain, pathogenic or apathogenic, can survive under natural conditions only if it has an optimal gene constellation. Thus, there must be yet a specific factor that discriminates pathogenic from apathogenic viruses, and we know that a specific role in determining pathogenicity can be attributed to the haemagglutinin.

THE ROLE OF THE HAEMAGGLUTININ IN INFECTION

The haemagglutinin plays an essential role in initiation of infection. We know now that it has two essential functions in this process: (1) It is generally agreed that the haemagglutinin is responsible for adsorption of the virus to the cell surface. (2) There is increasing evidence that the haemagglutinin is involved in penetration, by triggering fusion of the viral envelope with cellular membranes. Thus, cellular membranes exposed to influenza virus show fluidity changes similar to those observed after exposure to paramyxoviruses which are well-known fusing agents (Nicolau *et al.*, 1978). Exposure of cells results also in lysis by specifically sensitized cytotoxic T cells implying that the viral envelope has fused with the cell membrane (Kurrle *et al.*, 1979). It could also be shown that the haemagglutinin induces the fusion of liposomes with cell membranes (Huang *et al.*, 1980a, b), and, under appropriate conditions, cell fusion and haemolysis (Maeda and Ohnishi, 1980; Huang *et al.*, 1981; White *et al.*, 1981; Lenard and Miller, 1981). Structural aspects of the fusion capacity of the haemagglutinin are discussed in detail in the contribution of J. Skehel to this volume.

PROTEOLYTIC ACTIVATION OF THE FUSION CAPACITY OF THE HAEMAGGLUTININ

The biosynthesis of the haemagglutinin, like that of other integral membrane proteins, involves translation at membrane-bound ribosomes, insertion into the membranes of the rough endoplasmic reticulum, and transport to the plasma membrane (for review see Klenk and Rott, 1980). In the course of transport, the haemagglutinin precursor HA undergoes post-translational proteolytic cleavage into the amino-terminal fragment HA1 and the carboxy-terminal fragment HA2. Cleavage of HA is essential for the fusing capacity, and, thus, for the infectivity of the virus (Klenk *et al.*, 1975; Lazarowitz and Choppin, 1975). The observations that proteases of different specificities are able to cleave HA, but that activation is observed only after cleavage with trypsin or trypsin-like enzymes (Lazarowitz and Choppin, 1975; Klenk *et al.*, 1977) suggested that cleavage of a specific peptide bond is required for activation. It was also of interest to find out, if the same peptide bonds are cleaved either *in vivo* or *in vitro* using proteases of various specificities, and these studies gave insight into the mechanism of proteolytic activation.

The results obtained from the haemagglutinin of strain A/chick/Germany/49 (H10N7) are shown in Fig. 1. The amino termini of HA2 and the carboxy termini of HA1 are identical after *in vivo* and after *in vitro* cleavage with trypsin or the trypsin-like enzyme acrosin. When cleaved by the non-activating enzymes thermolysis and chymotrypsin, the cleavage site is

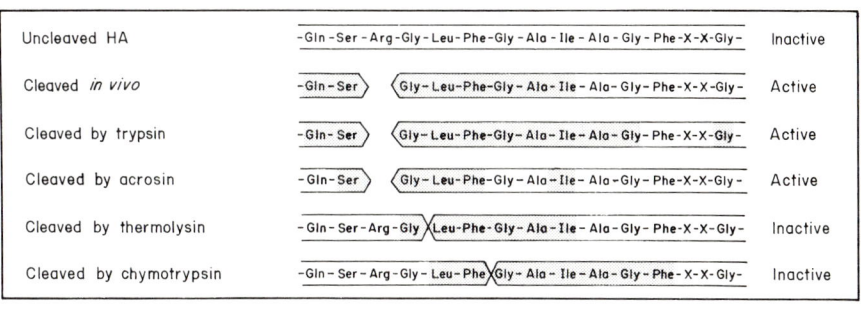

Fig. 1 The cleavage site of the haemagglutinin of strain A/chick/Germany/49 (H10N7). The sequence of the uncleaved precursor has been derived by analogy with the sequences determined on the cleaved haemagglutinin. "Active" and "Inactive" refer to the expression of the fusing capacity of the haemagglutinin. For further details see Garten *et al.* (1981).

shifted by one or three amino acids in carboxy-terminal direction. The data show also that only a single peptide bond is affected by the non-activating cleavage, whereas two bonds are affected by the activating cleavage resulting in the elimination of arginine. The loss of the basic residue can also be demonstrated when one analyses the haemagglutinin by isoelectric focussing. Haemagglutinin cleaved *in vivo* or cleaved by trypsin has a more acidic isoelectric point than uncleaved HA. Such a shift is not observed after cleavage with the non-activating enzyme thermolysin (Garten et al., 1981).

The observations made on the cleavage site of the H10 haemagglutinin allowed the following conclusions. Since trypsin can cleave only the arginine–glycine bond, but not the serine–arginine bond, it appeared that after the initial action of trypsin or a trypsin-like endoprotease, a carboxypeptidase of the B type is involved in the cleavage reaction as had been suggested before by us and by others (Dopheide and Ward, 1978; Klenk et al., 1980). The observation that arginine is eliminated, when the haemagglutinin is cleaved *in vitro* with trypsin added as the only enzyme to purified virus, indicates that carboxypeptidase is present in the virion. In recent studies the enzyme has been isolated and characterized in some detail. It appears to be a host component incorporated into the viral envelope and resembles in many respects carboxypeptidase N (Garten and Klenk, 1983).

TABLE I
Effects of *D*,L-2-mercaptomethyl-3-guanidinoethyl-thiopropanoic acid on the carboxypeptidase activity and on the haemolytic capacity of strain A/chick/Germany/49 (H10N7)

Virus[a]	Carboxypeptidase activity[b] (release of ^{3}H-arginine from matrix-bound ε-aminocaproyl-isoleucyl-(^{3}H)arginine, dpm)	Haemolysis at pH 5·0 (OD540 nm) Virus amounts (HAU)				
		50	100	200	400	800
Inhibitor treatment *before* trypsin treatment	30/51	0·075	0·145	0·295	0·500	0·875
Inhibitor treatment *after* trypsin treatment	28/35	0·068	0·153	0·330	0·571	0·871
No inhibitor, no trypsin	8806/8543	0·000	0·020	0·068	0·163	0·191

[a] Virus was treated with the inhibitor (1 mM) for 30 min at 37°C and with trypsin (10 μg/ml) for 20 min at 37°C. Trypsin treatment was stopped by the addition of TLCK (20 μg/ml). [b] Double determination. Data from Garten and Klenk (1983).

The results obtained with chymotrypsin and thermolysin (Fig. 1) demonstrate that a shift of the cleavage site by only three or even a single amino acid is enough to yield inactive haemagglutinin. This observation is compatible with the studies of Richardson and co-workers (1980) who, by a different approach, found that activation of infectivity requires a specific sequence at the amino terminus of HA2. Structural specificity at the carboxy terminus of HA1 appears to be not so important as a precondition for infectivity, because in this area the haemagglutinin exhibits substantial strain-specific variations. This concept is supported by the observation that specific inhibition of the carboxypeptidase which prevents elimination of the arginine does not interfere with the fusion activity of the haemagglutinin (Table I).

THE SUSCEPTIBILITY OF THE HAEMAGGLUTININ TO CLEAVAGE DETERMINES PATHOGENICITY

The haemagglutinins of influenza virus show differences in the susceptibility to proteolytic cleavage and, in the case of the avian viruses, without exception these differences correlate with pathogenicity. The haemagglutinin of the apathogenic strains is cleaved only in a few host cells, because only these cells have a suitable protease to cleave these haemagglutinins. Most cells lack such an enzyme. Therefore non-infectious virus with uncleaved haemagglutinin is formed. The haemagglutinin of the pathogenic strains is cleaved in all cells analysed, because it is susceptible to an enzyme present in all cells. Thus, there are differences in host range resulting from differences in cleavability (Bosch et al., 1979). It has been known for some time that the differences in cleavability are due to differences in the structure of the haemagglutinin. There is now good reason to believe that it is the cleavage site itself where these structural differences are located. As has been pointed out above, the haemagglutinin of strain A/chick/Germany/49 (H10) which is a prototype of an apathogenic virus has probably a single arginine residue that is eliminated in the cleavage reaction. This holds also true for the haemagglutinins of all human strains analysed so far (for references see Ward, 1981). In contrast, the elucidation by Porter and co-workers (1979) of the primary structure of the haemagglutinin of fowl plague virus (A/FPV/-Rostock/34 (H7N1)) which is the prototype of the pathogenic viruses, revealed that HA1 and HA2 are linked by a whole series of basic amino acids (Fig. 2.). That this may be a common property of pathogenic strains is suggested by recent observations on a series of pathogenic and apathogenic viruses, which all contain haemagglutinins of the same serotype (H7) but, of course, of different cleavability (Bosch et al., 1981). As already mentioned, elimination of the basic linker is paralleled by a shift in charge, and it is

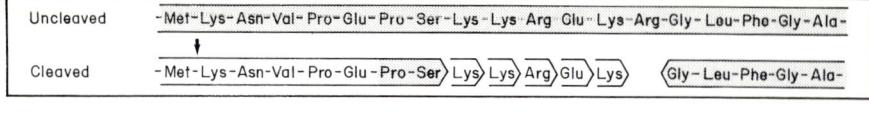

Fig. 2 The cleavage site of the haemagglutinin of fowl plague virus, strain A/FPV/Rostock/34 (H7N1). The sequence of the uncleaved precursor is from the work of Porter and co-workers (1979). The amino acid sequence between methionine-329 and alanine-347 is shown. For further details see Garten et al. (1982).

reasonable to assume that the extent of this shift depends on the number of basic residues eliminated. It was therefore interesting to see that, with one exception, the pathogenic strains show a larger charge shift than the apathogenic ones (Table II). Thus, it appears that the size of the basic intervening sequence is the essential structural determinant for the cleavability of the haemagglutinin.

Sequence analyses at the carboxy-terminus of HA1 and at the amino-terminus of HA2 have revealed that the FPV haemagglutinin is cleaved by

TABLE II
The charge shift paralleling proteolytic activation of H3 and H7 haemagglutinins

Virus	Haemagglutinin sub-type	Cleavability	Charge shift (pH units)
A/FPV/Rostock/34	H7	High	0·5
A/FPV/Dutch/27	H7	High	0·7
A/fowl/Victoria/75	H7	High	0·2
A/turkey/England/63	H7	High	0·9
A/Carduelis/Germany/72	H7	High	0·5
A/parrot/Ulster	H7	Low	0·2
A/turkey/England/77	H7	Low	0·2
A/turkey/Oregon/71	H7	Low	0·2
A/Victoria/3/75	H3	Low	0·2
A/Port Chalmers/73	H3	Low	0·2

Data from Bosch et al. (1981).

the same general mechanism as are the haemagglutinins with a single arginine at the cleavage site (Garten et al., 1982). The basic amino acids are gradually removed by the carboxypeptidase after the initial action of a trypsin-like endoprotease (Fig. 2). It has to be assumed, however, that differences exist in the specificity of the endoproteases involved in the activation of pathogenic and non-pathogenic viruses. The haemagglutinin of the pathogenic strains appears to be activated by a trypsin-like protease present in all host cells that requires at least a pair of basic amino acids at the cleavage site. On the other hand, the haemagglutinin of the non-pathogenic strains which is activated only in a few host cells, is cleaved by an enzyme that can act at a single arginine. This concept (Garten et al., 1982) is supported by the observation that other viral glycoproteins which also have pairs of basic amino acids at their cleavage sites, such as the precursor glycoproteins of murine leukaemia virus (Oroszlan et al., 1980) and the PE2 precursor glycoproteins of Semliki Forest virus (Garoff et al., 1980) and Sindbis virus (Rice and Strauss, 1981), are cleaved in all host cells, too.

The concept that infection with a pathogenic strain, which readily produces virus of full biological activity in a wide spectrum of different cells, spreads more rapidly in the organism than infection with an apathogenic strain, which has a narrow host range, was confirmed by studies carried out in an intact organism, namely, the chick embryo. The site of primary infection in the embryonated eggs is usually the chorio-allantoic membrane which consists of three tissue layers: endoderm, mesoderm, and ectoderm. It was found that the haemagglutinin of the pathogenic strain was activated in all three germinal layers, whereas the haemagglutinin of the apathogenic virus was cleaved only in the endoderm. Accordingly, there are differences between pathogenic and apathogenic viruses in the spread through the membrane as indicated by immune histology. Multiplication of the apathogenic strains was restricted to the cell layer that was inoculated. Spread of newly synthesized virus was inhibited as soon as the virus reached the barrier of the non-permissive mesoderm. On the other hand, the pathogenic viruses spread through the whole membrane and gained entrance into the blood vessels (Rott et al., 1980). A similar mechanism appeared to function in the chicken host. Pathogenic as well as non-pathogenic avian influenza viruses are produced in infectious form with uncleaved haemagglutinin in the epithelial cells which line the respiratory and intestinal tracts of birds. Spread of non-pathogenic viruses is inhibited as soon as the virus reaches the *lamina propria mucosa* which is non-permissive for these viruses. Only the very few pathogenic avian influenza viruses which possess a cleavable haemagglutinin pass this barrier and cause generalized infection.

CONCLUSIONS

The studies on which we report here have shown that proteolytic activation of the haemagglutinin proved to be of decisive importance for the pathogenicity of the avian influenza viruses. In order to become pathogenic, i.e. to induce systemic infection by our definition, a virus strain must have a haemagglutinin which is cleavable in a broad range of different host cells. Such a situation permits rapid production of a great many virus particles which can flood the host organism before defence mechanisms, in particular a potent immune response, can block the spread of the virus. If a certain haemagglutinin gene product is only cleaved in a restricted number of cell types, the infection will be confined to localized areas in the bird. This type of infection is likely to be clinically inapparent. The available evidence indicates that the structural variations of the haemagglutinin responsible for the differences in cleavability are confined to the cleavage site. i.e. to a small but functionally important part of the molecules.

ACKNOWLEDGMENTS

Work carried out in the authors' laboratory has been supported by the Deutsche Forschungsgemeinschaft (SFB 47, Virologie).

REFERENCES

Bosch, F. X., Orlich, M., Klenk, H.-D. and Rott, R. (1979). The structure of the hemagglutinin, a determinant for the pathogenicity of influenza viruses. *Virology* **95**, 191–207.

Bosch, F. X., Garten, W., Klenk, H.-D. and Rott, R. (1981). Proteolytic cleavage of influenza virus hemagglutinins: Primary structure of the connecting peptide between HA1 and HA2 determines proteolytic cleavability and pathogenicity of avian influenza viruses. *Virology* **113**, 725–735.

Dopheide, T. A. A. and Ward, C. W. (1978). The carboxyl-terminal sequence of the heavy chain of a Hong Kong influenza hemagglutinin. *Eur. J. Biochem.* **85**, 393–398.

Easterday, B. C. (1975). Animal influenza. *In* "The Influenza Viruses and Influenza" (Ed. E. D. Kilbourne). Academic Press, New York and London, pp. 449–482.

Garoff, H., Frischauf, A. M., Simons, K., Lehrach, H. and Delius, H. (1980). Nucleotide sequence of cDNA coding for Semliki forest virus membrane glycoproteins. *Nature* (Lond.) **288**, 236–241.

Garten, W. and Klenk, H.-D. (1983). Characterization of the carboxy-peptidase involved in the proteolytic cleavage of the influenza haemagglutinin. *J. Gen. Virol.* **64**, 2127–2137.

Garten, W., Bosch, F. X., Linder, D., Rott, R. and Klenk, H.-D. (1981). Proteolytic activation of the influenza virus hemagglutinin. The structure of the cleavage site and the enzymes involved in cleavage. *Virology* **115**, 361–374.

Garten, W., Linder, D., Rott, R. and Klenk, H.-D. (1982). The cleavage site of the hemagglutinin of fowl plague virus. *Virology* **122**, 186–190.

Hinshaw, V. S. and Webster, R. G. (1982). The natural history of influenza viruses. *In* "Basic and Applied Influenza Research" (Ed. A. S. Beare). CRC Press, Boca Raton, Florida, pp. 79–104.

Hinshaw, V. S., Webster, R. G. and Rodriguez, R. J. (1981). Influenza A viruses: combination of hemagglutinin and neuraminidase subtypes isolated from animals and other sources. *Arch. Virol.* **67**, 191–201.

Huang, R. T. C., Wahn, K., Klenk, H.-D. and Rott, R. (1980a). Fusion between cell membrane and liposomes containing the glycoproteins of influenza virus. *Virology* **104**, 294–302.

Huang, R. T. C., Rott, R., Wahn, K., Klenk, H.-D. and Kohama, T. (1980b). The function of the neuraminidase in membrane fusion induced by myxoviruses. *Virology* **107**, 313–319.

Huang, R. T. C., Rott, R. and Klenk, H.-D. (1981). Influenza viruses cause hemolysis and fusion of cells. *Virology* **110**, 243–247.

Klenk, H.-D. and Rott, R. (1980). Cotranslational and posttranslational processing of viral glycoproteins. *Curr. Topics Microbiol. and Immunol.* **90**, 19–48.

Klenk, H.-D., Rott, R. and Orlich, M. (1977). Further studies on the activation of influenza virus by proteolytic cleavage of the hemagglutinin. *J. Virol.* **36**, 151–161.

Klenk, H.-D., Rott, R., Orlich, M. and Blödorn, J. (1975). Activation of influenza A viruses by trypsin treatment. *Virology* **68**, 426–439.

Klenk, H.-D., Garten, W., Keil, W., Niemann, H., Schwarz, R. T. and Rott, R. (1980). Processing of the influenza virus hemagglutinin. *In* "Biosynthesis, Modifications, and Processing of Cellular and Viral Polyproteins" (Eds G. Koch and D. Richter). Academic Press, New York and London, pp. 175–184.

Kurrle, R., Wagner, H., Röllinghoff, M. and Rott, R. (1979). Influenza virus-specific T cell-mediated cytotoxicity: integration of the virus antigens into target cell membrane is essential for target cell formation. *Eur. J. Immunol.* **9**, 107–111.

Lazarowitz, S. G. and Choppin, P. W. (1975). Enhancement of the infectivity of influenza A and B viruses by proteolytic cleavage of the hemagglutinin polypeptide. *Virology* **68**, 440–454.

Lenard, J. and Miller, D. K. (1981). pH-Dependent hemolysis by influenza, Semliki Forest virus, and Sendai virus. *Virology* **110**, 479–482.

Maeda, T. and Ohnishi, S. (1980). Activation of influenza virus by acidic media causes hemolysis and fusion of erythrocytes. *FEBS-Letters* **122**, 283–287.

Nicolau, C., Klenk, H.-D., Reimann, A., Hildenbrand, K. and Bauer, H. (1978). Molecular events during the interaction of myxo- and RNS-tumor viruses with cell membranes. A270 MHZ^{1}H nuclear magnetic resonance study. *Biochim. Biophys, Acta* **51**, 83–92.

Oroszlan, S., Henderson, L. E., Copeland, T. D., Schultz, A. M. and Rabin, E. M. (1980). Processing and structure of murine leukemia virus *gag* and *env* gene-encoded polyproteins. *In* "Biosynthesis, Modification, and Processing of

Cellular and Viral Polyproteins" (Eds G. Koch and D. Richter). Academic Press, New York and London, pp. 219–232.

Porter, A. G., Barber, C., Carey, N. H., Hallewell, R. A., Threlfall, G. and Emtage, J. S. (1979). Complete nucleotide sequence of an influenza virus haemagglutinin gene from cloned DNA. *Nature* (Lond.) **282**, 471–477.

Rice, C. M. and Strauss, J. H. (1981). Nucleotide sequence of the 26S mRNA of Sindbis virus and deduced sequence of the encoded virus structural proteins. *Proc. Nat. Acad. Sci. USA* **78**, 2062–2066.

Richardson, C. D., Scheid, A. and Choppin, P. W. (1980). Specific inhibition of paramyxovirus and myxovirus replication by oligopeptides with amino acid sequences similar to those at the N-termini of the F_1 or HA_2 viral polypeptides. *Virology* **105**, 205–222.

Rott, R., Reinacher, M., Orlich, M. and Klenk, H.-D. (1980). Cleavability of hemagglutinin determines spread of avian influenza viruses in the chorioallantoic membrane of chicken embryo. *Arch. Virol.* **65**, 123–133.

Rott, R., Scholtissek, C. and Klenk, H.-D. (1983). Alterations in pathogenicity of influenza virus through reassortment. *In* "Modern Approaches to Vaccines" (Eds R. Lerner and R. Chanock). Cold Spring Harbor, (in press).

Scholtissek, C. (1983). Genetic relatedness of influenza viruses (RNA and protein). *In* "Genetics of Influenza Viruses" (Eds P. Palese and D. W. Kingsbury). Springer-Verlag, Wien, pp. 99–126.

Ward, C. W. (1981). Structure of influenza virus hemagglutinin. *Current Topics. Microbiol. Immunol.* **94**, 1–74.

White, J., Matlin, K. and Helenius, A. (1981). Cell fusion by Semliki Forest virus, influenza virus, and vesicular stomatitis virus. *J. Cell. Biol.* **89**, 674–679.

DISCUSSION

Laver Hans, what about the other three basic residues? Do you think they are essential, or are they just appendages?

Klenk I do not know yet. In order to answer this question I think a whole series of more pathogenic haemagglutinins has to be sequenced at the cleavage site. I should like perhaps to give this information at this stage that in fact we know of two more avian influenza strains which both happen to belong to the H7 serotype of the sequence at the cleavage site.

From the work of Naeve and Webster (1983) we know the entire sequence of the seal virus haemagglutinin and the sequence of this haemagglutinin at the cleavage site contains only a single arginine. With respect to this virus's cleavability and its pathogenicity for birds it behaves completely like an avirulent avian virus.

The other sequence concerns the H7 haemagglutinin of the Carduelis virus which was also on one of the slides I showed, and this is a pathogenic virus. With this virus, Dr Bosch has just sequenced the cleavage site and there the intervening sequence consists of the same number of basic amino acids as with fowl plague virus. So the sequences of these two additional haemagglutinins which are now known fit completely into the hypothesis which we would like to offer.

Skehel There was a suggestion that it might be the haemagglutinin that was involved as the carboxypeptidase, and you mentioned that it does not look as it is now. What is the evidence that it is not?

Klenk When we observed that the carboxypeptidase activity was present in purified virus, we of course thought that it might be a virus-specific activity and that it might be associated most likely with one of the two envelope proteins of the virus. However, according to the data which we have, this appears not to be the case. Dr Garten was able to separate the carboxypeptidase activity from the haemagglutinin as well as from the neuraminidase and he could show by polyacrylamide gel electrophoresis that he got a fairly pure preparation which did not correspond to any of these two viral proteins. Furthermore, there were host cell specific differences in the carboxypeptidase bands and this suggested to us that it was an enzyme of host origin.

Skehel Is it still conceivable that although there is a host carboxypeptidase around, there is also a virus-specific one?

Klenk I would not be able to exclude that possibility by 100%, but I would be willing to exclude it by 99%.

Webster The seal virus, as you know, spreads to the brain in the mammal, so cleavability in this case cannot be the only factor involved in the pathogenicity.

Klenk We never said and I hope I made it clear that we do not believe that cleavability of a viral glycoprotein is the only factor responsible for pathogenicity.

Palese Can you give us a model why two cleavage sites should make the haemagglutinin more pathogenic? Can you give us some kind of mechanistic model for that?

Klenk I did not actually want to say that we needed two cleavage sites. I think what happens is that in both cases, with the pathogenic and the apathogenic haemagglutinins, there is a prime action of the endoprotease. It cleaves between the glycine, which later on forms the amino terminus of HA_2 and the adjacent basic amino acid, which in all the cases we know of so far is an arginine. The only difference is that, with the apathogenic viruses, only a single arginine is being removed by the carboxypeptidase, whereas with the pathogenic viruses a whole stretch of basic amino acids appears to be removed with more or less high fidelity. We also think that different endoproteases are involved in the cleavage. In the case of the pathogenic viruses we believe that there is an endoprotease which must have at least two basic amino acids that it recognizes, whereas in the case of the apathogenic viruses a single arginine appears to be sufficient for recognition.

Palese Why should that help?

Tyrrell Can I try and clarify the question in a slightly different way? I think the picture you gave us first of all was that this was all related to fusion and therefore to the ability of a virus to infect cells.

Klenk That is right.

Tyrrell Why should it be that these particular chemical characteristics of the cleavage site make a virus better at fusing to some cells than others? Is that right?

Klenk No. This is not the point. The pathogenic and the apathogenic viruses, once they are activated, cleave with exactly the same efficiency. It is just that the pathogenic viruses are activated in a much larger amount of host cells. Practically all host cells do have an appropriate enzyme to activate them, whereas the apathogenic viruses find such an enzyme only in a few host cells. The apathogenic viruses are, therefore, activated in a smaller range of host cells.

Tyrrell The cells involved reflect the different distribution of the carboxypeptidase?

Klenk No. The cells involved reflect the differences in the endoproteases, in the trypsin-like enzymes involved.

H. Smith I wondered whether there was any connection between this cleavage and tissue specificity in the adult animal. I am not familiar with the spread of infection in the adult animal. Is there any tissue localization, and if there is, does this in any way connect with the ability of the cells in that site to cleave the haemagglutinin?

My other question is: do you get strain resistance in chickens against fowl plague, and, if you do get resistant chickens, in those chickens are the cells there unable to cleave the haemagglutinin?

Klenk To answer your second question first, I do not know of any case where resistance to fowl plague virus has been observed with chickens. Would you repeat your first question?

H. Smith Is there any localization in the adult animal of the virus in any particular tissue, or is it a generalized infection? For example, does it settle down at the lung or any other site? If so, is there a connection between the ability of the cells of that tissue to cleave and the cells in other areas of the body not to cleave?

Klenk Infection with fowl plague is, in the strict sense, a generalized infection, so you practically find the virus everywhere. From the original target it is rapidly disseminated by the blood stream. It is practically found in every tissue. That fits the concept that we find this activating protease which does the job with fowl plague virus haemagglutinin in practically all cells.

Laver If the second protease is a virus-specific enzyme, then you should be able to inhibit it with convalescent anti-serum.

Klenk Right. We have not been able to do that.

Scholtissek I have just a short correction on the intervening sequence which might help you to understand what has been said. We have re-examined this. Bosch has done this and we have done this in our group, too, using the specific primer obtained by Skehel. We found that the glutamic acid—the only acidic amino acid in the intervening sequence—is no longer glutamic acid but is lysine, so it is even more basic. It might be that the fowl plague virus has mutated in the meanwhile but we do not know. At least in our hands, it does not have glutamic acid at the cleavage site any more.

Klenk I am glad you mentioned this because this might help Dr Palese to understand a little better that the carboxypeptidase alone can remove the entire basic intervening sequence once the initial scission has been made by the endoprotease.

Mahy I have a question about the A/Seal/Mass/1/80 H7 sequence which Dr Webster has mentioned. Obviously it is of great interest to know where this additional sequence at the cleavage site comes from in the fowl plaque HA but I wondered what the homology was between the avian and seal viruses in the rest of the molecule. Do you have a figure for that?

Webster I do not have the data with me but I think there are fifty amino acid differences in the total sequence as compared with the fowl plague sequence as determined by Porter *et al.* (1979).

Scholtissek We have studied the genetic relatedness of the haemagglutinin of the various H7 strains by hybridization and we found that H7 haemagglutinins which could be cleaved were sometimes less well related than those haemagglutinins of the H7 sub-type which could not be cleaved. In other words, for example, Turkey/England virus haemagglutinin and the fowl plague virus haemagglutinin genes are not very much related relatively speaking but both could be cleaved. But then there were other strains where the RNase protection was very high between the two strains investigated but one could be cleaved and the other one not, so it looks as if there would be a difference in evolution of the cleavage sites compared with the rest of the molecule.

Tyrrell And the cleavage site, you feel, is critical because that is what correlates with pathogenicity?

Scholtissek Yes.

Kilbourne I wonder whether that kind of evidence really answers that question, because you could have differences in many other parts of the molecule, could you not? It does not necessarily localize it to the cleavage site.

Scholtissek No, I mean two strains which, concerning the haemagglutinin gene, exhibit a relatively low RNase protection after hybridization and might have a cleavable haemagglutinin. But sometimes two strains are highly related, one of them has a cleavable haemagglutinin and the other one does not. I think it is then quite clear that there is a difference in the evolution of the cleavage site and the rest of the molecule.

Klenk This supports the view that there is a close similarity between the seal virus haemagglutinin and the fowl plague virus haemagglutinin.

Chu Since the structure of the cleavage site is so important, has anyone tried to modify or change it from a pathogenic to an apathogenic one and vice versa by whatever method, chemical or genetic engineering? Would that prove your thesis?

My second question is has anybody produced an antibody against that particular fragment of peptide? It should be neutralizing if the antibody binds to the fusion site.

Klenk In answer to your first question, of course, alteration of the cleavage site by site-specific mutagenesis would be a crucial experiment to prove the hypothesis—actually, I think we would rather like to call it a concept. Since this is now a technique available to many labs, I am sure this will be done in the near future with us, but also in other labs.

Palese Site specific mutagenization is not yet possible with infectious influenza virus.

Klenk You can do it with a eucaryotic vector carrying the haemagglutinin gene. Such an experiment would not tell you whether the cleavability is necessary for the pathogenicity but it would provide further proof that the cleavage site is the only determinant for cleavability.

The second question was whether there are specific monoclonal antibodies available to the cleavage site and I do not know of any, but maybe somebody else does. There are however, HA2-specific antibodies. These antibodies did not inhibit haemagglutinin or haemolysis, did not prevent virus release, and did not neutralize infectivity (Becht *et al.*, 1984).

Potter For the record, Mr Chairman, may I ask Klenk whether any of his observations have been extended to the human influenza viruses?

Klenk From what we have heard this morning from several speakers, I think it is quite clear that with the human influenza strains around, we have a localized infection. All of these viruses have a haemagglutinin with a single arginine at the cleavage site and low cleavability. The situation is therefore quite compatible with our concept derived from the avian system.

Tyrrell I think the other general point to be made, is that although you have shown this crucial importance, it does depend on that particular piece of haemagglutinin being present as part of a virus which has a number of other genes which co-operate with it in a way which we cannot yet define precisely.

Klenk Pathogenicity as a multifactorial event is a valid and well-established concept; what we have to know now is how these different factors operate. I think this system provides a very good model to understand how one of these factors operates at the molecular level. I do not know of any other factor determining pathogenicity which is really understood as to how it operates mechanically. I have to stress that we do not consider this to be a model to explain in general the pathogenicity of human influenza virus. However, the model has certainly several aspects of significant impact for human disease.

It may have some relevance to human disease different from influenza virus. In this context one has to mention other systemic infections such as the haemorrhagic fevers, like Lassa fever, Ebola or Marburg disease. We do not know but it may have some relevance.

It also may have relevance to future human influenza strains. Whenever a haemagglutinin comes up in a natural human strain with an intervening sequence as it occurs in the FPV haemagglutinin, I would be worried. I think one also should be aware that such haemagglutinins should not be incorporated into live vaccines.

REFERENCES

Becht, H., Huang, R.T.C., Fleischer, B., Boschek, C.B. and Roth, R. (1984). Immunogenic properties of the small chain HA_2 of the haemagglutinin of influenza viruses. *J. Gen. Virol.* **65,** 173–183.

Naeve, C. W. and Webster, R. G. (1983). Sequence of the haemagglutinin gene from A/Seal/Mass/1/80. *Virology* **129,** 298–308.

Porter, A. G., Barber, C., Carey, N. H., Hallewell, R. A., Threlfall, G. and Emtage, J. S. (1979). Complete nucleotide sequence of an influenza virus haemagglutinin gene from cloned DNA. *Nature* (Lond.) **282,** 471–477.

The Basis of Attenuation of Virulence of Influenza Virus for Man

BRIAN R. MURPHY[a], MARY LOU CLEMENTS[b], HUNEIN F. MAASSAB[c], ALICIA J. BUCKLER-WHITE[a], SHU-FANG TIAN[a], WILLIAM T. LONDON[d], ROBERT M. CHANOCK[a]

[a]Laboratory of Infectious Diseases, National Institute of Allergy and Infectious Diseases, Bethesda, Maryland, USA,
[b]Center for Vaccine Development, Department of Medicine, University of Maryland, Baltimore, Maryland, USA,
[c]Department of Epidemiology, School of Public Health, University of Michigan, Ann Arbor, Michigan, USA,
[d]National Institute of Neurological and Communicative Disorders and Stroke, National Institutes of Health, Bethesda, Maryland, USA

THE FUNCTIONAL INTEGRITY OF EACH GENE IS NEEDED FOR VIRULENCE

The influenza virus, like most animal viruses, is an economical microorganism; each of its limited number of genes is essential for virus replication and dissemination. Therefore, the full expression of viral

"The Molecular Virology and Epidemiology of Influenza" (Eds Sir Charles Stuart-Harris and Professor C.W. Potter). Academic Press, London, New York and Orlando, 1984.

virulence is usually dependent on the functional integrity of each gene. Conversely, a mutation or alteration that results in reduced function of any gene can cause a decrease in the virulence of the virus for its host. Three lines of experimental evidence indicate that this is indeed the case for the influenza A virus.

The first line of evidence comes from the study of reassortant viruses produced by mating the highly virulent fowl plague virus (FPV) with a virus apathogenic for chickens (Scholtissek et al., 1977). When an RNA segment of the apathogenic virus was substituted for the corresponding PB1, PB2, PA, HA, NA, NP, or NS gene of FPV the resulting single gene substitution reassortant virus exhibited reduced virulence for chickens. Reduction of virulence was not the result of mutation, rather it resulted from substitution of a wild type gene from another virus. The substituted gene did not function as efficiently in chickens as the corresponding FPV gene. Incompatibility of its product(s) with those of the FPV genes may also have played a role in attenuation. How much of a decrease in virulence occurred depended on the particular foreign gene that was exchanged at each locus, but clearly, virulent virus could be rendered avirulent by single gene exchange at the seven different loci tested.

The second line of evidence that demonstrated the contribution of each gene to virulence came from an analysis of the effect of a conditional lethal, temperature-sensitive (*ts*) mutation on virulence (Chanock and Murphy, 1980). Viruses that exhibited a decreased ability to replicate at the body temperature of the host were attenuated for that host. At a given locus, the level of attenuation correlated with the level of temperature-sensitivity of replication of the virus *in vitro*, i.e. the lower the temperature to which a virus was restricted in replication *in vitro* the more attenuated it was *in vivo*. The *ts* viruses with a mutation in the gene coding for the PB1, PB2, PA, NP, NA, or M protein were attenuated for experimental animals or birds (Chanock and Murphy, 1980; Ghendon and Markushin, 1980). It is reasonable to assume that attenuated *ts* viruses representing each of the eight segments could be identified if enough mutants were examined. Thus, any gene can serve as a target for attenuation.

The third line of evidence is derived from *in vitro* studies of temperature-dependent host range (*td-hr*) mutants (Shimizu et al., 1983). The *td-hr* mutants were restricted in their replication at 40°C in MDCK cells, but not in monkey kidney cells. By complementation analysis on MDCK cells at 40°C, it was found that the *td-hr* mutants fell into eight complementation groups. These findings suggested each of the eight RNA segments of the influenza A virus genome can undergo mutation leading to an altered host range and, conversely, that host factors influence the functioning of each gene.

SPECIFIC GENES AFFECT VIRULENCE IN MAN

Trials in man by Dr Beare in the 1960s established that H2N2 viruses sensitive to inhibitors of haemagglutination that are present in horse or guinea pig serum were more virulent than the inhibitor-resistant strains (Beare and Bynoe, 1969). Recently Carroll and co-workers demonstrated that inhibitor-sensitive and inhibitor-resistant strains attached to different cell receptors (Carroll et al., 1981). The sensitive strains attached to a receptor that could not be cleaved by viral neuraminidase, whereas the cell receptors for resistant strains were cleaved by neuraminidase. Considering Dr Beare's and Carroll's findings together, the haemagglutinin gene is clearly implicated as one determinant in virulence of influenza H2N2 viruses for man.

Dr Beare has presented additional evidence that the HA and/or NA glycoproteins of another influenza virus, A/PR8/34 (H1N1) virus, are important determinants of virulence (Beare, 1982). The high-passage, egg-adapted influenza A/PR8/34 virus was found to be attenuated for man. However, a reassortant of PR8 virus and an H3N2 wild type virus that possessed the HA and NA genes of the H3N2 virus and the other six RNA segments from the PR8 virus exhibited a moderate level of virulence for man (Florent, 1980). The finding that substitution of H3N2 genes coding for HA and NA surface proteins conferred virulence on a virus that contained predominantly PR8 genes identifies the PR8 HA and/or NA genes as determinants of attenuation of the PR8 virus for man.

Initial studies from Doctors Scholtissek's and Rott's laboratories introduced the important concept that specific gene constellations are associated with virulence or attenuation (Scholtissek et al., 1977). Dr Florent has demonstrated this to be true for man as well (Florent, 1980). Florent compared the genotype and virulence of a series of reassortant viruses derived by mating PR8 and an H3N2 wild type virus. The reassortant England/69 clone 6 retained moderate virulence for man although it received all six genes that code for non-surface proteins from its PR8 parent. In contrast to clone 6 that derived all of its polymerase genes from PR8, six other independently derived H3N2 reassortants were suitably attenuated for susceptible adults. Each of the latter reassortants possessed a mixed polymerase gene constellation with one polymerase gene derived from the H3N2 parent and other polymerase genes derived from PR8 virus. Thus, full attenuation of the wild type influenza A virus required the restriction of viral replication imposed by incompatibility of mutant, (i.e. PR8), and wild type human influenza viral polymerase proteins in cells of the human respiratory tract. This is clearly an example of incompatibility of gene products rather than a simple host range effect because both PR8 and H3N2 polymerase genes function efficiently in the respiratory tract of man, but a specific mixed constellation of PR8 and H3N2 polymerase genes functions poorly, and this serves to restrict virus replication.

Conditional lethal, temperature-sensitive (*ts*) mutants of influenza A virus have also been evaluated in man for their level of attenuation and immunogenicity (Chanock and Murphy, 1980). These mutants were studied with the expectation that their *ts* defect would restrict virus replication in the warmer lower respiratory tract, the major site of disease, without interfering significantly with growth in the cooler upper respiratory tract. The *ts* mutants bearing *ts* mutation in the PB2, PB1, and/or NP genes were observed to be attenuated in man. As discussed earlier, it is likely that *ts* mutants bearing a mutation in any gene would be attenuated for man if the mutants were restricted in replication in the temperature range of the respiratory tract.

STUDIES WITH AVIAN INFLUENZA VIRUSES

Although squirrel monkeys are lower primates, their response to influenza A virus infection mimics that of man in many respects, and this allows us to evaluate virulence of influenza A viruses in this species prior to studies in man. Avian influenza A viruses exhibit a spectrum of replication in the lower respiratory tract of squirrel monkeys with several avian influenza A viruses growing at least 1000 times less efficiently than human influenza A viruses (Table I) (Murphy *et al.*, 1982a). We initiated the studies with avian influenza A viruses with the intent of producing avian–human reassortant viruses that are attenuated for man and that could be used as live virus vaccine strains (Murphy *et al.*, 1982b). Restriction of replication of an avian–human reassortant virus in the primate respiratory tract is effected by naturally occurring avian influenza virus genes rather than by mutant genes selected by limited passage of virus in an unnatural host. Many of the influenza A virus genes that have evolved over a long period in birds differ significantly in nucleotide sequence from the corresponding genes of human influenza A virus. Because of these marked differences, we would expect that (1) some avian influenza A viruses would not replicate efficiently in primate cells and (2) that this property of attenuation would be stable during infection of primates.

An avian influenza A virus, A/Mallard/New York/6750/78 (H2N2), that was markedly restricted in replication in the trachea of squirrel monkeys was evaluated as a donor of its six non-surface protein "internal" genes for attenuation of virulent human influenza A viruses. Avian–human influenza

TABLE I
Efficiency of plaque formation of avian and human influenza A viruses in tissue culture and their level of replication in squirrel monkeys

Influenza A Virus[b]	Antigenic sub-type	Reduction of plaque formation[a] at 42°C compared to 37°C ($\log_{10}$)	Mean $\log_{10}$ Titre of virus ($TCID_{50}$/ml) in tracheal lavage fluid
Avian			
MAL/573/78	H1N1	0.2	1.5
MAL/6750/78	H2N2	0.0	2.4
PIN/286/78	H4N8	0.0	2.4
PIN/358/79	H3N6	0.0	2.8
MAL/827/78	H8N4	0.6	2.9
PIN/119/79	H4N6	−0.1	3.0
TUR/5/79	H10N7	−0.1	3.1
MAL/88/76	H3N8	0.2	4.3
MAL/6874/78	H3N2	0.0	4.4
PIN/121/79	H7N8	0.0	5.0
Human			
Udorn/307/72	H3N2	>4.6	6.5
Wash/897/80	H3N2	>5.8	5.7

[a] On MDCK or primary chicken kidney cell culture. [b] Each virus tested in at least four squirrel monkeys.

reassortant viruses were produced by mating the avian influenza virus and a virulent human influenza virus at 37° and selecting progeny at 42° in the presence of antibodies to the surface antigens of the avian parent virus. As seen in Table I, 42°C is restrictive for replication of human influenza A viruses. In matings involving three different virulent human influenza viruses, each reassortant virus isolated derived its surface antigen genes from its human influenza virus parent and its "internal" genes from its avian parent virus (Fig. 1). Like their avian influenza parent virus, each of the avian–human influenza reassortant viruses produced plagues efficiently at 42°C indicating that one or more of the avian influenza genes that code for non-surface proteins specify growth at 42°C. The level of replication of two avian–human influenza reassortant viruses in the lower respiratory tract of the squirrel monkey was compared to that of their parental viruses (Table II).

The two avian–human influenza reassortant viruses were as restricted in growth in the monkey's trachea as their avian influenza parental virus. In each instance the reassortant viruses were shed in lower titre and for a shorter duration than the human influenza virus parent. These findings

Genotype of avian–human influenza reassortants from mating of avian influenza virus with indicated wild type human influenza virus[d]			
Gene	A/Udorn/72(H3N2)	A/Washington/80(H3N2)	A/California/78(H1N1)
PB2	c	c	c
PB1	c	c	c
PA	c	c	c
HA	b	b	b
NA	b	b	b
NP	c	c	c
M	c	c	c
NS	c	c	c

[a] Avian virus was A/Mallard/New York/6750/78(H2N2). [b] Gene derived from human wild type virus. [c] Gene derived from avian virus. [d] Progeny from indicated mating selected in the presence of antisera to avian influenza virus surface antigens at 42°C, a temperature restrictive for human influenza virus.

Fig. 1 Consistent transfer of six "internal" avian influenza virus genes to avian–human influenza virus reassortants with H1N1 or H3N2 surface antigens.

indicate that restriction of replication of the avian influenza virus is a function of one or more of its "internal" genes. To investigate which of the avian genes was responsible for restricted replication in primates, reassortant viruses were produced that contained the human influenza virus surface antigens from the A/Udorn/72 (H3N2) virus and one or more of the internal genes derived from the avian influenza virus parent (Fig. 2). Avian–human reassortant viruses that contained only an RNA 1, RNA 3, or NS RNA segment of avian influenza origin did not exhibit restriction (i.e. they grew to the same level as their human influenza A/Udorn/72 parent). In contrast, avian–human influenza reassortants that contained only the avian NP or M gene were as restricted in their growth as their avian influenza parent. Avian–human influenza reassortant viruses containing two or more genes derived from their avian influenza parent virus were restricted in replication if they possessed an NP or M gene from the avian parent. Thus, the avian influenza NP and M genes appear to play a major role in the host range restriction exhibited by avian viruses and by reassortants containing their six "internal" genes. Since M and NP genes are able to effect restriction, restoration of virulence of six-gene avian–human influenza reassortants for man would require appropriate genetic changes in both genes or suppression of both genes. The extent of the nucleotide differences between the avian

TABLE II
Restriction of avian–human influenza reassortant viruses in squirrel monkeys

Influenza A virus	Number of monkeys	Virus replication in trachea	
		Average duration of virus shedding (days)	Mean peak titre ($\log_{10}$ TCID$_{50}$/ml) of tracheal lavage fluid
Avian			
A/Mallard/6750/78	7	2·6^a	2·7^a
Reassortant^b			
A/Udorn/72	6	2·0^a	2·2^a
A/Washington/80	8	2·3^a	2·7^a
Human wild type			
A/Udorn/72	15	5·2	5·9
A/Washington/80	14	5·6	5·7

Note: Monkeys received $10^{7·0}$ TCID$_{50}$ of virus (0·5 ml intratracheally) and were infected in each instance. ^{a} Avian virus and reassortants significantly restricted in growth compared to wild type human influenza viruses. ^{b} Each reassortant contains six "internal" avian influenza virus genes.

NP and M genes and the corresponding human genes are currently under investigation. Significant resistance to challenge with wild type human influenza virus was observed in monkeys previously infected with the avian–human influenza reassortant viruses (Table III). Thus, despite restricted replication of the avian–human influenza reassortant viruses, significant resistance was induced to virulent virus.

In monkeys, the avian–human A/Washington/80 reassortant virus was found to retain its growth restriction after serial passage and to be non-transmissible. Furthermore, the virus did not spread to infect the gut or other non-respiratory tract tissues of the monkeys. Because of these encouraging findings a clinical trial was initiated with an avian–human influenza reassortant virus that possessed the six "internal" genes of its avian influenza virus parent (Table IV). This reassortant which contains the A/Washington/80 (H3N2) surface antigens was attenuated and immunogenic, but not transmissible. Satisfactory attenuation was reflected in a greatly diminished replication of virus in the nasal passages of susceptible adult volunteers. Importantly, we were unable to detect viraemia or growth of virus in the intestinal tract. These preliminary trials are encouraging because they demonstrate that avian–human reassortant viruses can be

Influenza virus[b]	Parental origin of genes in avian–human influenza reassortant viruses								Virus replication in trachea	
	RNA1	RNA2	RNA3	HA	NA	NP	M	NS	Average duration of virus shedding (days)	Mean peak titre ($\log_{10}$ TCID$_{50}$/ml) of tracheal lavage fluid
Human	e	e	e	e	e	e	e	e	5·3	5·1
Avian–Human reassortant										
(a) Six "internal" avian virus genes	f	f	f	e	e	f	f	f	0·3[c]	0·7[c]
(b) Single substitution of an avian virus gene	f	f	e	e	e	e	e	e	6·0	5·2
	e	e	f	e	e	e	e	e	5·0	5·4
	e	e	e	e	e	f	e	e	0·0[c]	0·5[c]
	e	e	e	e	e	e	f	e	3·3[c], 2·0[cd]	2·6[c], 1·6[cd]
	e	e	e	e	e	e	e	f	5·0	4·4

[a] Avian virus was A/Mallard/New York/6750/78(H2N2). Human virus was A/Udorn/307/72(H3N2). [b] Each virus tested in at least four squirrel monkeys. [c] Statistically significant difference from wild type human influenza virus. [d] Two independently derived reassortants with this gene constellation. [e] Gene derived from human virus. [f] Gene derived from avian virus.

Fig. 2 Effect of substitution of a single avian influenza virus gene on growth of human influenza A virus in monkeys[a].

TABLE III
Infection with avian–human influenza reassortant virus induces resistance to challenge with wild type human influenza virus parent

Monkeys administered 10^7 TCID$_{50}$ of indicated influenza virus intratracheally four weeks pre-challenge	Number of monkeys	Virus replication in trachea after intratracheal administration $10^{7 \cdot 0}$ TCID$_{50}$ of wild type human influenza virus	
		Average duration of virus shedding (days)	Mean peak titre ($\log_{10}$ TCID$_{50}$/ml of tracheal lavage fluid)
Human wild type virus[a]	6	0	≤0·5
Avian–Human reassortant	5	0·4	1·0
Avian virus[b]	2	6·0	3·8
Placebo	6	5·3	5·8

[a] Human virus was A/Washington/897/80(H3N2). [b] Avian virus was A/Mallard/New York/6750/78(H2N2).

given safely to man and that these reassortants are attenuated by virtue of their reduced replication in the respiratory tract. We are currently evaluating a series of avian–human influenza reassortant viruses derived from different avian influenza A donor viruses. By evaluating these reassortants in primates and man, it should be possible to identify an avian influenza virus donor whose "internal" genes specify an acceptable balance between attenuation and immunogenicity. By evaluating a series of single gene reassortants (i.e. one avian gene—the rest human) in man, it should be possible to identify avian influenza genes that confer attenuation on influenza A virus for man.

COLD-ADAPTED VIRUSES

Influenza A viruses also can be attenuated for man by the transfer of genes from the influenza A/Ann Arbor/6/60 cold-adapted (*ca*) donor virus to virulent human influenza A virus (La Montagne *et al.*, 1983). The A/Ann Arbor/60 virus was adapted to grow well at the suboptimal temperature of 25°C by serial passage at successively lower temperatures in primary chick kidney cell cultures (Maassab 1967, 1968). This temperature is restrictive for wild type viruses. During this process of cold-adaptation, the virus sustained one or more *ts* mutations and acquired a *ts* phenotype, as indicated

TABLE IV

Response of seronegative adults to influenza A/Washington/80 (H3N2) avian–human reassortant or wild-type virus

Influenza A virus administered	Dose of virus (TCID$_{50}$)	Number in group	Percent infected	Virus shedding (nasal wash)		Percent with immunological response			Percent with indicated illness	
				Percent shedding	Peak mean[a] log$_{10}$ titre (TCID$_{50}$/ml)	Serum HI, NI, and/or IgG ELISA antibody	Nasal wash ELISA IgA haemagglutinin antibody		Febrile, systemic or both	Any illness[b]
Avian–human reassortant	10$^{5 \cdot 0}$	12	17	17	1·0	8	8		0	0
	10$^{6 \cdot 0}$	13	67	8	0·6	46	25		0	0
	10$^{7 \cdot 0}$	19	84	11	0·6	74	37		0	0
	10$^{7 \cdot 5}$	20	80	10	0·5	79	47		0	0
	10$^{8 \cdot 0}$	19	100	49	0·7	89	74		11[c]	11
Wild type	10$^{6 \cdot 0}$	24	96	88	3·6	91	93		38	46

[a] Data from each infected volunteer were used for calculations. [b] This category also includes upper respiratory tract illnesses. [c] Afebrile illness of less than 24 h duration. Notes: Transmission of reassortant virus to six contact controls was not observed. Virus was not recovered from blood or rectal swabs. HI = haemagglutination-inhibiting; NI = neuraminidase-inhibiting; and ELISA = enzyme linked immunosorbant assay.

by an *in vitro* shut-off temperature for plaque formation of 38°C (Murphy *et al.*, 1981a). When the A/Ann Arbor/6/60 *ca* donor virus is mated with a virulent human influenza A H1N1 or H3N2 wild type virus at 25°C and progeny are selected at this temperature in the presence of antibodies to surface antigens of the *ca* parent, the majority of reassortants bear the surface antigens of the virulent human virus while the six "internal" RNA segments are derived from the *ca* parent (Cox *et al.*, 1979). Reassortants possessing the six internal genes of the *ca* donor virus have consistently been attenuated in ferrets and in man (Fig. 3) (Maassab *et al.*, 1982; La Montagne, 1983). Each of the four *ca* reassortants shown in Fig. 3 was attenuated compared to wild type virus. The *ca* reassortants also grew in the respiratory tract for a shorter period of time and in greatly reduced amounts compared to wild type virus. The few systemic illnesses observed were generally less than 24 h duration and were less severe than those seen following infection with wild type virus. The human infectious dose$_{50}$ (HID$_{50}$) of the four *ca* reassortants was approximately $10^{5.5}$ to $10^{6.1}$ TCID$_{50}$ (Table V).

Since these viruses grow in eggs to titres of $10^{8.0}$ to $10^{8.5}$ TCID$_{50}$ per ml of allantoic fluid, it is possible to produce enough virus to administer greater than 50 HID$_{50}$ to adult vaccinees. Doctors Peter Wright and Robert Belshe estimate the HID$_{50}$ for completely susceptible children to be about $10^{4.0}$ TCID$_{50}$ (personal communication). At doses of 50 to 100 HID$_{50}$s the *ca* reassortant viruses are satisfactorily immunogenic in adults and children. Furthermore, their *ca* and *ts* phenotypes are stable even in the susceptible young children studied by Doctors Wright and Belshe and are non-

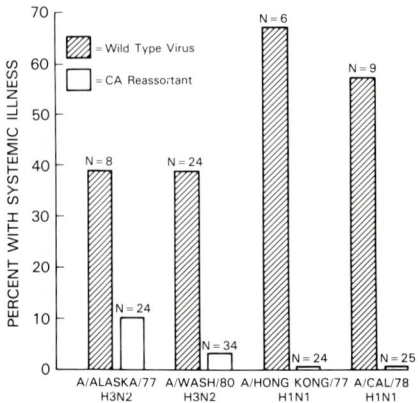

Fig. 3 Response of susceptible (serum HI ≤ 1 : 8) adult volunteers to four cold-adapted (CA) influenza A reassortant viruses.

TABLE V
Human infectious dose $_{50}$ (HID$_{50}$) of cold-adapted influenza A H3N2 or H1N1 reassortant viruses

Cold-adapted reassortant virus[a]	HID$_{50}$ (TCID$_{50}$)
A/Alaska/6/77/(H3N2)	$10^{5.7}$
A/Washington/897/80(H3N2)	$10^{6.0}$
A/Hong Kong/123/77(H1N1)	$10^{5.5}$
A/California/10/78(H1N1)	$10^{6.1}$

Note: HID$_{50}$ of each wild type virus was $10^{3.5}$ TCID$_{50}$ or less.
[a] Virus administered intranasally to seronegative volunteers and infection detected by recovery of virus and/or development of local and/or serum antibody response.

transmissible in adults and children (Chanock and Murphy, 1980, Wright et al., 1982).

The genetic basis of the attenuation of the *ca* virus remains unclear. It appears from studies of *ca* viruses in ferrets and man that the level of temperature-sensitivity of the virus *in vitro* is not the primary determinant of attenuation as was shown to be the case for *ts* viruses whose mutations were induced by chemical mutagenesis. These results suggest the influenza A/Ann Arbor/6/60 virus sustained host range mutations during its passage at low temperature in heterologous avian kidney tissue culture. These host range mutations permit efficient replication in the allantoic cavity of eggs but restrict growth in the human respiratory tract. *ca* reassortant viruses possessing the internal genes of the *ca* donor virus except for the PB1, M, or NS gene were as attenuated for man as those reassortants possessing all six internal *ca* genes. Thus, the PB1, M, and NS genes do not appear to be primary determinants of attenuation of the *ca* donor virus for man (Murphy et al., 1979; Murphy et al., 1981b).

The influenza A/Washington/80 (H3N2) *ca* reassortant virus with six "internal" genes from the *ca* parent was recently compared with commercially available inactivated vaccine for protection against experimental challenge with homologous wild type virus (Table VI). The live virus vaccinees exhibited greater resistance to infection than individuals who received inactivated vaccine parenterally. The *ca* vaccinees had a significantly lower rate of infection and shed significantly less virus. Following challenge with virulent H3N2 virus, the live virus vaccinees failed to develop systemic illness, but this was not statistically different from the low frequency of illness observed among inactivated vaccine recipients. Live virus vaccinees, however, did exhibit significant resistance to illness when compared to unvaccinated control volunteers.

TABLE VI

Resistance[a] of vaccinees to experimental challenge with wild type influenza A/Washington/80(H3N2) virus

Vaccine previously administered	Number of volunteers	Percent infected	Virus shedding (nasal wash)			Percent with systemic illness
			Percent shedding	Average duration (days)[b]	Peak mean titre ($\log_{10}$ TCID$_{50}$/ml)[b]	
Live, cold-adapted reassortant	16	19 ⎫ $P<0.03$	13 ⎫ $P<0.01$	0.7 ⎫ $P<0.02$	1.3 ⎫ $P<0.02$	0 ⎫ $P=0.0$
Inactivated, subvirion	16	63	63	4.4	4.3	13
None	24	96	83	4.0	3.6	38

[a] Vaccine administered four to six weeks before challenge with $10^{6.0}$ TCID$_{50}$ of A/Washington/80(H3N2) wild type virus. Live virus vaccine was a cold-adapted A/Washington/80(H3N2) reassortant; inactivated vaccine contained A/Bangkok/79(H3N2) antigens that are similar to those of A/Washington/80 virus. [b] Only data from infected volunteers used for calculations.

Based on these observations it appears the six "internal" genes of the *ca* donor virus reproducibly confer a satisfactory level of attenuation and immunogenicity upon virulent H3N2 and H1N1 viruses. For this reason the A/Ann Arbor/6/60 cold-adapted virus represents a promising donor of genes for attenuation of new epidemic or pandemic influenza A viruses. It will be important to identify the gene or genes in the *ca* donor virus responsible for attenuation of the *ca* reassortants for man. It is likely that more than one gene plays a significant role in attenuation, otherwise it would be difficult to explain the phenotypic stability of this virus during infection of susceptible individuals. Nucleotide sequence analysis of the A/Ann Arbor/6/60 parental genes and the cold-adapted genes that specify attenuation should further our understanding of the mechanism of attenuation of this virus for man.

ACKNOWLEDGMENTS

Tables I, II and IV and Figs 1 and 2 have been simultaneously submitted to be published in the Proceedings of the Negative Strand Viruses Conference, held at Hilton Head, S.C., September 1983. Tables I, IV, and Fig. 3 were also simultaneously submitted to be published by the Cold Spring Harbor Symposium on Modern Approaches to Vaccines, held at Cold Spring Harbor, New York, August 1983.

REFERENCES

Beare, A. S. (1982). Research into the immunization of humans against influenza by means of living viruses. *In* "Basic and Applied Influenza Research" (Ed. A. S. Beare). CRC Press, Inc., Boca Raton, Florida, pp. 211–234.

Beare, A. S. and Bynoe, M. L. (1969). Attenuation of human influenza A viruses. *Br. Med. J.* **4**, 198–201.

Carroll, S. M., Higa, H. H. and Paulson, J. C. (1981). Different cell-surface receptor determinants of antigenically similar influenza virus hemagglutinins. *J. Biol. Chem.* **256**, 8357–8363.

Chanock, R. M. and Murphy, B. R. (1980). Use of temperature-sensitive and cold-adapted mutant viruses in immunoprophylaxis of acute respiratory tract disease. *Rev. Infect. Dis.* **3**, 421–432.

Cox, N. J., Maassab, H. F. and Kendal, A. P. (1979). Comparative studies of wild-type and cold-mutant (temperature-sensitive) influenza viruses: nonrandom reassortment of genes during preparation of live virus vaccine candidates by recombination of 25° between recent H3N2 and H1N1 epidemic strains and cold-adapted A/Ann Arbor/6/60. *Virology* **97**, 190–194.

Florent, G. (1980). Gene constellation of live influenza A vaccines: brief report. *Arch. Virol.* **64**, 171–173.

Ghendon, Y. Z. and Markushin, S. G. (1980). Studies on mutation lesions and physiology of fowl plague virus *ts* mutants. *Phil. Trans. R. Soc. Lond.* **288**, 383–392.

La Montagne, J. R., Wright, P. F., Clements, M. L., Maassab, H. F. and Murphy, B. R. (1983). Prospects for live, attenuated influenza vaccines using reassortants derived from the A/Ann Arbor/6/60 (H2N2) cold-adapted (*ca*) donor virus. *In* "The Origin of Pandemic Influenza Viruses" (Ed. W. G. Laver). Elsevier Science Pub. Co., Amsterdam, pp. 243–257.

Maassab, H. F. (1967). Adaptation and growth characteristics of influenza virus at 25°C. *Nature* (Lond.) **213**, 612–614.

Maassab, H. F. (1968). Plaque formation of influenza virus at 25°C. *Nature* (London.) **219**, 645–646.

Maassab, H. F., Kendal, A. P., Abrams, G. D. and Monto, A. S. (1982). Evaluation of a cold-recombinant influenza virus vaccine in ferrets. *J. Infect. Dis.* **146**, 780–790.

Murphy, B. R., Holley, H. P. Jr., Berquist, E. J., Levine, M. M., Spring, S. B., Maassab, H. F., Kendal, A. P. and Chanock, R. M. (1979). Cold-adapted variants of influenza A virus: evaluation in adult seronegative volunteers of A/Scotland/840/74 and A/Victoria/3/75 cold-adapted recombinants derived from the cold-adapted A/Ann Arbor/6/60 strain. *Infect. Immun.* **23**, 253–259.

Murphy, B. R., Maassab, H. F., Wood, F. T. Jr. and Chanock, R. M. (1981a). Characterization of the A/Ann Arbor/6/60 cold-adapted virus and its recombinants. *Infect. Immun.* **32**, 960–963.

Murphy, B. R., Chanock, R. M., Clements, M. L., Anthony, W. C., Sear, A. J., Cisneros, L. A., Rennels, M. B., Miller, E. H., Black, R. E., Levine, M. M., Betts, R. F., Douglas, R. G. Jr., Maassab, H. F., Cox, N. J. and Kendal, A. P. (1981b). Evaluation of A/Alaska/6/77 (H3N2) cold-adapted recombinant viruses derived from A/Ann Arbor/6/60 cold-adapted donor virus in adult seronegative volunteers. *Infect. Immun.* **32**, 693–697.

Murphy, B. R., Hinshaw, V. S., Sly, D. L., London, W. T., Hosier, N. T., Wood, F. T., Webster, R. G. and Chanock, R. M. (1982a). Virulence of avian influenza A viruses for squirrel monkeys. *Infect. Immun.* **37**, 1119–1126.

Murphy, B. R., Sly, D. L., Tierney, E. L., Hosier, N. T., Massicot, J. G., London, W. T., Chanock, R. M., Webster, R. G. and Hinshaw, V. S. (1982b). Influenza A reassortant virus derived from avian and human influenza A viruses is attenuated and immunogenic in monkeys. *Science* **218**, 1330–1332.

Scholtissek, C., Rott, R., Orlich, M., Harms, E. and Rohde, W. (1977). Correlation of pathogenicity and gene constellation of an influenza A virus (fowl plague). 1. Exchange of a single gene. *Virology* **81**, 74–80.

Shimizu, K., Mullinix, M. G., Chanock, R. M. and Murphy, B. R. (1983). Temperature sensitive mutants of influenza A/Udorn/72 (H3N2) virus III. Genetic analysis of temperature-dependent host range mutants. *Virology* **124**, 35–44.

Wright, P. F., Okabe, N., McKee, K. T. Jr., Maassab, H. F. and Karzon, D. T. (1982). Cold-adapted recombinant influenza A virus vaccines in seronegative young children. *J. Infect. Dis.* **146**, 71–79.

DISCUSSION

Scholtissek   I have several comments and questions. You mentioned that you can decrease pathogenicity by reassortment but you forgot to mention that you can also create pathogenic properties by reassortment. We have shown this with the mouse system just by mating two harmless viruses and then creating a reassortant which became highly neurotropic for mice and killed all the mice within a short time. That is one point and you might comment on it later.

The other point is that we have also studied recently *ts* mutants for being possible live vaccines just by looking for reversion. We have found that the reversion rate of our *ts* mutants depends very much upon where the *ts* mutation is located. For example, all mutants which had the *ts* mutation located in segments 1 and 2 especially—and also 3 and 5—had a relatively high reversion rate and they are almost as pathogenic as the wild type when we checked them in chickens. A mutant which had the *ts* lesion in neuraminidase did not show much reversion and it was also quite safe. The same holds true for the mutations in the haemagglutinin gene. This presumably is due to the fact that gene products co-operate with each other, and the gene products of the polymerase complex especially co-operate very well with each other. You might then get suppressor mutations or suppressor recombinations very easily with such genes and, therefore, the reversion to the *ts* + phenotype is much higher than would be expected from a normal reversion. In other words, in most cases with these mutants you are dealing with presumably suppressor mutations rather than real reversions.

Then we have also checked double mutants. Here we found again that, if the shut-off temperature of double or multiple mutations is relatively low, these were relatively safe. However, during multiple passages of such mutants which had an intermediate shut-off temperature, after three, four or five passages we finally found that these mutants—despite the fact that they had two or more mutations—reverted and the revertants then overgrew everything very rapidly. Only if the shut-off temperature was relatively low did we lose this mutant after a few passages at high temperatures, but at intermediate temperatures again these mutants reverted, at a temperature where they multiplied to a certain extent. This is in agreement with your observation that the shut-off temperature is very important.

We also found that the route of infection was very important because if you do it intranasally there is a relatively low temperature in the respiratory tract and, therefore, reversion to wild type is much more frequent. In this sense, the mutants which had a relatively low shut-off temperature were again safer than the others. By intra-muscular injection these mutants were completely safe. The safest one was a double mutant with a low shut-off temperature in which the mutation was located in segments 1 and 4. We can imagine that the haemagglutinin and the PB2 protein do not co-operate well and therefore we cannot expect much reversion by suppressor mutation.

This is just a comment. One can study some parameters which might help us by measurement to pick out a relatively safe temperature-sensitive mutant.

Murphy I think that is a very convincing argument for not using *ts* viruses as the basis for attenuation of vaccine viruses for man. I agree with you that and it is precisely for that reason that we are no longer using these *ts* viruses that have been generated by mutagenesis as vaccine strains. We felt that their instability was basically an insoluble problem.

As to the *ts* property of the cold-adapted virus, I wanted to make the point in the paper that I do not believe that this is the only reason that this virus is attenuated. I think that there are, in addition to *ts* mutations in the cold-adapted virus, host range mutations and these are limiting the replication of the reassortant vaccine viruses in the respiratory tract. Even if the *ts* mutations revert in this particular cold-adapted virus there would be other host range mutations that act as governors on the replication of the virus in the respiratory tract.

Getting back to Scholtissek's first point which raised the possibility of an increase in virulence of viruses generated through reassortment, I am very much aware of the important studies that you have conducted in this area. These and other studies have actually formed the basis for us to recommend the production of reassortant viruses that have a limited gene constellation. I think that with both the cold-adapted virus and with the avian–human reassortant viruses you will have noticed that we have been requiring that the six internal genes all come from the same parent. In this way a reproducible phenotype can be best achieved. The alterations in the virulence that have been reported have been mediated by interactions of internal genes but not by interactions of surface antigens and internal genes.

I think therefore, that with the procedure for generating the six-gene reassortants as outlined above problems associated with unanticipated effects on replication such as unexpected decrease in replication or an increase in replication, would be minimized.

Palese I noticed on one of your slides that for the avian recombinants the dose used was 10^8 PFU. This dose was required to infect 100% of the volunteers. Is that not a great amount in terms of antigenic mass? You are almost approaching the amount one gives with killed vaccines.

Murphy That was part of a dose/response curve that we were studying. The purpose of doing that study was to determine the human infectious dose/50. 10^8 is indeed a large amount of virus. It would probably represent about 10–20% of the quantity of haemagglutinin that is contained in a regular inactivated vaccine; i.e. it would probably contain about one microgram of haemagglutinin.

Palese Thus one would forego one advantage of live virus vaccines, which is that one could give less virus vaccine preparations than with inactivated vaccine.

Murphy   As currently formulated you can make perhaps two or three doses of inactivated vaccine per egg. For live virus vaccines in adults you are able to obtain probably 20 to 30 doses per egg, which is an increase in efficiency of about tenfold. I am not sure that we are going to do much better than this but we do not require as much egg material. We are still talking about a substantial amount of virus. In contrast, doubly sero-negative children can be readily infected with the virus at a level of about 10^5 or 10^6 TC ID50. So for children one egg would yield 100 to 1000 doses of vaccine.

Tyrrell   Can I add a small point before we go on? There is one problem, namely that the dose/response curves are very flat. A one hundredfold increase in concentration does not produce a total shift always from all negative to all positive. So it is a little arbitrary to talk about only a 50% dose if you are thinking about vaccination policy and how many people you want to protect with a particular amount of virus.

Murphy   You simply have to determine the dose response of these viruses in man. There is no other way of being able to evaluate viruses that are given to people unless you can estimate the infectious dose/50. What you also need to know is the dose of virus required to induce resistance to either natural or experimental challenge. We have done that as presented in the talk and we find that you need approximately 50–100 human infectious dose/50s in order to induce in adult vaccinees a level of resistance that is acceptable.

Potter   I would like to go back to the original question about the basis of pathogenicity. We have used a different laboratory model for assessing the virulence of virus strains by inoculation of viruses into infant rats. We have found that virulent strains allow a systemic infection by *Haemophilus influenzae* to occur following challenge whereas attenuated strains do not. We have now examined a large number of strains of viruses in this way and have sufficient confidence in the system to distinguish strains; indeed, not only can we assign to strains the property of virulence or attenuation for man, but determine degrees of virulence as well.

Using this model we have tested for virulence a number of the cold-adapted recombinants, given to us by Dr Maassab. All the strains with the two external antigens of the wild type and the six internal antigens of the cold-adapted type were clearly avirulent. But if there is any further enrichment of any wild type virus then the virus is more virulent. This is a progressive phenomenon.

Dr Murphy has spoken about incompatibility of components and this may be a quantitative factor: the more wild type genes you have the less attenuated is the strain. Looking at this data, I wonder if specific genes are ever responsible for virulence. One possibility is that a progressive incompatibility of components related to the number of attenuated genes present, can cause conformational changes which are reflected in decreased replication; and this may be due to translation of change and distortion to the polymerase enzymes.

Maassab We have been trying to see if we could obtain two or even three strains from the double infection. Our experience—in ferrets, not in man—is that for the last ten years I have tried and tried using two or three viruses which have the 6/2 configuration and by infections at a high dose in the ferret. We have not been able to get a pathogenic reassortant.

The other point I would like to make is that in these viruses at least the *ca* and *ts* markers always help to evaluate and monitor the system in which we have additional genes from the wild type. Our experience is that you need a minimum of three genes from A/Ann Arbor/6/60 donor to achieve at least an acceptable level of attenuation; we have reassortants with one gene from A/Ann Arbor/6/60 and the one single gene does not seem to confer attenuation. My impression, although I do not have any empirical data, is that you can transfer cold-adaptability to a wild type even with a single gene from A/Ann Arbor/6/60 without altering too much the pathogenicity. But you need a minimum of three gene constellations to achieve attenuation of some sort. With the six genes, so far as predictibility and reproducibility are concerned, we have achieved at least reasonable data to say that the cold reassortants are genetically stable with no evidence of reversion.

Couch What we learned from volunteers in the kind of studies that we presented to you, is that they are guidelines for evaluation in the field against naturally occurring diseases. Any conclusions that we draw from challenge studies in volunteers would certainly have to be considered tentative.

Schild The current consensus about design of live vaccines is that they should not be shed at all, or should be shed minimally and certainly not transmitted. Did you look at this for your human–avian recombinants?

Murphy We do see shedding. Anyone who has made a rule that they cannot be shed is perhaps a bit unrealistic.

Schild I said shed minimally.

Murphy Shed minimally is something that these viruses definitely are, both the cold-adapted and the avian–human reassortants. With both of these strains there has been no evidence of transmission to date. With the avian–human reassortant virus we have not measured transmission in children but transmission was not seen in adults. With the cold-adapted viruses which are shed in slightly higher quantities transmission in adults and children has not been detected.

Chu I want to say a few words about the virulence of naturally occurring *ts* viruses on which we have worked for some years. We found the first strain of natural *ts* virus in 1973. I want to explain that we were then testing our temperature-sensitivity in chick embryos and in chick cell systems, plaquing in chick cells. Subsequently we found that you can detect naturally-occurring *ts* virus among all sub-types, although the frequency varies quite a lot. For instance, with the old H1N1 it was less than 10%; while with the recent post-1977 H1N1, it was over 50%. They occur in all sub-types including H2N2 and H3N2. We have tested H1N1 strains in a human trial in 1977, that is after the first wave of H1N1 was over. We picked out youngsters around 20 with no antibody, presumably they had never been exposed to H1N1. We tested seven strains. One was the wild type strain. That gave a quite bad reaction with about 40% with a temperature reaction above 37·6°. We had two strains with a shut-off temperature of 39° which also gave a reaction from 20% to 40%. Then we tested four strains with a shut-off temperature of 38°; two did not give rise to any temperature reaction, while the other two only caused minimal reactions. Mind you, the groups were small; there were about ten to 20 people per group.

At that time it looked as if we had confirmed Murphy's finding, that temperature-sensitivity is an indicator of virulence in man. Later, we found that they were in reality temperature-dependent host range mutants—we tested 13 strains—the two wild type, including PR8, and one H2N2 were wild type in chick cells as well as in MDCK. Of the other 11 strains, only one strain appeared to be *ts* in both systems; the other ten were wild type on MDCK and *ts* in chick cells. Whether you call them "temperature-dependent host range" or "host-dependent temperature-sensitive" is just the same. It looks as if most of these viruses are not temperature-sensitive by the MDCK test. We know that that contradicts Murphy's finding that temperature-sensitivity in MDCK is an indicator for human virulence. I do not know how to explain it. At least for H1N1 we think that the human trial seems to be valid. If that is valid, it means that viruses do occur in nature which are in different degrees of temperature-sensitivity and different degrees of virulence for man. It is difficult to test with H3N2 however, because of immunity levels.

Chanock I would like to respond to Dr Schild's comment. I think a more reasonable standard to apply would be where one would insist on the human infectious dose/50 being considerably less than the amount of virus shed. I think Dr Murphy indicated that that was the case with the two viruses. The human infectious dose/50 is about 10^5, 10^6; the amount of virus shed is only about 10^2, or 10^3. I would propose that you consider this rather than an absolute prohibition on any virus shed.

The second point is the question raised by Scholtissek—that of enhanced virulence or *de novo* appearance of virulence, when one mates two viruses both of which are avirulent. It should be pointed out that in the studies which he described one of the parents was the fowl plague virus, which we learned earlier from Dr Klenk's presentation is a virus which has the property of disseminating in its natural host. It has a haemagglutinin which can be cleaved not only in endodermal tissue, but in mesodermal and ectodermal tissue as well. This virus is not neurotropic in suckling mice, possible because of a limitation imposed by one or more of its internal genes. When this virus is reassorted with a human virus, which is also not neurovirulent, reassortants are produced which are highly neurovirulent.

This unusual phenomenon may result from combining the haemagglutinin of fowl plague (which is cleaved in mesodermal and ectodermal cells) with certain mammalian internal influenza virus genes which are needed for efficient replication of reassortment viruses in mammalian cells. In this way, reassortant viruses are able to grow well enough in a variety of tissues to invade the brain and produce devastating results.

In the reassortants described by Murphy the haemagglutinin is always derived from a new human influenza virus that does not disseminate beyond the respiratory tract. Following the mating of an avian virus or a *ca* virus donor with a new human influenza virus, reassortants are selected which possess the surface proteins of the new human influenza virus. Under these conditions it is unlikely that virulence would be enhanced.

Scholtissek I agree with you that the particular properties of fowl plague virus could contribute to what you have said. But we also have done a mating between two human strains and we obtained neurovirulent recombinants from an H2N2 virus and the WS strain—the non-neurovirulent WS strain. This is also in our paper.

I would like to reply to Maassab's suggestion. He said that he was unable to increase pathogenicity by doubly or triply infecting ferrets. We tried to do the same with mice and we did not succeed, but this might be due to some kind of interference. If you have a lot of non-virulent virus this might interfere with the appearance of something which is dangerous. You have to do the recombination in tissue culture or somewhere else in order to obtain a reassortant with increased pathogenicity.

Maassab We tried to do that *in vitro* also but we were not able to. I do not know if there is some kind of technical gimmick we could use in the combination, in order to be able to do that. We have tried by reassortants *in vitro* or *in vivo* but we have not been able to derive reassortants which reverted to virulence. We tried to see if we could create a monster from two avirulent viruses, but we have not been able to do that.

H. Smith I think I should say here what I might have said this morning—that in the system which I described this morning we found with regard to ferret virulence (and I should stress here the measurement of fever) the heightened extent of fever and the measurement of lower respiratory tract infection, with the two clones 7a and 64c, that were more virulent for the ferret than both parents—more virulent than PR8 and A/England/69. We would confirm that system in ferrets—I do not know about humans—that recombinants were more virulent.

I should also emphasize what I said this morning, that we had in another system, A/Okuda and another H3N2 virus, two recombinants with exactly the same gene structure, the same genes from the two parents, and there was a definite difference in lower respiratory tract infection.

Kilbourne I think the picking of the parental viruses in this kind of recombination and reassortment experiment may be crucial, particularly if one is looking for an end-point like neurovirulence. A while back, when I looked at the detailed lineage of neurotropic viruses, I remember there being essentially only two, the WSN and NWS variants. There does seem to be something potentially intrinsically neurovirulent about WS, even before it is put into brains. That has to be said. In terms of PR8 in the ferret model, if I may say so, it was isolated in the ferret—as we all know. There again, you have a latent potential of some of the genes there. The comment I really wanted to make was in relation to the interesting concept of the fixation of genes in the species, that is with the idea that by stultifying a potential for transfer into it specifically.

We heard yesterday from Webster about an avian virus that went into a mammal and created an epizotic in the seal. I wonder what your response to that would be? The seal virus is essentially proved as an avian virus by a lot of criteria.

Murphy This question can fortunately be studied in animals. Our avian–human reassortant viruses that we generate in the laboratory are evaluated extensively in squirrel monkeys to determine if they have any unusual pathogenic properties. We are now serially passaging avian–human reassortant viruses in squirrel monkeys to assess what changes occur as a result of replication of the reassortant virus in the primate respiratory tract. Dr Chanock will be talking about that in his paper.

Kilbourne Only one base change is necessary.

Murphy We do not know whether one base is necessary for the pathogenicity of the seal virus. We do not know the parents that would be perhaps speculating a little too much with this particular virus. We do not know the nature of the changes that occurred in the generation of the seal virus.

Both I think we were getting to a very interesting point in the discussion which stemmed from Kilbourne's comment about the avian virus being able to infect seals, and also the observations that we are now at the point where it is apparent that single mutations can quite dramatically change the growth capabilities of the virus. I think we ought to continue this discussion, particularly since I noted some fairly animated conversation between Dr Kilbourne and Dr Chanock which most of us were not a party to. Perhaps Dr Chanock would like to comment.

Chanock Kilbourne and I had a little discussion in the coffee room about the origin of the so-called "avian genes" in the seal virus. At this point it was not clear from whence these genes came. I suggested one experiment to Webster which might be helpful in determining whether the internal genes of the seal virus were of recent avian origin. The proposed experiment involves reassorting genes of the seal virus with another avian virus which grows well in birds; selection could be for reassortants bearing the surface antigens of the authentic avian virus. The reassortants would then be tested for their capacity to grow in avian cells. It may well be that the seal virus internal genes have diverged significantly from their ancestral avian influenza genes. Webster makes this point very clearly in his presentation when he indicated that the seal virus is highly restricted in birds.

Both The simplest way to assess whether these are avian genes is to determine the sequence, which seems to me to be the best way of approaching it. The hydridization data does not take into account silent base changes, and you would know then how many amino acid changes you are dealing with. I think that is a very important objective that should be achieved to really understand the genetic variation of these genes.

Chanock You would have to know which avian influenza genes should be compared with the seal virus genes. There are so many avian genes in nature that this type of comparison might require a lengthy search.

Scholtissek I would like to suggest a functional test which would show whether the gene is derived from an avian strain or from a human strain. For example, we have one test running for segment number 5. For example our *ts* mutants of FPV which have a defect in segment number 5, cannot be rescued on chick embryo cells by the Hong Kong virus or the H2 viruses because their gene 5 does not fit into the gene constellation of FPV. In order to get recombinants we have to choose another cell system, for example MDCK cells. Ken Shortridge and I want to do some experiments next week in Giessen. Ken has sent a lot of strains which he obtained in Hong Kong: the H3N2 viruses isolated from ducks, from swine and from humans. You will forgive me, Ken, when I say that I was very curious to start an experiment already. We found that the duck virus could contribute its segment 5 to establish recombinants but the swine viruses could not, and the human virus also could not. It was just a very preliminary experiment and we have to await more data when Ken is in Giessen. This is a functional test where you can say whether a gene can function in such a constellation.

Tyrrell On the other hand, would you not agree that, if a biological model system were available in which there were a fairly small number of choices rather than the large number of choices which Murphy has alluded to, the sequencing approach would give you a really definitive answer?

Scholtissek Not necessarily. You can change host range by a single mutation. I think a function test is much better.

Kendal We heard, as part of the discussion today, by Dr Murphy on the difficulties of interpreting McMichael and his collaborators' studies on the basis for human response to infection. I think one of the things that we have to be very cautious about in the work thus far with all of the attenuated virus derivatives is that they are being tested usually in very selective groups of the population. It would certainly be very valuable to know what will happen when these viruses with different genetic backgrounds are given to populations with defined differences in cellular immunity and different levels of humoral immunity.

Secondly, when Drs Couch and Cate and collaborators conducted a rather large open field study with cold-adapted virus at Texas A & M University several years ago there was a curious observation of isolation of a virus from a recipient of placebo which at the time had unclear genetic background since it appeared to have some properties of wild type and some properties of vaccine strain. Subsequently, Dr Cox in my laboratory has managed to identify at least seven of the eight genes in this virus and it clearly is a recombinant between a field strain of H1N1 virus then circulating and the vaccine strain.

Particularly with respect to viruses with avian genes, one has to ask the question, what would be the potential for producing various diverse reassortants during the use of live vaccines? Bearing in mind the propensity for nature to select successful genetic stock, would there be a possibility to select the virus that would contain a mixture of human and avian genes that would transmit readily to man?

Perhaps this type of question could be approached by experiments in a small primate model by mixedly infecting the animals with the vaccine candidate strain and prevalent wild type strains and seeing what types of viruses are selected for and whether they have novel biological properties? There are systems apparently available that would enable us to start looking at this question.

I was asked by the person facing me across the table to comment on the situation in the Soviet Union, for the record. Again, many people around the table know that the Soviet scientists have for many years worked with live vaccine strains and in fact were presumably the first to investigate the possibility for attenuating influenza viruses, inhibitor-resistant strains being the first and cold-adapted strains subsequently. Although we find it difficult to know what the exact experiences are, there is no doubt that in practice many millions of doses of cold-adapted virus vaccines have been given with apparently no untoward effects that anyone is aware of. However, the prime developers of the vaccines in the Soviet Union feel quite strongly that two types of vaccine are needed, one for children and one for adults. This, perhaps, takes us around in a full circle to where I started my comments; that presumably the level of background immunity in the host can indeed affect the replication of the virus to the extent that this approach needs to be looked at.

To add one final point, which also relates to other items that have been discussed at the meeting in terms of local immunity versus humoral immunity, again many people here are aware of the proposals that peroral live vaccine would be in fact a safe and effective option for attenuation of influenza viruses. I think we probably know enough to believe that there may indeed be opportunities to develop influenza strains that can pass into, and replicate in, the gut of man as they do in animals and produce IgA memory cells that can migrate to the upper respiratory tract and be of some value.

There are very many aspects in terms of attenuation of virulence of influenza virus, and we have only scratched the surface, even with the vast amount of information we have so far.

Kilbourne Having started the fight, I would like to add another note. If Emerson was right that "a foolish consistency is the hobgoblin of little minds" I find myself surrounded by great men! I am somewhat baffled. As a simple-minded fellow, I hear one day that we are talking about avian genes and the next day they are seal genes, although they are indistinguishable by present testing.

The other point is that Dr Schild has told us very compellingly about the heterogeneity of virus populations in isolates, and we have to remember that the minute that tern or whatever it was, infected the seal, that seal selected a population of particles ostensibly quite different from that carried by the bird—at least in a number of respects—so that constantly as we think about these interspecies transfers—and I would agree that there are no "avian" genes, no "horse" genes or anything else—we have to be very concerned about the changes occurring with the host transfer. That is the only point I wanted to make.

Prospects for Stabilization of Attenuation

ROBERT M. CHANOCK, BRIAN R. MURPHY,
CHING-JUH LAI, LEWIS J. MARKOFF
and BOR-CHIAN LIN

Laboratory of Infectious Diseases, National Institute of Allergy and Infectious Diseases, National Institutes of Health, Bethesda, Maryland, USA

Unlike many other viruses that have a complex pathogenesis which can be interrupted at several different sites in the body, human influenza virus initiates infection and causes disease in the same site, namely the respiratory tract. This property of the human influenza viruses limits the region in which attenuation can be achieved to this site. Probably for this reason, every attenuated human influenza virus studied thus far grows less well in the respiratory tract than does its wild-type parent. Thus, the common pathway for attenuation appears to be diminished growth in the target organ. The usefulness of a live influenza virus vaccine depends upon the balance that is achieved between its restriction of growth and its immunogenicity.

"The Molecular Virology and Epidemiology of Influenza" (Eds Sir Charles Stuart-Harris and Professor C.W. Potter). Academic Press, London, New York and Orlando, 1984.

Polygenic Nature of Virulence

Attenuation can be achieved by mutation or sequence divergence that diminishes the capacity of virus to replicate in the human respiratory tract (Murphy *et al.*, this volume pp. 211–225). Because the efficient functioning of every viral gene is required for virulence, a defect in any viral function can impair replication and bring about attenuation. For example, a *ts* mutation in any of seven viral genes tested thus far can lead to attenuation of influenza A virus for experimental animals or birds (Richman and Murphy, 1979; Ghendon and Markushin, 1980). Evidence for the polygenic nature of virulence also comes from the gene substitution studies of Scholtissek and Rott (Scholtissek *et al.*, 1977). The genes of fowl plague virus, which is highly virulent for chickens were reassorted with those of other influenza A viruses apathogenic for chickens. At seven separate loci substitution of a gene from the attenuated parent for the corresponding fowl plague virus gene resulted in a decrease in virulence for chickens. The preceding observations indicate that attempts at attenuation of influenza virus can be made across a broad genetic front.

Strategy for Attenuation

Present efforts to attenuate influenza A virus are focused primarily on genes that code for non-surface viral proteins, the so-called "internal" genes. These genes can be transferred by reassortment into viruses bearing the surface glycoprotein antigens of new epidemic or pandemic viruses. In this manner, a satisfactory level of attenuation can be achieved rapidly and reproducibly to meet an epidemic or pandemic threat. Attenuation can also be achieved by mutations in the haemagglutinin (HA) and neuraminidase (NA) genes; however, such mutations are generally not useful for construction of live vaccine strains because these attenuating genes can not be transferred into vaccine reassortant viruses when antigenic shift or drift occurs.

Stability of Genetic Determinants of Attenuation

To date, it has been easier to achieve a satisfactory level of attenuation and immunogenicity than to stabilize this phenotype so that it is not altered during growth of vaccine virus in susceptible individuals. Viruses with a single-stranded RNA genome are transcribed by viral polymerases that are not completely faithful, and there is no mechanism available to correct mistakes (Holland et al., 1982). For influenza A virus, the frequency of mutation at any single nucleotide appears to be $10^{-5.5}$ per replication. This estimate is derived from the frequency of spontaneous mutants that are resistant to neutralizing monoclonal antibodies directed at a variety of epitopes on the viral haemagglutinin or neuraminidase (Portner et al., 1980; Webster et al., 1982). This estimate can be extrapolated to a frequency of mutation of $10^{-1.5}$ for the entire viral genome. Furthermore, this frequency is several orders of magnitude higher than for DNA genomes of similar complexity. As a consequence, many mutants are generated during every cycle of replication and these mutants are available for selection during subsequent cycles of growth in infected vaccinees. Since the phenotype imposed on attenuated live influenza vaccine viruses is poor growth in the respiratory tract, there is strong pressure for selection of mutants that grow better than their vaccine parent. For this reason it is unrealistic to expect the RNA sequences responsible for attenuation to remain unaltered by reversion or suppression. Viable deletion mutants might be an exception, since they would not be subject to reversion. Also, it is likely that such mutations would be difficult to modify by suppression, but this remains to be determined.

Except in the case of deletion mutants, our goal should be to stabilize the attenuation phenotype by constructing vaccine strains that contain as many independent genetic determinants of attenuation as is consistent with viability and satisfactory immunogenicity. The more independent mutations or sequence divergences in a vaccine virus, the more new mutations required for restoration of virulence.

In any case, it is likely that the ultimate live virus vaccine strains will bear genes of defined nucleotide sequence that specify a satisfactory level of attenuation and immunogenicity. Once the nucleotide sequences responsible for attenuation have been identified, it will be possible to monitor attenuation in the laboratory during all phases of vaccine development, manufacture and utilization in man.

TEMPERATURE-SENSITIVE *ts* MUTANTS

The problem of genetic instability of live attenuated influenza viruses was highlighted during the clinical evaluation of viruses bearing *ts* mutations. Initially *ts* mutations were induced in donor viruses by chemical mutagenesis. These *ts* genes were then transferred to reassortant viruses bearing the surface antigens of new epidemic strains. Reassortant viruses prepared in this manner from two different *ts* donor viruses were satisfactorily attenuated for susceptible adults (Murphy and Chanock, 1981). Furthermore, these reassortants retained their *ts* phenotype during infection of susceptible adults. One donor, *ts*-1[E], had *ts* mutations on its PB2 and NP genes, while the other, *ts* 1A2, had *ts* mutations on its PB1 and PB2 genes. The *ts* 1[E] reassortants retained a low level of virulence for susceptible young children, whereas *ts* 1A2 reassortants were satisfactorily attenuated for such individuals (Kim *et al.*, 1976; Wright *et al.*, 1982). Nonetheless, both *ts* 1[E] and *ts* 1A2 reassortants lost their *ts* phenotype during infection of susceptible young children (Kim *et al.*, 1976; Murphy *et al.*, 1980).

Escape of a *ts* 1A2 reassortant from its *ts* phenotype was studied in some detail, and this led to the first demonstration that an influenza virus mutation could be suppressed by a new mutation on another gene (Table I). At least three new mutations were identified in a *ts* + isolate recovered from a young child infected with a *ts* 1A2 reassortant (Murphy *et al.*, 1980; Tolpin *et al.*, 1981). A new mutation developed on the PB2 gene that decreased, but did not abolish its temperature-sensitivity. A new mutation on the PB1 gene, that represented intragenic suppression or reversion, led to loss of temperature-sensitivity of its product, the PB1 protein. Finally, a "suppressor" mutation developed on the PA gene and this corrected the temperature-sensitivity of the PB2 gene product.

The response of susceptible adult volunteers to the *ts* + isolate from the *ts* 1A2 was similar to that observed with wild-type virus, indicating that the *ts* phenotype was a major determinant of attenuation and loss of this phenotype led to restoration of virulence (Tolpin *et al.*, 1982). Although a limited number of *ts* mutations, such as those present in the *ts* 1[E] and *ts*

TABLE I
Escape of an influenza A (H3N2) *ts* 1A2 reassortant from its *ts* phenotype during infection of a susceptible young child

Influenza A/Alaska/77 (H3N2) virus	Shut off temp. for plaque formation	Phenotype specified by indicated gene		
		PB1	PA	PB2
ts 1A2 reassortant	37°C	*ts* (38–39°C)		*ts* (37–38°C)
ts + isolate[a]	40°C	*ts* +[b]	Mutation that suppresses *ts* of PB2	*ts* (39°C)[b]
Wild type	>40°C			

[a] Recovered from susceptible young child who underwent asymptomatic infection with *ts* 1A2 reassortant. [b] Phenotype determined by back cross to wild type virus.

1A2 donor viruses, can restrict replication *in vivo* sufficiently to bring about a satisfactory level of attenuation, the use of this approach can not be recommended because of the problem of genetic instability.

HOST RANGE RESTRICTION

Attenuation can also be achieved by the substitution of influenza virus "internal" genes which function efficiently in a nonhuman host but are restricted in the human respiratory tract. Genes bearing host range mutations can be selected by "adaptation" of a human influenza virus to an unnatural host such as the chick embryo or avian cell culture. Alternatively, avian influenza virus genes that have undergone evolutionary divergence from their corresponding human influenza virus genes can be used to restrict growth of reassortant viruses in man.

The best studied example of human influenza virus genes bearing host range mutations is the influenza A/PR8/34 virus that had been adapted to embryonated eggs (Beare, 1982). The total complement of six "internal" genes of PR8 virus did not confer satisfactory attenuation on a reassortant prepared by mating this virus with a virulent influenza A H3N2 virus. Satisfactory attenuation of virulent human influenza A H3N2 viruses by substitution of internal PR8 genes required a mixed constellation of PR8 and virulent human influenza virus polymerase genes (Florent, 1980). Since one cannot be certain that future human influenza polymerase genes will exhibit incompatibility with PR8 polymerase genes, this approach has been abandoned.

Current efforts to use avian influenza virus genes for attenuation of human influenza viruses employ the entire complement of "internal" avian influenza genes and hence gene incompatibility is not required for success. Transfer of the six "internal" genes also favours a more uniform phenotype for the resulting avian–human influenza virus reassortants. The possibility of suppressing the attenuation phenotype of vaccine viruses by gene reassortment was recently raised when it was observed that the *ts* phenotype specified by a *ts* NS gene was suppressed by a wild type polymerase gene derived from another virus (Scholtissek and Spring, 1981). Also, generation of reassortant viruses neurovirulent for mice has been observed following coinfection by two distinct non-neurovirulent viruses (Scholtissek *et al.*, 1979; Vallbracht *et al.*, 1980). Transfer of the six "internal" genes of the avian influenza donor virus into avian–human influenza virus reassortants should minimize the possibility of these occurrences, since suppression of attenuation or acquisition of virulence usually involves a reassortment of internal genes derived from different viruses.

Using RNA–RNA hybridization, Scholtissek compared two avian influenza A viruses (FPV and virus N) with human influenza A viruses of the three known sub-types (Scholtissek et al., 1978). Five of the six internal genes of the two avian influenza viruses differed significantly from the corresponding human influenza virus genes. In addition, using the technique of RNA hybridization competition, Bean recently observed that the NP gene of a variety of avian influenza viruses tested, including those currently being evaluated as vaccine donor strains, differed significantly from the corresponding NP genes of human influenza viruses (W. Bean, personal communication, 1983). These findings are not surprising because the genes of avian influenza viruses have been selected over a long period to function efficiently in avian cells, particularly in cooperative activities, some of which involve host cell functions. The many sequence divergences between corresponding human and avian influenza virus genes suggests that the attenuation phenotype specified by avian influenza virus "internal" genes should be stable during infection of vaccinated individuals. It should also be noted that gene substitution experiments indicate that the NP and M genes of our avian influenza donor virus each specify significant restriction of viral replication in simian respiratory epithelium (Murphy et al., this volume pp. 211–225). Furthermore, the avian PB2 and NS genes act cooperatively to restrict virus growth in monkeys. This means that at least four of the six internal avian influenza virus genes contribute to attenuation.

TABLE II

Stability of growth restriction phenotype of avian–human influenza A virus reassortant following five passages in squirrel monkeys

Influenza A virus— $10^{7.0}$ TCID$_{50}$ inoculated intratracheally	Number of monkeys	Peak level of virus recovered (Mean log$_{10}$ TCID$_{50}$ per ml)	
		Nasopharyngeal washing[c]	Tracheal lavage[d]
Human A/Wash/80	14	3·9	5·7
Avian A/Mallard/78	7	2·6	2·7
Avian–human reassortant with 6 "internal" avian genes[a]	8	0·9	2·7
Reassortant[b] following 5 passages in monkeys	6	2·5	3·6

[a] Two surface glycoprotein genes from human influenza virus parent and remaining 6 genes from avian influenza virus parent. [b] Alternating passage in monkeys and eggs. [c] Monkeys sampled daily for 10 days. [d] Monkeys sampled on 2nd, 4th, and 6th days.

Preliminary evaluation of stability of the attenuation phenotype has been performed in squirrel monkeys (Table II). An avian–human influenza virus reassortant derived from the avian A/Mallard/78 donor was subjected to five serial passages in squirrel monkeys. Virus recovered at each passage was amplified by passage in eggs because the amount of virus recovered from tracheal lavage fluid was insufficient to infect squirrel monkeys. Following five alternating monkey-egg passages the avian–human influenza virus reassortant retained its restriction of growth in the monkey's respiratory tract.

HOST RANGE PLUS COLD-ADAPTATION MUTATIONS

Another approach to attenuation involves selection of a mutant that grows well at sub-optimal temperature in primary chick kidney cell culture (Maassab et al., 1981). In this manner there is selection for both host range mutations and mutations that shift the temperature optimum for certain viral functions. This procedure yielded a virus, the A/Ann Arbor/6/60 donor strain, which acquired one or more detectable mutations on each of its six "internal" genes (Cox et al., 1981). Some of these mutations conferred the cold-adapted (ca) and ts phenotypes on the A/Ann Arbor/6/60 virus. Mutations on the PB1 and M genes appear to be responsible for the ts phenotype, while mutations affecting the PB2, PA and NP genes appear to play a major role in conferring the ca phenotype. Reassortants bearing five "internal" genes from the ca donor and a PB1, M or NS gene derived from a virulent human influenza A virus were attenuated for susceptible volunteers, suggesting that the PB1, M and NS genes of the ca donor do not play an essential role in attenuation (Murphy and Chanock, 1981; Murphy et al., this volume pp. 211–225). These observations further suggest that mutations affecting the PB2, PA and NP genes of the ca donor virus are responsible for satisfactory attenuation of ca reassortants. Although the PB2, PA and NP genes appear to play the major role in attenuation, the other three ca "internal" genes may be needed for stability of the ca phenotype. Loss of the ca phenotype has been observed only when ca reassortants lacking the PB1 or NS gene of the ca donor were administered to susceptible volunteers (Murphy and Chanock, 1981; La Montagne et al., 1983).

To ensure maximum stability of the ca and ts phenotypes, it is necessary to use ca reassortants that possess all six "internal" genes of the ca donor virus. When such reassortants were administered to susceptible children and adults, every isolate from infected vaccinees retained the ca phenotype (Table III) (Murphy and Chanock, 1981; La Montagne et al., 1983). However, an occasional H3N2 isolate recovered from young children exhibited a partial loss of the ts phenotype in MDCK cell culture, but this

TABLE III
Stability of *ca* and *ts* phenotypes of influenza A *ca* reassortant viruses during infection of susceptible individuals (serum H1 antibody ≤1:8)

Vaccinees	*ca* reassortant sub-type	*ca* phenotype in primary chick kidney cells		*ts* phenotype in MDCK cells	
		No. isolates	No. *ca*+	No. isolates	No. *ts*+
Adults	H3N2	75	0	122	2[a]
	H1N1	91	0	111	0
Young children	H3N2	Not tested	—	69	9[a,b]
	H1N1	Not tested	—	129	0

[a] *ts*+ in MDCK cells but *ts* in primary chick kidney cells. [b] Four of 9 *ts*+ isolates recovered directly in MDCK cells at 39°C, a temperature restrictive for original reassortant. One *ts*+ isolate tested in ferrets and found to be attenuated.

alteration was not observed in primary chick kidney cell culture (Wright et al., 1982). Because the genetic basis of attenuation of the *ca* reassortants is not completely understood at this time, it is not possible to interpret the significance of this temperature-dependent, host range genetic alteration with respect to virulence for man. In one instance an isolate that was *ts*+ in MDCK cells and *ts* in chick kidney cells was evaluated in ferrets and found to be attenuated. This is reassuring but this observation hardly constitutes a definitive test for stability of attenuation. Clearly, additional *ts*+ isolates must be evaluated in ferrets and ultimately in man. Because transmission of *ca* reassortants from infected vaccinees to susceptible contacts has not been demonstrated it is likely that we will find that attenuation is not altered by loss of the *ts* phenotype. If this view is correct, stability of attenuation can be explained by the many independent mutations on the six "internal" genes of the *ca* donor virus that were selected by growth at sub-optimal temperature in an unnatural host, chick kidney cells (Cox et al., 1981).

DELETION MUTANTS

Deletion mutations offer an attractive alternative to other approaches to stabilization of attenuation. Such mutations should be stable because they are not subject to reversion and it is unlikely that they would be easily suppressed by a new mutation at another site on the viral genome. For these reasons we have initiated efforts to isolate or construct stable deletion mutations that will render influenza A virus sufficiently defective that it becomes attenuated but not so defective that it loses viability (Lai *et al.*, 1984). The feasibility of this approach is indicated by the recent identification of a viable deletion mutation in the coding region of the NS gene that restricts growth in mammalian cells but is permissive for growth in eggs and avian cells in culture (Maassab and De Borde, 1984). This viable, host range restriction, deletion mutation was identified and characterized by Maassab, DeBorde and Palese. Although this mutation does not appear promising for use in a live vaccine virus because it markedly restricts growth in mammalian cells, its existence suggests that other less restrictive deletions may occur naturally. A strategy for the identification of such naturally occurring, less restrictive deletion mutations will be described later.

Defined regions of an influenza A virus gene can also be deleted using recombinant DNA techniques. This type of genetic surgery can only be performed on DNA. Hence, the RNA genes of influenza virus must be transcribed into complementary DNA and manipulated in this form (Lai *et al.*, 1984). This presents us with the difficult problem of transcribing mutant DNA into an RNA form that can be transferred back into an infectious virus. This transfer has not been a problem with poliovirus which contains positive strand genomic RNA that is infectious. Cloned, full-length poliovirus cDNA was recently shown to be infectious in tissue culture (Racaniello and Baltimore, 1981). Unfortunately, influenza virus has a negative-strand RNA genome that is not infectious.

Our efforts to produce stable deletion mutations in influenza virus genes began with cloning full-length DNA copies of six of the eight virus genes—PB2, HA, NA, NP, M and NS (Lai *et al.*, 1980; Lamb and Lai, 1980, 1981; Markoff and Lai, 1982; Lin and Lai, 1983). Each of these cloned genes retained the conserved 5′ and 3′ terminal sequence (Table IV). In addition, the NA, M and NS clones were sequenced and shown to contain the complete nucleotide sequence of their respective genes (Markoff and Lai, 1982; Lamb and Lai, 1980, 1981). Thus, these clones contain all the sequences required to derive corresponding RNA transcripts that possess the control signals for replication of viral genes.

Next, the full-length cloned HA, NA, NP, M or NS DNA was inserted in the sense orientation into an SV40 vector in place of a portion of the late region that codes for SV40 capsid proteins (Fig. 1). These SV40-influenza DNA recombinants expressed functional influenza protein when introduced into permissive monkey cell cultures together with an early *ts* A mutant of SV40 that provided the late SV40 functions defective in the SV40-influenza DNA recombinants (Sveda and Lai, 1981; Markoff *et al.*, 1984 and unpublished observation). Sequence analysis indicated that complete influenza RNA transcripts of positive polarity were produced in cells infected with an SV40-M or SV40-NS recombinant. Subsequently,

TABLE IV
Cloning complete cDNA of influenza A virus genes

Synthesis of double stranded DNA		Linker	Gene	Terminal sequences of cloned DNA(+) strand
(+) cDNA	(−) cDNA			
vRNA template and primer complementary to 3′ conserved terminal sequences of vRNA	(+) cDNA template and primer complementary to 3′ conserved terminal sequences of (+) cDNA	Bam HI	NS[a], M[a], NA[a], NP and PB2	5′ Bam HI linker—conserved 3′ vRNA 12 base sequence . . . . conserved 5′ vRNA 13 base sequence—Bam HI linker 3′
As above	Viral mRNA template and oligo-(dT) primer	GC tail	HA	5′ Oligo G–host mRNA sequence—conserved 3′ vRNA 12 base sequence . . . . conserved 5′ vRNA 13 base sequence—Oligo C 3′

[a] Completeness confirmed by sequencing of the entire cloned DNA.

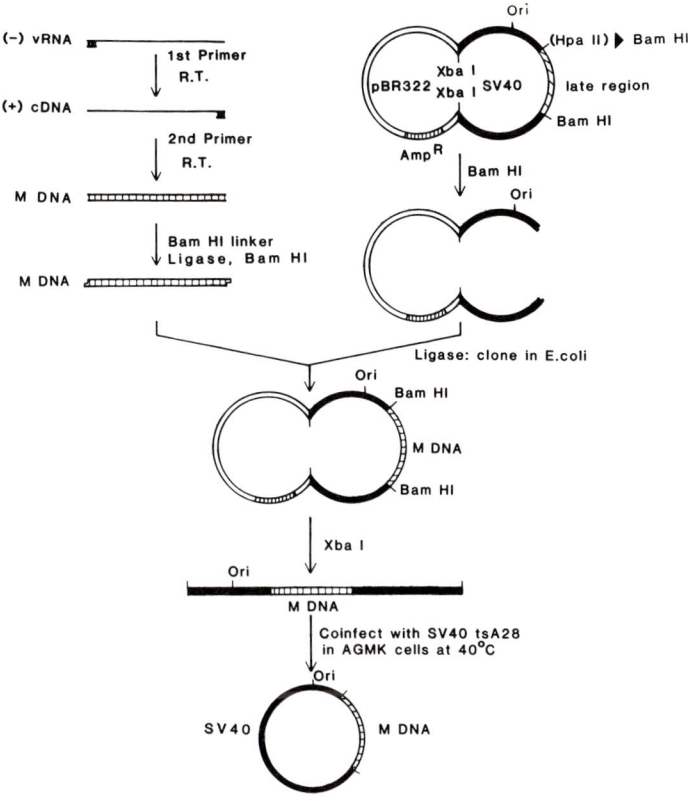

Fig. 1 Construction of SV40-influenza M recombinant that expresses M_1 protein in African green monkey kidney cells (reprinted from Lamb and Lai, 1982).

the influenza DNA present in certain SV40-influenza recombinants was subjected to deletion at different sites and the effect of these deletions on structure and function of the expressed influenza virus protein was characterized (Sveda et al., 1982; Sekikawa and Lai, 1983; Markoff et al., 1984). For example, deletion of sequences near the amino or carboxy terminus of the HA gene resulted in an alteration in the pattern of glycosylation of HA. Also, in some instances, there was an alteration of the insertion or anchorage of HA in the outer cell membrane. Similarly, deletion of sequences within the amino terminus of the NA gene affected insertion of its product into the outer cell membrane, as well as pattern of glycosylation. These observations indicated that defined deletions affecting structure and function of influenza proteins could be produced in cloned DNA.

To determine whether cloned influenza DNA could be converted back to viral RNA (vRNA) and packaged in the virion, influenza gene rescue experiments (so-called allele replacement) were attempted (Lai et al., 1984). Initially recombinant SV40-HA and SV40-NA DNA were used in allele replacement attempts because of the ease of identification of the two surface antigens coded by these genes. Also specific antiserum which effectively neutralized virus bearing the HA or NA of the coinfecting virus could be used to facilitate detection of reassortant viruses that had undergone allele replacement. Permissive African green monkey kidney cells (AGMK) were infected sequentially with an SV40-HA (H3) or SV40-NA (N2) recombinant and influenza A/WSN/1933 (H1N1) which bears surface antigens of another sub-type. Infected cell lysates were passaged once and incubated with WSN antiserum to neutralize progeny virus bearing H1 or N1; this was done to favour the detection of reassortant virus that had undergone allele replacement. Heterogeneous WSN antiserum (anti-H1N1) was used in the attempt at allele replacement of the H1 gene, while monoclonal antibody capable of neutralizing virus bearing N1 was used in the attempt at replacement of the N1 gene. This protocol should allow detection of reassortant virus that had acquired an RNA segment derived from a HA or NA DNA insert resulting in replacement of the corresponding WSN gene. We were unable to detect gene rescue with an SV40-HA or SV40-NA recombinant that produced positive strand RNA transcripts. We were also unsuccessful using an SV40-NA recombinant which produced negative strand RNA transcripts.

SV40-NP recombinants with their influenza insert in the positive or negative orientation were also tested for their ability to replace an NP gene bearing a non-leaky *ts* mutation. AGMK cells were coinfected with an SV40-NP recombinant and a NP *ts* mutant and then incubated at a temperature restrictive for the *ts* mutant. These attempts at allele replacement were also unsuccessful because we did not detect influenza virus plaques in the coinfected cultures (Lin and Lai, unpublished observations).

Previous analysis of transcripts produced during infection with an SV40-M recombinant indicated that full-length, positive strand influenza RNA sequences were transcribed from an insert in the appropriate orientation, but these influenza sequences were flanked at both ends by SV40 sequences (5′ late SV40 transcription initiation sequences and 3′ polyadenylation signals) (Fig. 2) (Lamb and Lai, 1982). It is likely that the viral replicase provided by the coinfecting influenza virus did not recognize the 3′ terminal influenza sequences in the RNA transcripts because of flanking SV40 sequences and was thus unable to initiate influenza vRNA synthesis. Similarly, failure to rescue negative strand influenza RNA transcripts produced during infection by an SV40-NA or SV40-NP

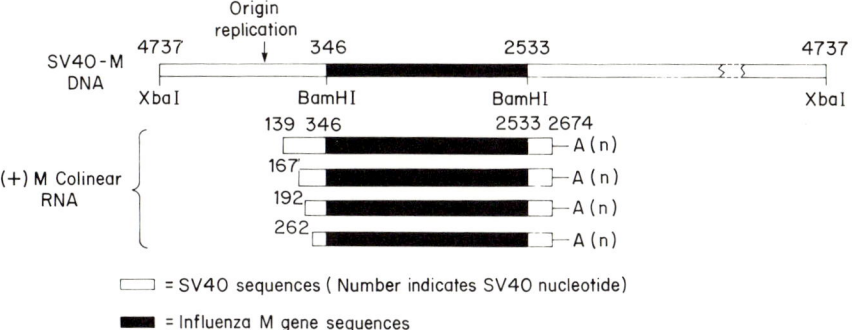

Fig. 2 Complete influenza A virus (+) RNA transcripts produced from SV40-M recombinant in African green monkey kidney cells are flanked by 5′ late SV40 transcription initiation sequences and 3′ SV40 polyadenylation signals (adapted from Lamb and Lai, 1982).

recombinant with an influenza insert in the opposite orientation, suggests that these influenza transcripts, presumably flanked by SV40 sequences, were neither replicated nor encapsidated and packaged in virions. Precise terminal sequences may be required for replication and encapsidation of full-length influenza RNA. If this is the case, the 5′ and 3′ flanking SV40 sequences contained in RNA transcripts from the recombinant influenza DNA may have prevented rescue. In order to provide specific terminal sequences in the RNA transcripts that are recognized by the influenza replicase complex, it may be necessary to remove the flanking SV40 sequences.

Ultimately, "rescue" of RNA transcripts derived from cloned mutant influenza DNA may require the expression of cloned genes in persistently infected, stably transformed cells. For example, one obstacle to achieving complementation and rescue during lytic infection by an SV40 vector may be the cytolytic effect of SV40 infection. To circumvent this difficulty and to provide a continuous source of RNA transcripts from cloned influenza DNA, a collaborative effort was initiated with Doctors Peter Howley and Ming-fan Law (NCI) in an effort to exploit their bovine papilloma virus (BPV) vector for the expression of cloned influenza viral genes (Lin, Law, Howley and Lai, unpublished observation). Bovine papilloma virus is a large DNA virus that replicates autonomously and extrachromosomally during persistent infection of animal cells. Recently, a BPV recombinant that incorporated the influenza nucleoprotein (NP) gene was successfully constructed. This BPV-NP recombinant DNA was used to transform mouse C127 cells. Transformed cells produced what appeared to be functional NP as judged by its size, specific immunoprecipitation, localization in the nucleus and finally, phosphorylation.

The mouse cell line (C127) used in the initial studies is not permissive for influenza virus replication and hence can not be employed for gene rescue ("allele replacement"). For this reason, other host cell systems were examined to determine if they would support both influenza virus replication and transfection by BPV. Simian CV-1 cells show some promise in this regard. CV-1 cells were co-transfected with the BPV-NP recombinant and a neomycin resistance gene cloned in the pSV-2 vector (Lin, Law, Howley and Lai, unpublished observations). Neomycin selection was then used to facilitate detection of NP protein expressed in cotransformed neomycin resistant CV-1 cells. Using indirect immunofluorescence for detection of antigen it was observed that the NP protein was synthesized in a small percentage (approximately 2–3%) of neomycin resistant cells. It should be noted that neomycin-resistant CV-1 cells were found to be permissive for influenza virus infection.

Cell lines persistently expressing a cloned influenza gene might be suitable for selection of genes bearing naturally occurring deletion mutations. It should be possible to propagate viruses bearing such deletion mutations using a cell line that persistently expresses a cloned gene that corresponds to the gene bearing the deletion mutation. This type of complementation should allow us to screen for a variety of spontaneous deletion mutations and provide a permissive system for the growth of such mutants which can then be assessed for evidence of restriction and attenuation. In this manner, it may be possible to select stable, naturally occurring genes carrying deletion mutations that can be used to confer attenuation on epidemic or pandemic strains of influenza virus by gene reassortment.

REFERENCES

Beare, A. S. (1982). Research into the immunization of humans against influenza by means of living viruses. In "Basic and Applied Influenza Research" (Ed. A. S. Beare. CRC Press, Inc., Boca Raton, Florida, pp. 211–234.

Cox, N. J., Konnecke, I. and Kendal, A. P. (1981). Genetic and biochemical analysis of the A/Ann Arbor/6/60 cold-adapted mutant. In "Genetic Variation Among Influenza Viruses" (Ed. D. P. Nayak). Academic Press, New York and London, pp. 639–652.

Florent, G. (1980). Gene constellation of live influenza A vaccines. *Arch. Virol.* **64**, 171–173.

Ghendon, Y. Z. and Markushin, S. G. (1980). Studies on mutation lesions and physiology of fowl plague virus *ts* mutants. *Phil. Trans. R. Soc. Lond.* **288**, 383–392.

Holland, J., Spindler, K., Horodyski, F., Grabau, E., Nichol, S. and VandePol, S. (1982). Rapid evolution of RNA genomes. *Science* **215**, 1577–1585.

Kim, H. W., Arrobio, J. O., Brandt, C. D., Parrott, R. H., Murphy, B. R., Richman, D. D. and Chanock, R. M. (1976). Temperature-sensitive mutants of influenza A virus: response of children to the influenza A/Hong Kong/68 ts-1 (E) (H3N2) candidate vaccine viruses and significance to neuraminidase antigen. *Pediat. Res.* **10**, 238–242.

La Montagne, J. R., Wright, P. F., Clements, M. L., Maassab, H. F. and Murphy, B. R. (1983). Prospects for live, attenuated influenza vaccines using reassortants derived from the A/Ann Arbor/6/60 (H2N2) cold-adapted (*ca*) donor virus. In "The Origin of Pandemic Influenza Viruses" (Ed. W. G. Laver). Elsevier Science Publishing Co., Inc., Amsterdam, pp. 243–257.

Lai, C.-J., Markoff, L. J., Zimmerman, S., Cohen, B., Berndt, J. A. and Chanock, R. M. (1980). Cloning DNA sequences from influenza viral RNA segments. *Proc. Nat. Acad. Sci. USA* **77**, 210–214.

Lai, C.-J., Markoff, L. J., Lin, B.-C. and Chanock, R. M. (1984). Engineering the genome of influenza viruses for immunoprophylaxis: progress and obstacles. In "Cold Spring Harbor Conference on Modern Approaches to Vaccines" (Eds R. Chanock and R. Lerner). Cold Spring Harbor, New York (in press).

Lamb, R. A. and Lai, C.-J. (1980) Sequence of interrupted and uninterrupted mRNA's and cloned DNA coding for the two overlapping nonstructural proteins of influenza virus. *Cell* **21**, 475–485.

Lamb, R. A. and Lai, C.-J. (1981). Conservation of the influenza virus membrane protein (M_1) amino acid sequence and an open reading frame of RNA segment 7 encoding a second protein (M_2) in H1N1 strains. *Virology* **112**, 746–751.

Lamb, R. A. and Lai, C.-J. (1982). Spliced and unspliced messenger RNA's synthesized from cloned influenza virus M DNA in an SV40 vector: expression of the influenza virus membrane protein (M_1). *Virology* **123**, 237–256.

Lin, B.-C. and Lai, C.-J. (1983). The influenza virus nucleoprotein synthesized from cloned DNA in a simian virus 40 vector is detected in the nucleus. *J. Virol.* **45**, 434–438.

Maassab, H. F. and DeBorde, D. C. (1983). Characterization of an influenza A host range mutant. *Virology* **130**, 342–350.

Maassab, J. F., Monto, A. S., DeBorde, D. C., Cox, N. J. and Kendal, A. P. (1981). Development of cold recombinants of influenza virus as live virus vaccines. In "Genetic Variation Among Influenza Viruses" (Ed. D. P. Nayak). Academic Press, New York and London, pp. 617–637.

Markoff, L. and Lai, C.-J. (1982). Sequence of the influenza A/Udorn/72 (H3N2) virus neuraminidase gene as determined from cloned full-length DNA. *Virology* **119**, 288–297.

Markoff, L., Lin, B.-C., Sveda, M. M. and Lai, C.-J. (1984). Glycosylation and surface expression of the influenza virus neuraminidase requires the N-terminal hydrophobic region. *J. Mol. Cell. Biol.* **4**, 8–16.

Murphy, B. R. and Chanock, R. M. (1981). Genetic approaches to the prevention of influenza A virus infection. In "Genetic Variation Among Influenza Viruses" (Ed. D. P. Nayak). Academic Press, New York and London, pp. 601–615.

Murphy, B. R., Tolpin, M. D., Massicot, J. G., Kim, H. Y., Parrott, R. H. and Chanock, R. M. (1980). Escape of a highly defective influenza A virus mutant from its temperature-sensitive phenotype by extragenic suppression and other types of mutation. *Ann. N.Y. Acad. Sci.* **354**, 172–182.

Portner, A., Webster, R. G. and Bean, W. H. (1980). Similar frequencies of antigenic variants in Sendai vesicular stomatitis, and influenza A viruses. *Virology* **104**, 235–238.

Racaniello, V. R. and Baltimore, D. (1981). Cloned poliovirus complementary DNA is infectious in mammalian cells. *Science* **214**, 916–919.

Richman, D. D. and Murphy, B. R. (1979). The association of the T-S phenotype with viral attenuation in animals and humans: implications for the development and use of live virus vaccines. *Rev. Infect. Dis.* **1**, 413–433.

Scholtissek, C. and Spring, S. B. (1981). Suppressor recombinants and suppressor mutants. *In* "Genetic Variation Among Influenza Viruses" (Ed. D. P. Nayak). Academic Press, New York and London, pp. 399–413.

Scholtissek, C., Rott, R., Orlich, M., Harms, E. and Rohde, W. (1977). Correlation of pathogenicity and gene constellation of an influenza A virus (fowl plague). 1. Exchange of a single gene. *Virology* **81**, 74–80.

Scholtissek, C., Rohde, W., von Hoyningen, V. and Rott, R. (1978). On the origin of the human influenza virus subtypes H2N2 and H3N2. *Virology* **87**, 13–20.

Scholtissek, C., Vallbracht, A., Flehmig, B. and Rott, R. (1979). Correlation of pathogenicity and gene constellation of influenza A viruses. *Virology* **95**, 492–500.

Sekikawa, K. and Lai, C.-J. (1983). Defects in functional expression of an influenza virus hemagglutinin lacking the signal peptide sequence. *Proc. Nat. Acad. Sci. USA* **80**, 3563–3567.

Sveda, M. M. and Lai, C.-J. (1981). Functional expression in primate cells of cloned DNA coding for the hemagglutinin surface glycoprotein of influenza virus. *Proc. Nat. Acad. Sci. USA* **78**, 5488–5492.

Sveda, M. M., Markoff, L. J. and Lai, C. J. (1982). Cell surface expression of the influenza virus hemagglutinin requires the hydrophobic carboxy-terminal sequences. *Cell* **30**, 649–656.

Tolpin, M. D., Massicot, J. G., Mullinix, M. G., Kim, H. W., Parrott, R. H., Chanock, R. M. and Murphy, B. R. (1981). Genetic factors associated with loss of the temperature-sensitive phenotype of the influenza A/Alaska/77-*ts*-1A2 recombinant during growth *in vivo*. *Virology* **112**, 505–517.

Tolpin, M. D., Clements, M. L., Levine, M. M., Black, R. E., Saah, A. J., Anthony, W. C., Cisneros, L., Chanock, R. M. and Murphy, B. R. (1982). Evaluation of a phenotypic revertant of the A/Alaska/77/*ts*-1A2 reassortant virus in hamsters and in seronegative adult volunteers: further evidence that the temperature-sensitive phenotype is responsible for attenuation of *ts*-1A2 reassortant viruses. *Infect. Immun.* **36**, 645–650.

Vallbracht, A., Scholtissek, C., Flehmig, B. and Gerth, H.-J. (1980). Recombination of influenza A strains with fowl plague virus can change pneumotropism for mice to a generalized infection with involvement of the central nervous system. *Virology* **107**, 452–460.

Webster, R. G., Hinshaw, V. S. and Laver, W. G. (1982). Selection and analysis of antigenic variants of the neuraminidase of N2 influenza viruses with monoclonal antibodies. *Virology* **117**, 93–104.

Wright, P. F., Okabe, N., McKee, K. T. Jr., Maassab, H. F. and Karzon, D. T. (1982). Cold-adapted recombinant influenza A virus vaccines in seronegative young children. *J. Infect. Dis.* **146**, 71–79.

DISCUSSION

Mahy Could I just mention one sort of deletion mutant, perhaps we might call it, which you have not referred to and ask whether you have any information on this. It is simply to put the HA gene alone into the vaccinia virus by the technique developed by Doctors G. Smith and Moss. I believe that some work has been done in this area with influenza and I should be interested to know what the results are.

Chanock I will refer the question to Dr Murphy who has done a collaborative study with Doctors Smith and Moss.

Murphy Doctors Smith and Moss constructed a vector in which the H2 gene, which had been cloned by M. J. Gething, was inserted into vaccinia under the control of a vaccinia promoter (Smith et al., 1984). This virus was immunogenic in terms of inducing the formation of HA1 antibody in rabbits. Geoff and I injected hamsters with the vaccinia-HA recombinant virus intradermally. We were able to induce levels of antibody that were comparable to that achieved with a wild type H2N2 virus. Following challenge with a wild type H2N2 virus both the vaccinia-infected animals and the wild type animals resisted infection, whereas control animals readily replicated the virus. Thus, this approach has some promise in terms of stimulating protective antibodies.

Tyrrell Can I ask for just one point of clarification? Was the vaccinia inactivated or live when it was injected?

Murphy The vaccinia recombinant was live when it was injected.

Scholtissek I just want to make a comment on the genetic stability of mutants which carry deletions and which have extended replacements of amino acids. In most of the cases where we obtained non-pathogenic recombinants of FPV they were temperature-sensitive, almost all, and we have developed a very fast test by means of which we can isolate very rapidly temperature-sensitive recombinants in which many genes have been replaced. We also thought that these would be genetically very stable and could be used as vaccines, but unfortunately this was not the case. We have also obtained temperature-sensitive mutants by undiluted passage of FPV and at least in one case we know already that we have a deletion mutant and yet presumably with other mutants also we might have deletions, but we have not yet sequenced the corresponding genes. Unfortunately these *ts* mutants are not more stable than those obtained by normal mutagens. The *ts* recombinants with many replacements of genes can be reactivated to become highly pathogenic again by undiluted passages at the non-permissive temperature as shown by Rott (Rott et al., 1983). Sometimes we needed up to ten passages, so it may be that five passages are not sufficient to demonstrate stability. I doubt whether you really will end up with completely stable recombinants, or even deletion mutants which are stable genetically. In any case, if they are stable enough, so that the immune system is faster than reversion, they might be useful.

Chanock What Murphy has described are two different types of reassortant viruses which do not grow to a level which would permit these viruses to infect other individuals. Thus, we are discussing viruses that produce a dead-end infection. Five passages would certainly be more than an avian–human influenza reassortant could ever hope to attain.

Scholtissek I was referring to the monkey/egg passages.

Chanock Growing the virus to high titre between successive monkey passages was necessary in order to provide sufficient virus to infect monkeys and to amplify any mutants that arose during the preceding passage in monkeys. In other words, the probability of detecting mutants was increased by administering a large amount of virus to monkeys at each passage. Our intent was to increase the opportunities for spontaneous mutants to be selected because of the very strong selective pressure for highly restricted viruses to grow well *in vivo*. A more stringent test might be ten or 20 passages, but it is to be noted that we are dealing with viruses which are not able to spread. They are not transmissible because they are produced in a quantity that is insufficient to infect another monkey.

Tyrrell It is a very severe test of stability.

Maassab I would like to add a few additional points. Dealing with what Dr Chanock says about the reassortant deletion mutant we have tried to infect ferrets and mice and giving 10^8 EID 50 intranasally to ferrets we have not been able to recover the virus even 24h after inoculation or infection, but we were able to show some immune response to it.

In addition, if we infect mice or hamsters intranasally no virus can be isolated even 18h after infection. I thought there should be some residual virus, but there was not, in the turbinates, in the trachea or in the lungs. So the deletion has created at least biologically speaking some changes in the behaviour of the virus.

Kilbourne I have to be cranky this afternoon but every time you do a so-called sawtooth passage and bring it back into the egg, you again have a potential attenuating step. So you are between Scylla and Charybdis with this type of experiment. I am referring not to your comment but I am going back to Dr Chanock's story. He has a need for amplifying the squirrel monkey virus which is appropriate but then every time he takes it back into that alien host, the chick embryo, he has a chance of attenuation.

Chanock It is not possible to infect other animals with the amount of virus that is produced by an infected squirrel monkey. That is the problem.

Couch Then you are saying that in the squirrel monkey system you cannot go squirrel monkey to squirrel monkey.

Kilbourne Another point for clarification is that when you talk about levels which are inadequate to infect, is this based on the wild type model, because that is important? Again, the virus coming out from the infected individual is going to be potentially different, so that even if there is a small amount shed, it might be qualitatively different. I would accept that, if you get 10^2 ID 50 coming out of a squirrel monkey and infected with the most infectious virus, the equivalent of wild type, that this, then, is not contagious.

Chanock No, I referred to the avian–human influenza reassortant. For clarification it is this attenuated virus that replicates to a very low level in monkeys. So it is necessary to amplify the virus in order to perform the next passage.

Both As a molecular biologist I was interested in the approach you mentioned in the last part of your talk concerning virus rescue from cells expressing cloned genes. If I have understood, I believe you have not successfully been able to do that so far. Have you actually looked in any of the experiments to see if you are actually synthesizing any negative stranded RNA?

Chanock Negative strand transcripts have not been characterized. However, positive strand transcripts were characterized and sequenced by Lamb and Lai (1982). In experiments involving recombinant SV40-influenza DNA that produces negative strand RNA transcripts we only looked for the emergence of a reassortant virus that bears the influenza gene present in the SV40-influenza recombinant DNA.

You are correct, it is important to characterize the negative strand RNA transcripts.

Both Obviously you have to get positive strands synthesized to express the proteins, but effectively you are asking the polymerase of influenza virus to recognize the sequences it normally sees, but in the context of flanking sequences as well. That would seem to me to be the step on which you should perhaps concentrate your efforts.

Chanock Both positive and negative orientation recombinant molecules were tested; in other words, the NP or NA gene was inserted into SV40 in a positive or negative orientation and we failed to detect gene rescue in either orientation. Of course, the flanking sequences should be present in either orientation.

Scholtissek I have a very short question for Dr Chanock concerning the NP gene expression. Did you look by fluorescent antibodies to see whether this was restricted to the nucleus?

Chanock Yes, the NP was produced in the nucleus of cells previously infected with a recombinant bovine virus vector containing the influenza NP gene insert. NP was localized to the nucleus. It was immunoprecipitated by specific monoclones directed against this protein.

Scholtissek But then it might be that you are facing the problem of abortive infection because in abortively infected cells the nucleoprotein does not leave the nucleus. This might be the reason why you could not rescue the virus.

Chanock We were not asking to rescue the nucleoprotein, we were attempting to rescue the RNA that was produced by the influenza DNA insert in the recombinant. Nucleoprotein was also present in lower concentration in the cytoplasm of cells transfected with the bovine papilloma—NP recombinant.

REFERENCES

Lamb, R. A. and Lai, C.-J. (1982). Spliced and unspliced messenger RNA's synthesized from cloned influenza virus M-DNA in an SV40 vector; expression of the influenza virus membrane protein (M_1). *Virology* **123**, 237–256.

Rott, R., Orlich, M. and Scholtissek, C. (1983). Pathogenicity reactivation of non-pathogenic influenza virus recombinants under von Magnus conditions. *Virology* **126**, 459–465.

Smith, G. L., Murphy, B. R. and Moss, B. (1984). Construction and characterization of an infectious vaccinia virus recombinant that expresses the influenza haemagglutinin gene and induces resistance to influenza virus infection in hamsters. *Proc. Nat. Acad. Sci. USA* **80,** 7155–7159.

Molecular Determination of the Epidemiology of Influenza—a Reconciliation of Approaches

EDWIN D. KILBOURNE

Department of Microbiology, Mount Sinai School of Medicine, of the City University of New York, New York, USA

When I was invited by Sir Charles to present a paper on, "Reconciliation of the Epidemiology and Molecular Biology of Influenza", I was pleased to accept the assignment having boldly talked of the molecular epidemiology of influenza a decade ago (Kilbourne, 1973), before haemagglutinin and neuraminidase had become household words and their portraits had embellished magazine covers. However, I demurred somewhat from the suggested title, writing to Sir Charles that I believed no reconciliation was needed because in the field of influenza research, epidemiologists are painfully aware of molecular changes and molecular biologists cannot refrain from drawing epidemiologic conclusions. But, of course, Sir Charles was right. The tremendous progress in the last few years in physicochemical characterization of the virus, as well as increased understanding of its replication mechanisms, have occurred while many of our traditional

"The Molecular Virology and Epidemiology of Influenza" (Eds Sir Charles Stuart-Harris and Professor C.W. Potter). Academic Press, London, New York and Orlando, 1984.

epidemiological concepts have been shattered or at least badly shaken by the caprices of a disease which defies simplistic generalizations. Perhaps, then, some reconciliation is needed in the sense of attempting a "removal or explanation of inconsistency" (Webster's New International Dictionary, 2nd Ed., 1958). Certainly, a "restoration to harmony or friendship" (ibid.) hardly seems necessary in the present atmosphere of international communication and cooperation exemplified by this meeting.

As a first step in reconciliation and as a reminder of the focus of this meeting, it should be recalled that we commemorate not the discovery of orthomyxoviruses, but the first recovery of a transmissible agent from the human disease, influenza. In 1933 influenza virus could be defined only as a filtrate of a human throat washing which produced disease in ferrets. So little changed was the virus in that host after 196 passages that ferrets, having been infected by one, S-H, three days before, returned the favour and infected *him*, an event duly recorded by W.S. (whence came the original virus) and by S-H (Smith and Stuart-Harris, 1936), if not by the ferrets. (Molecular biologists, please note the more tractable behaviour of the egg.)

But what of the viruses that molecular biologists study? Do these preparations which we prepare in multilitre batches and handle daily without special precautions bear much resemblance to the agent of disease which attacked S-H? For that matter, *that* virus after its isolation from him was clearly different from fresh human isolates in its enhanced virulence for ferrets and mice.

Quite properly, I think, we have concentrated our efforts on examination of a limited number of viruses during the past 50 years. Our *E. coli*'s have included WSN, PR8, and more recently X-31, in whose contributions to understanding of viral structure I take indirect satisfaction as its accoucheur, so to speak.

Let us look at these venerable and peripatetic viruses. WS, following hundreds of passages in ferrets and mice, and 194 transfers in minced chick embryo tissue culture was adapted to replication in the mouse brain as WSN prior to its more recent passage in the chick embryo (Fig. 1). Similarly, PR8, initially isolated in ferrets, was subjected to multiple mouse lung and chick embryo passages (Fig. 2). And which PR8 are we talking about, the "Cambridge" or the so-called "Mount Sinai" strain (which is known to those at Mount Sinai as the Ann Arbor strain from Rockefeller Institute!)? Indeed, these PR8 strains differ biologically and in haemagglutinin nucleotide sequences. X-31, of course, is about six-eighths Mount Sinai PR8 with haemagglutinin and neuraminidase genes from the Aichi strains of H3N2 (Kilbourne, 1969)—a blending of genes from the West Indies and Japan (Fig. 2).

Diverted to replication in a series of non-human hosts, these prototype

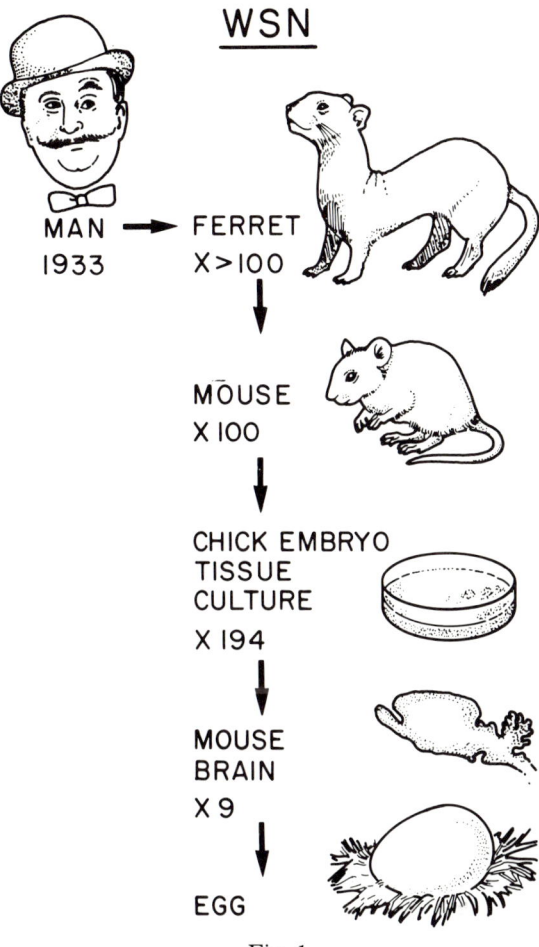

Fig. 1

influenza viruses would appear to be tame tabbies with little relation to the potentially lethal tigers circulating (and written about) in *Nature*. Beare's work in volunteers shows that PR8 is virtually unable even to replicate in man (Beare *et al.*, 1978). That not only virulence but antigenicity may be influenced by the nature of the laboratory host in which viruses are isolated has been recently demonstrated by studies of influenza B viruses in Schild's laboratory (Schild *et al.*, 1983).

But if the molecular biologist studies a few atypical strains intensively, and the epidemiologist many strains superficially, it is reassuring that within influenza A viral sub-types, strains are more notable for their similarities

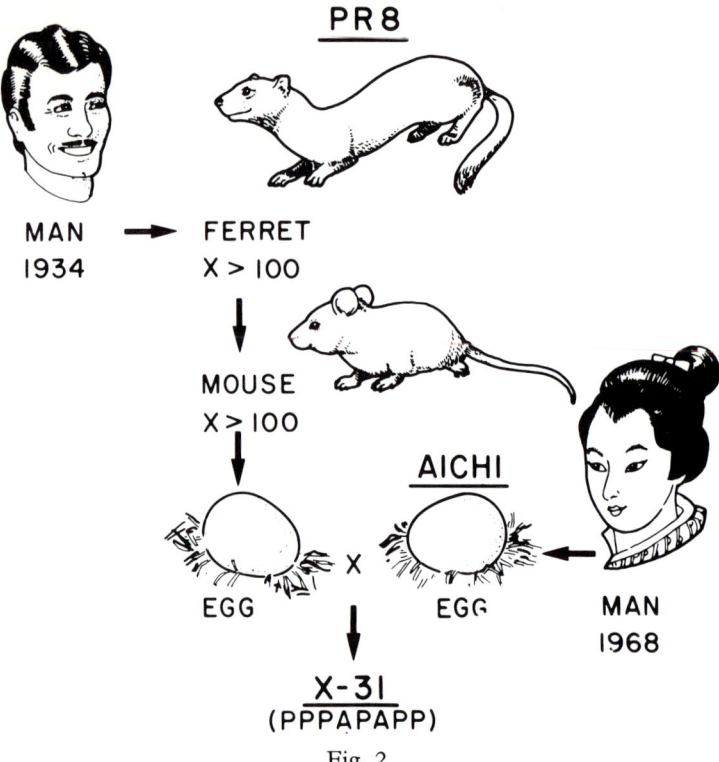

Fig. 2

than their differences. This is not surprising in view of structural similarities shared not only among sub-types but by types of influenza viruses. However, significant biological and antigenic differences may reflect only minimal (i.e. single base) changes in gene nucleotide sequences (Both *et al.*, 1983), some readily reversible.

Now, recognizing that influenza epidemiologists and molecular biologists are not necessarily poles apart, let us nevertheless polarize their views as follows (see Fig. 3).

The epidemiologist (EP) says: "I have here an acute, brief, febrile, prostrating, myalgic, highly communicable, usually self-limiting infection of the respiratory tract. It is characterized by sudden onset and a short incubation period. The incidence is sharply seasonal and morbidity rates are inconstant and unpredictable. Prevalence is sometimes pandemic. Mortality rates are low but lethal impact is significant because of high morbidity. The source of new pandemic viruses is unclear."   "Very interesting," says MB, the molecular biologist. "I have here an enveloped virus whose genome comprises eight pieces of RNA coding for at least 10 proteins, the replication

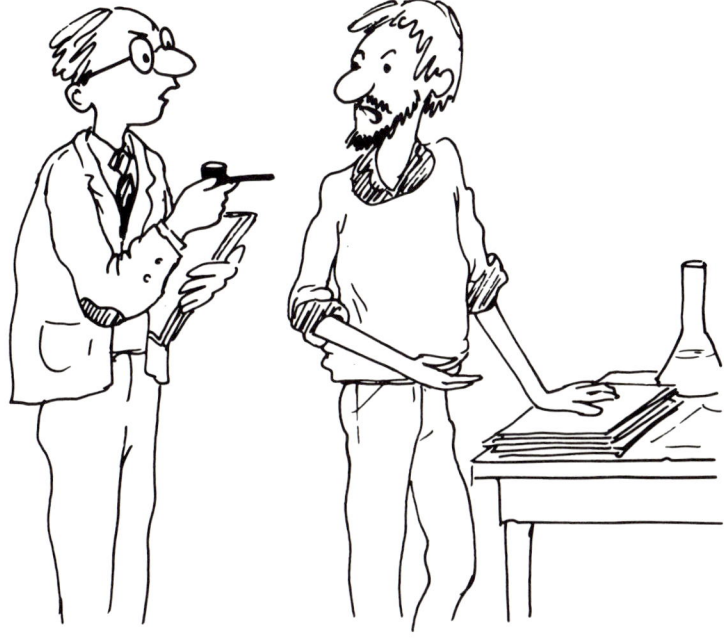

Fig. 3

of which depends on certain cellular functions. I know the size and nature of the proteins. I know the nucleotide sequence of many of the genes coding for these proteins, including the glycoproteins on the virion exterior. I know a fair amount about the comparative virology of the human and animal influenza viruses. I know that some of the genes of human viruses can be found in animals. I know something about virulence in experimental animals. I know something about the evolution and origin of these viruses."

There follows then a dialogue (by which device reconciliations are often reached). Here again is the epidemiologist.

EP: We both know that antigenic variation is the cardinal question and that variants seem to be selected by specific neutralizing antibody in the human population. Do antigenic variants arise in the absence of immunoselection?

MB: They may. Selection for host or for replication advantage may result coincidentally in antigenic change in the viral haemagglutinin.

EP: But such change might be too small to influence resistance of the virus to population antibody. Speaking of host effects, I need explanations for variation in individual susceptibility and for the species specificity of influenza viruses.

MB: Little is yet know but there are many promising approaches. Differences in endogenous host proteases might affect haemagglutinin cleavage and thereby viral infectivity (Lazarowitz and Choppin, 1975; Klenk *et al.*, 1975); variability in host-specific sialyl-oligosaccharide receptors might also alter susceptibility to virus—differences in H3 viral specificity have been related to the species of origin, human or non-human, of the virus (Rogers and Paulson, 1983). Clearly, the virion glycoproteins are critical in determining species specificity (Rott, 1980).

But now it's your turn. This virus has no known latency mechanisms—no reverse transcriptase. How do we explain its persistence between epidemics and the recycling of its antigens?

EP: Despite a large arsenal of antigens in animal reservoirs, only a few may be capable of infecting man in concert with the "human" genes for internal proteins with which they must reassort. This answer might explain the abortive reappearance of non-reassorted "swine flu" virus in 1976, and is reinforced by the reprise of H1N1 a year later. H1N1 as a virus antigenically and genetically unchanged since 1950 is inexplicable except as a resurrected dinosaur.

But let us speak of the future. How can we work together in the *next* 50 years to really understand influenza? Is another pandemic a certainty or has the virus put itself out of business with the premature return of H1N1 into a relatively resistant population?

MB: If and when another pandemic occurs, we shall have the techniques to isolate and characterize the genes and proteins of its causative virus, to compare them with those of recent strains, and to trace its origin, through oligonucleotide mapping, nucleic acid hybridization and sequence analysis. The structure of its haemagglutinin will be worked out quickly with reference to the H3 prototype.

EP: Very good. But the epidemiologist must sample widely and provide you with many isolates from many regions isolated in a variety of laboratory hosts. He must also define precisely the nature of the disease in various populations with different immunological experience. We must compare the viral glycoproteins with those of known animal viruses, and we must follow carefully the evolution of the virus and the disease.

MB: Will we still have some unanswered questions?

EP: Yes. Why is this a winter-time disease? What are the molecular determinants of virus transmission and the causation of systemic and myalgic symptoms in a non-viraemic disease?

MB: But there seem to be viruses structurally similar to influenza viruses that are carried by ticks (Clerx *et al.*, 1983). Where do they fit in? Is this another ecologic dimension for virus survival?

You tell me that influenza A, B and C viruses differ epidemiologically. I can tell you that they differ structurally and functionally. But can we correlate the absence of neuraminidase in influenza C virus and the newly discerned NB protein of influenza B virus (Shaw *et al.*, 1983) with epidemiological differences? What are the functions of the non-structural proteins? How are the genes assembled, and are mutation rates excessive even for an RNA virus?

EP: Perhaps your questions are related to mine.

MB: If not, then the answers surely are.

EP: We are united on one point at least. We can define neither the virus nor the disease at a single point in time. Rapid evolution is a way of life with

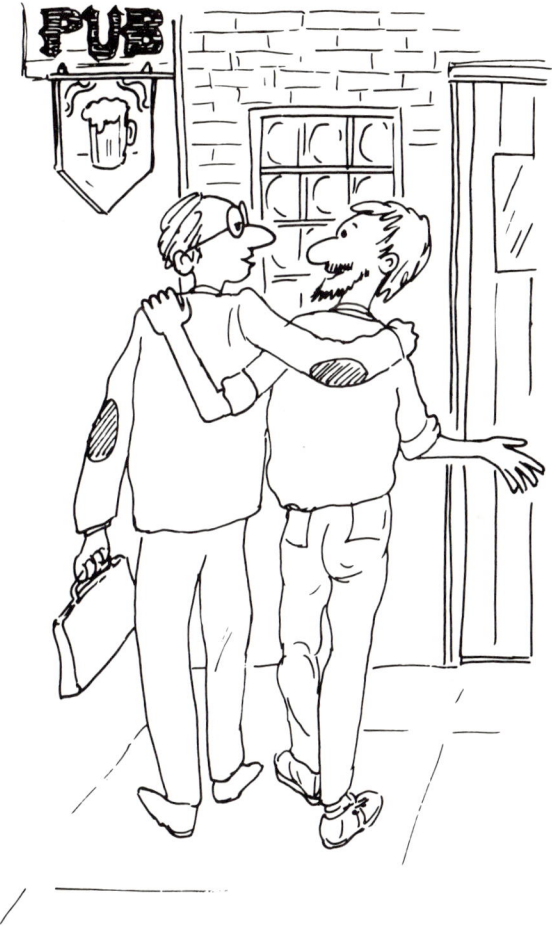

Fig. 4

this virus and its survival depends upon constant mutation. So, too, the disease is variable and unpredictable in its occurrence from year to year.

We now leave our friends walking arm in arm—if not into the sunset—probably into a nearby pub for continued discussions and refreshment (Fig. 4).

EPILOGUE

I have asked you to attend this rambling discourse only to remind you of the state of the art and some unsolved problems. Let me now try to identify more specifically new principles with epidemiological implications which have merged from the intensive studies of the last ten years, in particular.

Genetic Variation Involves all Viral Genes

Variation, antigenic or otherwise, occurs in all genes of the virus and can be sequential (reviewed by Palese and Young, 1982).

The Surface Glycoproteins have Critical Importance

The primary epidemiological role of the haemagglutinin is clear not only with regard to its antigenic mutability but with respect to its biologic function in infectivity and in defining the host range of the virus. As the *sine qua non* of infection, its effects can be polar and its mutations of overriding importance. It is clear that single point mutations can determine antigenicity (reviewed by Webster *et al.*, 1982), replication characteristics (sometimes concordantly) (Kilbourne, 1978; Both *et al.*, 1983), as well as receptor specificity (Rogers *et al.*, 1983).

The potential epidemiologic role of the neuraminidase is less well defined, but certainly antigenic drift and shift occur. Its demonstrated role in influencing cleavage of the haemagglutinin (Schulman and Palese, 1977) has obvious epidemiological implications.

Viral Genetic Reassortment Contributes to Viral Variation and Adaptability

The conjectures of more than a decade ago (reviewed by Kilbourne, 1975) about the origin of pandemic viruses from reassortment of human and animal virus genes have received strong support from molecular biological studies of both 1957 and 1968 viruses.

Genetic reassortment of human viruses in nature has recently occurred (Young and Palese, 1979).

Experimental reassortment in the laboratory has demonstrated not only attenuation (as expected) (Kilbourne, 1969) but occasional increase in viral virulence beyond that of either parental virus (Rott et al., 1979; Scholtissek et al., 1979). Thus, the ability of influenza viruses to trade their genes greatly enhances their epidemiological potential. Not only a reservoir of discrete *viruses*, limited in their transmission potential, but a reservoir of old and new viral *genes* await incorporation into the reassorting virus of influenza.

The context or constellation of such genes is important but can be overridden or suppressed by a single mutation.

The Influenza Viruses are Genetically Heterogenous (as derived from Individual Patients or within Epidemics)

Although influenza viruses are not unique in being genetically heterogeneous or polymorphic, there is now clear evidence that: (a) Antigenically identical mutants in human or animal isolates may be biologically dissimilar and distinguishable (reviewed by Kilbourne, 1979). (b) A mutation influencing viral biologic activity may concordantly change viral antigenicity. Thus, selection of antigenic variants may be non-immunological (Kilbourne, 1978). (c) Selection for host range, as in viral isolation, can concomitantly select for antigenic variants (Schild et al., 1983).

Recycling not only of Genes but of Complete Viruses can Occur

Although the reappearance of viral antigens has left a legacy of specific antibody in the human population, only recently has the molecular near identity of all returning viral genes been shown, in comparison of 1977 and 1950 H1N1 viruses (Nakajima et al., 1978).

Do these principles help in the explanation of recent epidemiological phenomena? While our conjecture is now better informed, conjecture it must remain. The pandemic viruses of 1957 and 1968 seem to owe their success to reassortment of genes for internal proteins adapted to man with genes for surface glycoproteins alien to recent human immunological experience. Accordingly, the failure of swine influenza virus to establish itself in 1976 may reflect its failure to hybridize with co-circulating H3N2 virus, or to undergo a critical mutation of its haemagglutinin.

On the other hand, reassortment does not insure the survival or ascendancy of a virus as shown by the recent decline of the H1N1–H3N2 reassortants which appeared in 1978. An apparent initial advantage here might have been aborted by a single unfavourable mutation in any gene or by ecological factors having nothing to do with the viral genotype.

Finally, molecular genetics has identified but not yet explained a new epidemiological problem—the reappearance not just of a recycled haemagglutinin but of a virtually unchanged 1950 virus in 1977 (Nakajima et al., 1978). The burden is now on the the epidemiologist to trace the source of this virus or upon the biologist to discover its mechanism of latency or persistence.

Molecular biology and epidemiology are not only reconciled; they are integral.

REFERENCES

Beare, A. S., Kendal, A. P. and Schild, G. S. (1978). Trials of live influenza A recombinants in man during natural antigenic change in 1971–1976. *Med. Microbiol. Immunol.* **166**, 91–98.

Both, G. W., Shi, C. H. and Kilbourne, E. D. (1983). The hemagglutinin of swine influenza virus: A single amino acid change pleiotropically affects viral antigenicity and replication. *Proc. Natl. Acad. Sci. USA.* **80**, 6996–7000.

Clerx, J. P. M., Fuller, F. and Bishop, D. H. L. (1983). Tick-borne viruses structurally similar to orthomyxoviruses. *Virology* **127**, 205–219.

Kilbourne, E. D. (1969). Future influenza vaccines and the use of genetic recombinants. *Bull. WHO* **41**, 643–645.

Kilbourne, E. D. (1973). The molecular epidemiology of influenza. *J. Infect. Dis.* **127**, 478–487.

Kilbourne, E. D. (1975). Epidemiology of influenza. In "The Influenza Viruses and Influenza" (Ed. E. D. Kilbourne). Academic Press, New York and London, pp. 483–538.

Kilbourne, E. D. (1978). Genetic dimorphism in influenza viruses: Characterization of stably associated hemagglutinin mutants differing in antigenicity and biological properties. *Proc. Natl. Acad. Sci. USA* **75**, 6258–6262.

Kilbourne, E. D. (1979). Molecular epidemiology—Influenza as archetype. *The Harvey Lectures* **73**, 225–258.

Klenk, H.-D., Rott, R., Orlich, M. and Blodorn, J. (1975). Activation of influenza A viruses by trypsin treatment. *Virology* **68**, 426–439.

Lazarowitz, S. G. and Choppin, P. W. (1975). Enhancement of the infectivity of influenza A and B viruses by proteolytic cleavage of the hemagglutinin polypeptide. *Virology* **68**, 440–454.

Nakajima, K., Desselberger, U. and Palese, P. (1978). Recent human influenza A (H1N1) viruses are closely related genetically to strains isolated in 1950. *Nature* (Lond,) **274**, 334–339.

Palese, P. and Young, J. F. (1982). Variation of influenza A, B and C viruses. *Science* **215**, 1468–1474.

Rogers, G. N. and Paulson, J. C. (1983). Receptor determinants of human and animal influenza virus isolates: Differences in receptor specificity of the H3 hemagglutinin based on species of origin. *Virology* **127**, 361–373.

Rogers, G. N., Paulson, J. C., Daniels, R. S., Skehel, J. J., Wilson, I. A. and Wiley, D. C. (1983). Single amino acid substitutions in influenza hemagglutinin change receptor-binding specificity. *Nature* (Lond.) **304**, 76–78.

Rott, R. (1980). Genetic determinants for infectivity and pathogenicity of influenza viruses. *Phil. Trans. R. Soc. Lond.* **288**, 393–399.

Rott, R., Orlich, M. and Scholtissek, C. (1979). Correlation of pathogenicity and gene constellation of influenza A viruses. III. Non-pathogenic recombinants derived from highly pathogenic parent strains. *J. Gen. Virol.* **44**, 471–477.

Schild, G. C., Oxford, J. S., de Jong, J. C. and Webster, R. G. (1983). Evidence for host cell selection of antigenic variants of influenza virus. *Nature* (Lond.) **303**, 706–709.

Scholtissek, C., Vallbracht, A., Flehmig, B. and Rott, R. (1979). Correlation of pathogenicity and gene constellation of influenza A viruses. II. Highly neurovirulent recombinants derived from non-neurovirulent or weakly neurovirulent parent virus strains. *Virology* **95**, 492–500.

Schulman, J. L. and Palese, P. (1977). Virulence factors of influenza viruses. WSN virus neuraminidase is required for productive infection of MDBK cells. *J. Virol.* **24**, 170–176.

Shaw, M. W., Choppin, P. W. and Lamb, R. A. (1983). A previously unrecognized influenza B virus glycoprotein from a bicistronic mRNA that also encodes the viral neuraminidase. *Proc. Natl. Acad. Sci. USA* **80**, 4879–4883.

Smith, W. and Stuart-Harris, C. H. (1936). Influenza infection of man from the ferret. *Lancet* **ii**, 121–123.

Webster, R. G., Laver, W. G., Air, G. M. and Schild, G. C. (1982). Molecular mechanisms of variation in influenza viruses. *Nature* (Lond.) **296**, 115–121.

Young, J. F. and Palese, P. (1979). Evolution of human influenza A viruses in nature: Recombination contributes to genetic variations of H1N1 strains. *Proc. Natl. Acad. Sci. USA* **76**, 6547–6551.

Outlook for the Control of Influenza

D. A. J. TYRRELL

MRC Common Cold Unit, Harvard Hospital, Salisbury, UK

Previous papers at this meeting have covered comprehensively our knowledge of the influenza viruses, especially those of man, down to the fundamental level. These contributions have been well-based on experimental data and have in general drawn conclusions in a careful and logical fashion from the results available. This contribution is by nature much less securely based. In the first place it is generally accepted that influenza is not being controlled, and therefore the results to be drawn upon are mostly negative, and in the second I have been asked to look forward to the future and thus to add to the weakness of arguing from our present position by trying to extrapolate for at least a few years.

The Present Understanding

It is nevertheless sensible to start by looking in broad terms at what we now know about the factors involved in influenza epidemics. Although research

"The Molecular Virology and Epidemiology of Influenza" (Eds Sir Charles Stuart-Harris and Professor C.W. Potter). Academic Press, London, New York and Orlando, 1984.

workers and physicians give less attention to influenza B than to influenza A the overall situation is probably simpler and in principle more manageable in B than in A and so I propose to discuss it first—and to ignore influenza C altogether since it is apparently responsible for particularly mild and infrequent illnesses.

Influenza B virus apparently circulates only in human populations. It is highly communicable, infects particularly children and young adults, and can be regarded epidemiologically as differing only in detail from viruses such as the parainfluenza or adenoviruses. Presumably because of immunological selection pressure acting on genetic mutations there is a slow antigenic "drift" in the haemagglutinin which is the antigen which seems to play the greatest single role in determining immunity. Transmission seems to occur most readily in the winter in temperate countries, but there is little information about the status of the virus in the summer season or in the rather prolonged non-epidemic periods, but PHLS records suggest that infections may be detected in many months somewhere in England and Wales if specific tests are made on patients with acute respiratory infections. Well-made inactivated influenza B vaccines are readily available, usually formulated along with influenza A strains. They are known to stimulate antibody responses though there is less information about how good they are at protecting against infection. Prototype live influenza B vaccines based on recombinants with cold-adapted strains have been made and used but they have not been fully evaluated or licensed and are not generally available. The best studied anti-influenza drugs, amantadine and related compounds, are ineffective against influenza B, but there is now evidence that ribavirin is effective when given as an aerosol to cases of clinical disease (McClung *et al.*, 1983), and when given in this way it seems to be less likely to be toxic than by the oral route, though this has still to be demonstrated. Though influenza B is often regarded as a mild disease and indeed may not often kill patients it does produce the full picture of clinical influenza, and also initiates grave complicated diseases such as Reye's syndrome and staphylococcal pneumonia.

As is well known influenza A is a more serious problem and this seems to be mainly because antigen "shifts" occur at intervals of a decade or so and these increase the incidence of the disease above that of influenza B. The shifts enable the virus to evade the immunity produced by earlier infections so that it produces infection and disease in individuals infected only recently with the previous influenza A serotype. It thus attacks subjects of all ages, although its ill effects are most marked on certain sub-groups such as the very young, the very old and those with chronic illnesses, especially of the heart and lungs. This is not merely due to a greater effect of the virus itself but also to a greater frequency of complications, ranging from febrile convulsions in babies to pneumonia and cardiac failure in those with chest disease. There have been repeated efforts to understand and then explain and predict more of the detail of the epidemiology of influenza A. However, like predictions of the weather and the behaviour of the economy, they seem to work well only in retrospect(!) though there is a Russian computer model which uses data drawn from the beginning of an epidemic and apparently predicts the size and course of the rest of the outbreak in other cities of the Soviet Union. However there is no model which is generally accepted and used and this is probably because we understand too little about the structure and behaviour of various populations, and how to define them, and also about the influences which play on them, such as the weather. Furthermore although the importance of "shifts" of antigens are well recognized and quite easily measured there are also changes due to "drift" in the interpandemic period and the effect of these may only be understood if we look at a wide range of immune parameters, including for instance secretory antibody and cytotoxic T cells, and how a potential epidemic virus may interact with them rather than limiting our attention to circulating antihaemagglutinin antibody as is usual at present. Furthermore it may well be that other properties of the virus, such as the amount shed and its resistance to inactivation in air and also the type of disease it produces and particularly its effect on functions such as sneezing and coughing may all be important in deciding whether it will spread efficiently or not. It seems that there was a period in the nineteenth century when few influenza epidemics occurred and it is tempting to suggest that influenza A virus was unusually stable genetically during that period, so another parameter we need to understand better is the degree of stability or flexibility in the genome of a virus.

As is well known, influenza A is the only communicable disease which can have an impact on the community in a developed country great enough to interrupt normal life and produce a substantial peak in the statistics of morbidity and mortality. Further it can cause serious mortality among the elderly, particularly when they are gathered in residential homes.

A special feature of the epidemiology of influenza A appears to be that when a shift occurs the genetic information for the new antigens is derived from animal influenza viruses (Webster et al., 1980). It is now clear that many serotypes are circulating regularly in the wild, especially in water birds and these may well enter and infect domesticated animals in certain farming areas. The farm animals may then pass the virus on to man and if, by mutation or recombination, it acquires the ability to spread and cause disease in human beings, then a "shift" may have occurred and a new pandemic wave begun.

What Sort of Control?

It is important to define what we mean by control in relation to any disease, and in none more than influenza. For instance, we do not mean control of all influenza-like diseases since these are very heterogeneous and due to many etiological agents; but we could choose a number of other definitions such as:

(1) Eliminating or reducing the mortality due to or associated with infections with influenza A or B viruses.
(2) Preventing the occurrence of epidemic waves of influenzal disease reducing the incidence of disease.
(3) Preventing the circulation of the virus.

These possible targets for control will now be considered in turn.

REDUCING MORTALITY

This is probably the main component of our present efforts at control and taking a fairly long view of the statistics we could argue that we are having some success. It is well-known that the mortality rate from the great 1918–9 pandemic was very high, though it has been suggested that this might have been due to some unusual features of the virus or to the epidemics taking place in camps and refugee populations. However, the disease seems to have carried a high mortality in ordinary civilian populations as well. Since the 1930s death rates per million have continued to fall and the statistics of mortality rates per million at the time each of the new "shifted" strains appear, have fallen from the 1940s to 1968 (Stuart-Harris and Schild, 1976). We can assume that virtually all the population was infected on each occasion. Furthermore, a new influenza A virus appeared. All this implies that the denominator for calculating the lethality of infection has grown slowly with the population. In this period the infections have involved an increasing proportion of the more susceptible elderly subjects, so it seems a reasonable conclusion that the disease has in fact become gradually less lethal, though it would be unwise to put a figure on "how much" less lethal. It seems likely that the effectiveness of treatment has improved steadily, by the use of better antibiotics for, say, staphylococcal infections, better physiological support in the way of treatment of impaired gas exchange, cardiac failure or cardiovascular collapse. General health care may play an important role because it is likely that better referral of the very young and very old may be important in making it possible to start treatment relatively early and before irreversible physiological deterioration has occurred. Case-fatality rates mean little, as they depend so much on the criteria for the admission of patients, and are in any case not available in any comprehensive form. Thus it is plausible that improvements in medical care may have reduced influenza mortality. It is possible that other factors which have changed, including housing and nutrition, have been beneficial too but there are few plausible mechanisms to suggest and nothing like proof is available.

Mortality from influenza might be improved if we treated the virus infection and not just its secondary consequences. After many years of research we still have not got a really satisfactory anti-influenza drug, but there are also problems in working out how to apply whatever treatments are available. Some cases may not come for medical attention until after the virus infection is over, although in many cases virus is multiplying and being shed. Clinical diagnosis can be fairly confident in a typical case seen during an epidemic, but in others it is not, but rapid methods of diagnosis by immunofluorescence of respiratory secretions are available and have proved useful in clinical practice, for instance in the management of RSV infections in children. So in principle we can identify some patients in which infection is actively proceeding and be fairly sure that the virus is influenza A or B. Such patients could be given antiviral treatment. This was limited in the past to oral amantadine (Oxford and Galbraith, 1980) followed later by rimantadine. Ribavirin had been tried orally and was apparently not effective. However, ribavirin by small particle aerosol appears to be effective when given soon after the onset of uncomplicated influenza A and B (Knight et al., 1981; McClung et al., 1983). Anecdotal reports suggest it may be helpful in complicated influenza and severe RSV infection in children. This should be followed-up and if it were effective and could be applied in complicated and severe influenza it might enable us to reduce the mortality from influenza still further.

Although influenza infection alone can kill healthy young people the route to death is often by way of superadded bacterial infection and/or cardiorespiratory failure, or the metabolic or neurological disturbances of Reye's syndrome or even febrile convulsions, and many such cases are not recognized or certified as associated with influenza. Thus any improvements in the management of these are likely to curb the rises in general death rates that occur at the time of influenza epidemics.

However, it is generally agreed that it is better to control infectious disease by prevention than by treatment. This can be achieved either by preventing transmission or by immunizing and these will be dealt with later. However, it is worth pointing out now that the present policy of selective vaccination of risk groups, or future developments on the same lines, would closely complement improved methods of control by improved case management because the very groups in which vaccination is recommended are those from which most of the life-endangering infections are drawn and who would be receiving the benefits of improved treatment. When all this has been planned we should nevertheless ask ourselves whether what we are doing could be legitimately criticized as an unjustified application of technology, that interferes with a satisfactory aspect of the natural world; for example influenzal pneumonia may provide a fragile, elderly person with a quick and painless terminal illness instead of a possibly protracted and painful decay of the faculties and organs.

REDUCING INCIDENCE OF INFLUENZA—ALTERNATIVE VACCINES

The most likely way to reduce the occurrence of cases of influenza is to use immunization by vaccination either of target groups, or, in theory, of the whole population.

There are now rather numerous alternatives in this field, some of which we have reviewed quite recently (Tyrrell, 1980; Tyrrell et al., 1981). Briefly the first alternative is inactivated virus particle vaccine which can now be produced to a very high standard of purity and homogeneity. The purest product causing the least side-effects is made by extracting haemagglutinin and neuraminidase of the three current serotypes from virus grown in eggs and this induces good antibody responses when injected intramuscularly. Enhanced resistance to disease follows but is not complete. It may be that in effect infection is only deferred since in one study in children undertaken during years when the virus antigens were drifting the net result of such vaccination seemed to be to postpone infection for a few years (Hoskins et al., 1979); the final incidence of disease and infection was the same in the vaccinated and unvaccinated groups, whereas those who were *infected* at the beginning of the study period were apparently resistant to further infections and protected from further attacks of disease. It remains to be seen whether this is a general phenomenon, but it should not obscure the fact that standard vaccination, even of elderly persons, can apparently prevent disease.

We continue to learn more and more about the genetic basis of virulence and attenuation in influenza viruses and this is being applied as described elsewhere in this volume. Recombinants were made with *ts* mutants and with laboratory-adapted "master" strains such as PR8 and were found to be attenuated for man *if* they contained most or critical RNAs coding for internal components of the virus. However, there were difficulties in getting predictably stable, attenuated vaccines and other donors of attenuation are being explored. The experimental vaccines have been used for a number of clinical studies, and it has been shown repeatedly that they can confer resistance to infection and be sufficiently attenuated for used in children and elderly sick subjects. While this has been going on we have been learning more about the immunity to influenza (Freestone et al., 1972); antibodies against HA and NA in the serum and secretions do not adequately account for resistance to virus challenge and recent work has shown how cytotoxic T cells may confer resistance to virus infection in those who do not have specific antibody (McMichael et al., 1983). There is therefore room to examine how vaccines modify all these parameters of the immune response, as well as to continue to search for better manipulated attenuated strains using the approaches mentioned earlier. However, it would be desirable also to do more work of a practical type on how to administer live attenuated vaccines, at least to the target groups at increased risk of the disease. The present methods of giving drops, and of making up and delivering intranasal sprays, seem to me to be capable of significant improvement. We also need to explore whether viruses grown only in human cells would give better protection (Schild et al., 1983).

We are, of course, hopeful that understanding the immunochemistry of influenza virus haemagglutinins may enable us to devise better vaccines which can be manufactured without the limitations of supply and price imposed by the use of embryonated eggs. As other papers indicate it has proved possible to clone a copy DNA of influenza haemagglutinin RNA and this can be translated in bacteria, though in non-glycosylated form. If cloned into mammalian cells the peptide is glycosylated and produced in substantial amounts and indeed agglutinates red cells like the natural material. Though cloning and translation are becoming easier to do it is still not feasible, it seems, to produce by this means material for use as an antigen in clinical practice, but it would not surprise me if the position were to change at some time in the future. Because the chemical structures of haemagglutinins from a number of influenza A viruses and mutants have been solved it has become possible to synthesize short peptide sequences from the molecule for use as vaccines (Zuckerman, 1982). An obvious approach is to concentrate on those regions of the protein which seem to be concerned with antigenicity. By and large the results have not been what was hoped (Jackson et al., 1982; Müller et al., 1982). In the case of foot-and-mouth disease virus this approach yielded sequences 14 amino acid residues long which were used as an antigen (conjugated with keyhole limpet hemocyanin and incorporated into Freund's complete adjuvant). Specific antibodies were produced which not only bound to the synthetic antigen but also neutralized virus infectivity *in vitro* and protected guinea pigs from a fatal infection with infectious virus (Bittle et al., 1982). Antibodies against peptides from influenza virus haemagglutinin bind to the peptide but often fail to combine with specific virus haemagglutinin efficiently though antiviral antibodies may bind to peptide. It has been suggested that as an alternative target we should try to induce antibodies that are directed against a common determinant of many influenza A viruses (Green et al., 1982) and thus induce a much broader immunity than that from our present day vaccines. This possibility is still hypothetical but would bear more study. It should be remembered, however, that if we start inducing immune responses against an antigenic site to which, for some reason, the host does not respond during a natural infection, we might produce some unexpected and even adverse effects when patients, in whom this response has been induced become infected. It is only necessary to remind the reader of the serious effects of measles virus in patients who had been immunized with a vaccine lacking the F antigen. Another problem, common to all attempts to immunize with oligopeptides is that the antigen formulations used in animals are quite unacceptable for use in man. However, work with human chorionic gonadotrophin (HCG) has shown that antigen responses can be induced in monkeys using antigen conjugated to diphtheria or tetanus toxoid and combined with acceptable adjuvants (Stevens et al., 1981). We certainly need to know a lot more about the stereochemistry of the antigenic site of influenza viruses and about the details of the response of the immune system to this and other molecules. We may already be producing one sort of the broad immune response, that Green et al. (1982) want, by stimulating specific cytotoxic T cell responses with whole viruses but this phenomenon is ill understood at the moment. Practical success with synthetic vaccines is most likely to come in the wake of progress in the molecular biology of haemagglutinin and in basic studies on the processes of immunogenesis. I am sure such progress will occur and we should be ready to test it in the field when the time is ripe.

VACCINE STRATEGIES

I suspect that if a broadly antigenic killed vaccine or live vaccine became available we might want to change our strategy to one of trying to protect the population at large and ultimately prevent virus from circulating. In these cases we might wish to aim at vaccinating children even more than adults. Even if this is not practical yet there are still a number of unsolved questions about the most effective way of using our present vaccines. The obvious way to study this would be to undertake field experiments involving whole communities, and these would be very cumbersome and inevitably therefore few in number. I am therefore hopeful that work will be continued on mathematical modelling of epidemics. Several models and computational techniques are available (Fine, 1982), and if a model is even partly validated it can be used to study the effects of different sorts of intervention and the resources in medicaments, vaccines, staff and money could be estimated and the advantages and disadvantages of alternative proposals could be compared. Even if we do not wish to investigate some of these alternatives before their introduction becomes a live issue, epidemic modelling could be really valuable if it enabled us to predict an influenza epidemic in the drift period. Admittedly it is unlikely we could make a forecast which was sufficiently long-term to help the vaccine manufacturers, but it might be possible to give real assistance to those who need to decide whether to go ahead and give vaccine to vulnerable populations who might or might not be exposed in the next few months. An interesting new contribution on these lines uses data on the frequency of acute respiratory infections collected from general practice to predict an upswing in influenza later in the season (Smith, 1982). Presumably the data are a measure of how favourable meteorological and other conditions are for the transmission of such viruses but the consequences in the form of an influenza epidemic take some time to develop. This procedure is admittedly quite empirical and even naive but we should remember that something very similar was the starting-point of methods of forecasting crop disease which are now in regular use and commercially viable. Perhaps it can be developed by adding in a structured mathematical model, information from serum surveys, dates of public holidays and school terms, or additional weather recording. The practical advantages of forecasting the size and approximate time of an influenza epidemic could be quite considerable whatever methods of control are envisaged (Selby, 1982). A recent modelling study of various strategies for vaccinating against rubella and measles showed results which looked plausible in the light of experience and provided conclusions and predictions which were useful and not intuitively obvious (Anderson and May, 1983). Let us hope that earlier work on vaccination strategies for influenza will be developed similarly.

PREVENTING VIRUS CIRCULATION—ERADICATION

It is now confirmed that the smallpox virus has been eradicated from the globe and a recent meeting discussed the possibility of eradicating some other infectious diseases, and indeed suggested that measles and poliomyelitis might be suitable candidates (Stuart-Harris *et al.*, 1982). The thought is therefore in the air that influenza might be abolished in the same or a similar way. It is necessary to state that it could not be abolished on the model of smallpox. It is not a disease with a distinctive clinical picture, it is more readily and rapidly transmissible. Therefore, unlike smallpox, there is no possibility of following-up cases locally, nor is there any vaccine or other treatment that could have such a powerful effect as smallpox vaccination. If there is a model that might be followed it would be that of poliovirus infection in Scandinavia where, because universal vaccination has been agreed upon and achieved, transmission of all three polioviruses has declined until it has now effectively ceased, even though the method of vaccination does not make infection of the intestinal tract impossible, only more difficult. (This is to be expected and is a common feature of many epidemiological models, due to the fact that if on the average one infection gives rise to less than one further infection the causative organism will eventually cease to circulate.)

Even if effective community-wide influenza vaccination was possible and was introduced it would still render a country, say Britain, an influenza-free pool in a sea of virus circulation, for it is inconceivable that such vaccination could or would be introduced in most areas of the world. This is partly because of the lack of resources and the other priorities of developing countries, and partly to the impression that influenza is not an important cause of disease or death in rural areas. There are already some observations that indicate that this is not true and I look forward to seeing the results of studies now being stimulated by the WHO to determine the important causes of acute respiratory disease in children under five. Thus if influenza virus ceased to circulate in Britain it would be necessary to continue anti-influenzal control measures so that if virus was reintroduced it would not be able to circulate.

It would be a valuable step towards reducing the frequency of severe epidemics if we could prevent the successful introduction of genetic information from animal influenza viruses. This seems to be a rare event. It is likely that from time to time animal influenza viruses infect some human beings as in the case of swine influenza virus at Fort Dix. Only if a mutation or recombination occurs to enhance its pathogenicity can the virus really spread effectively. Thus if we could reduce the frequency with which virus in animals such as ducks, pigs or horses is inhaled by human beings, particularly children, then pandemics are less likely to start. It may well be that the new serotypes of viruses, are so often found in Asia, because that is where human beings and potentially infectious birds are most frequently in contact. There is a thrust to improve agricultural practices and the effect of many such changes would probably be to reduce the contact between farm animals and man. However, research should continue to try and identify the circumstances and places in which the virus enters the human population, and if this can be done successfully it may be possible by some relatively simple measures to reduce the risk of this occurring quite quickly and efficiently. If this were done we could expect the problem of influenza A to decline to the level of that of influenza B. There is even a possibility that, as has happened before with the H1N1 and H2N2 viruses the influenza A strains might immunize so many of the population that they would die out.

CONCLUSIONS

The control of influenza must still be regarded as a dream but one which may yet be realized. The diseases produced by the virus are part of the world-wide problem of acute respiratory infections and as such are best dealt with as part of that, namely, by providing to all areas a better quality of primary health care. Management by better antiviral therapy and prevention by better regimes of vaccination could reduce still further the impact of disease on the health and mortality of the population. Eradication of the viruses is too much to hope for but it is just possible that by accident or design we may delay or prevent new influenza virus genetic material being introduced into human viruses from the large collection being maintained in wild life. If so, this would be the best way of controlling the appearance of pandemic influenza.

REFERENCES

Anderson, R. M. and May, R. M. (1983). Vaccination against rubella and measles: quantitative investigations of different policies. *J. Hyg.* (Camb.) **90**, 259–325.

Bittle, J. L., Houghten, R. A., Alexander, H., Shinnick, T. M., Sutcliffe, J. G., Werner, R. A., Rowlands, D. J. and Brown, F. (1982). Protection against foot-and-mouth disease by immunization with a chemically synthesised peptide predicted from the viral nucleotide sequence. *Nature* (Lond.) **298**, 30–33.

Fine, P. (1982). "Applications of Mathematical Models to the Epidemiology of Influenza: a Critique in Influenza Models" (Ed., P. Selby). MTP Press Limited, Lancaster, pp. 15–86.

Freestone, D. S., Hamilton-Smith, S., Schild, G. C., Buckland, R., Chinn, S. and Tyrrell, D. A. J. (1972). Antibody responses and resistance to challenge in volunteers vaccinated with live attenuated, detergent split and oil adjuvant A2/Hong Kong/68 (H_3N_2) influenza vaccines. *J. Hyg.* (Camb.) **70**, 531–543.

Green, N., Alexander, H., Olson, A., Alexander, S., Shinnick, T. M., Sutcliffe, J. G. and Lerner, R. A. (1982). Immunogenic structure of the influenza virus haemagglutinin. *Cell* **28**, 477–487.

Hoskins, T. W., Davies, J. R., Smith, A. J., Miller, C. L. and Allchin, A. (1979). Assessment of influenza A vaccine after three outbreaks of influenza at Christ's Hospital. *Lancet* **i**, 33–35.

Jackson, D. C., Murray, J. M., White, D. O., Fagan, C. N. and Tregear, G. W. (1982). Antigenic activity of a synthetic peptide comprising the 'loop' region of influenza virus hemagglutinin. *Virology* **120**, 273–276.

Knight, V., McClung, H. W., Wilson, S. Z., Waters, B. K., Quarles, J. M., Cameron, R. W., Greggs, S., Zerwas, J. M., Couch, R. B. (1981). Ribavirin small-particle aerosol treatment of influenza. *Lancet* **ii**, 945–949.

McClung, H. W., Knight, V., Gilbert, B. E., Wilson, S. Z., Quarles, J. M. and Divine, G. W. (1983). Ribavirin aerosol treatment of influenza B virus infection. *J. Am. Med. Assoc.* **249**, 2671–2674.

McMichael, A. J. M., Gotch, F. M., Noble, G. and Beare, A. S. (1983). Cytotoxic T cell immunity to influenza. *New Engl. J. Med.* **309**, 13–16.

Müller, G. M., Shapira, M. and Arnon, R. (1982). Anti-influenza response achieved by immunization with a synthetic conjugate. *Proc. Nat. Acad. Sci. USA* **79**, 569–573.

Oxford, J. S. and Galbraith, A. (1980). Antiviral activity of amantadine—a review of laboratory and clinical data. *Pharmacology and Therapeutics* **2**, 181–262.

Schild, G. C., Oxford, J. S., de Jong, J. C. and Webster, R. G. (1983). Evidence for host cell selection of influenza virus antigenic variants. *Nature* (Lond.) **303**, 706–709.

Selby, P. (Ed.) (1982). "Influenza Models." MTP Press Limited, Lancaster.

Smith, L. P. (1982). Numerical forecasting of epidemics of influenza in Great Britain and Northern Ireland. *Rev. Epidem. et Santé Publ.* **30**, 413–422.

Stevens, V. C., Cinader, B., Powell, J. E., Lee, A. C. and Koh, S. W. (1981). Preparation and formulation of a human chorionic gonadotrophin antifertility vaccine: selection of adjuvant and vehicle *Am. J. Reprod. Immunol.* **1**, 315–321.

Stuart-Harris, C. H. and Schild, G. C. (1976). "Influenza. The Viruses and the Disease." Edward Arnold, London.

Stuart-Harris, C., Western, K. A. and Chamberlayne, E. C. (Eds) (1982). Can infectious diseases be eradicated? *Rev. Infect. Dis.* **4**, 912–984.

Tyrrell, D. A. J. (1980). Influenza vaccines. *Phil. Trans. Roy. Soc. Lond.* B **288**, 449–460.

Tyrrell, D. A. J., Schild, G. C., Dowdle, W. R., Chanock, R. M. and Murphy, B. (1981). Development and use of influenza vaccines. *Bull. WHO* **59**, 165–173.

Webster, R. G., Hinshaw, V. S., Bean, W. J. and Sriram, G. (1980). Influenza viruses: transmission between species. *Phil. Trans. Roy. Soc. Lond.* B **288**, 439–447.

Zuckerman, A. J. (1982). Developing synthetic vaccines. *Nature* (Lond.) **295**, 98–99.

DISCUSSION

J. W. G. Smith First, I should like to record the pleasure it has given us all here at Hampstead that Beecham's, and WHO who are co-sponsoring, and your Organizing Committee, decided to hold the meeting at this Institute. We are always very glad to have a well-behaved group here but I think that on this occasion you have done the Institute honour by celebrating this fiftieth anniversary with us.

I would like also particularly to record our delight that Sir Christopher Andrewes was able to join us. If he can speak as he did two days ago at the age of 86, I wonder what he must have been like 50 years ago—quite extraordinary I think!

Seeing so many distinguished guests from all over the world I could not let this occasion pass without remarking upon the invaluable presence of commanding figures in the field as Dr Chu from China and Dr Kilbourne of New York from whose papers I have learnt so much about influenza and its mysteries.

On a personal note, it has been most rewarding to see Sir Charles Stuart-Harris who, as I think you all recognize, has straddled the field of influenza from the laboratory to the clinical bedside and has made major contributions embracing all this wide area throughout his professional life. I think it is very fitting that this last session will attempt to do the same thing, to relate the clinical and field experience of influenza to the molecular biological findings to which so many of you have made fine contributions.

One last point I would like to mention is that we have been doing a little influenza research here in the Institute. The work I want to talk about was aimed at a distinct and clear object which was to identify the room in which Sir Christopher Andrewes did his work here 50 years ago. We established that it was in this building, not in any of the huts in the grounds, that it was on the second floor, and we worked out that it was in the last room on the right on the second floor. A critical experiment was conducted two days ago and we established that it was in this building, it was on the second floor, but it was quite the other end. I am sorry to say that the room is now the office of the Virology Department, so that a major laboratory has been changed into an office, although, in defence, we do sometimes change offices into laboratories.

If any of you are sentimentally inclined, you are very welcome to visit Geoffrey's departmental office and see where this work went on.

This critical experiment was conducted by the expedient of asking Sir Christopher where he worked. I had always thought that you could not do this with influenza but perhaps we shall learn from Dr Kilbourne that you can indeed ask the influenza virus critical questions in the same way.

Perhaps I could make one small comment on the two papers. I have a rather pessimistic attitude to influenza vaccines at present, because the people you want to protect vote with their feet, in England at any rate, and they do not come forward for the vaccine. If you offer it, for example, in a factory operation, or to the Post Office, in Britain, in my experience you eventually end up with an annual acceptance rate of around 15%. I suspect that that sort of experience is reflected in other countries. I think we are very much dependent on the molecular biologist coming up with better vaccines before the public are going to put their votes in favour of the vaccine.

Skehel One of the things which Dr Kilbourne mentioned in regard to vaccination concerned this business of Schild with obtaining antigenic variants simply by growth of virus in different cells. I wondered if that could be taken any further? What do you think the consequences are of the observation that you get antigenically different viruses depending on the cell system that you use to produce the virus for vaccine?

Kilbourne I think that ultimately the answer should come from Dr Schild, but my own feeling is that it is a very interesting phenomenon. However, it needs more work before we can really make the definitive correlations with the antibody response of egg-grown virus versus the virus grown in mammalian cells. I think that the preliminary evidence that Dr Schild showed us is very suggestive that we are looking at different antibody populations, but again we have the problem of making the field correlations in terms of what actually happens in the matter of protection.

Schild Obviously this is on our agenda to investigate. One of the first things to do would be to investigate protection in experimental animal systems. For example, to immunize ferrets with inactivated products made in various cell substrates and to challenge with different viruses prepared in mammalian cells or eggs. If this looks interesting, then it may be possible to go to small-scale experiments in human volunteers.

Another aspect of the same phenomenon interests me, and this is the relationship of selection by host cell to virulence. Again, that is a thing which can be readily studied in experimental animal systems. I would not like to predict at this moment whether this is going to turn out to be of importance in designing vaccines, but it is certainly something we should not leave untested.

Skehel Would you put it at the moment as one of the major reasons why influenza vaccine might not be particularly effective?

Schild That is a difficult question. I think there are possibly several factors contributing to the limited efficacy of inactivated vaccines.

Tyrrell I think that from the point of view of actually using vaccines, the problem can be focused around the fact that certain individuals are not apparently protected by vaccine. As Dr Schild has indicated, we think that vaccines probably do contribute to immunity in a number of different ways, and the central question is: would it make a big difference to that quarter or third of the population who are apparently not protected if they had this antigenic type of virus rather that the one they are getting at the moment? I do not think anybody can know the answer to that yet. I think one has to do the experiment and find out. It might even be different for live and killed vaccines. I think it has to be done with both.

Assaad I would like to mention one thing along these lines but from a completely different angle. We did not actually discuss the production of vaccines. One of the real problems you are having is that you produce under best conditions 1·3 dose per egg, which makes it prohibitively expensive for any but the very rich countries. If we add to this what has been discussed, I think we may have then to look not only at the vaccine itself but at the substrate. Recently we had a talk by John Beale on adjuvants, and it was most distressing. There is no promising one on the horizon. Therefore, it is the carrier system, adjuvants, and substrates that we have also to think of. So even with influenza, after all this time, we still have to go to basic research. Can we produce an efficient vaccine that will be antigenically effective and cheap, or reasonably cheap, to produce?

Murphy I just wanted to suggest to Dr Schild that it might be very interesting to study some of these viruses in primates rather than in human volunteers, because the viruses might grow a little bit more efficiently in monkeys because there would not be any immunity. It might be that after one or two cycles of replication of egg-passaged material you start generating the variants that have MDCK determinants. The implications for live virus vaccines would be studied in this way.

J. W. G. Smith One other aspect of the performance of influenza vaccine, is the short duration of immunity apparently given in contrast with the durable immunity that can follow natural infection, as we saw when the H1N1 reappeared. Dr Kilbourne, do you think this is just a reflection of the poor antigenic response generally, or is there some fundamental problem? I cannot quite see why you cannot produce a durable immunity with killed vaccine as you can with other antigens. It does not seem to occur with influenza.

Kilbourne I am not sure I would accept that generalization to begin. I think it has been the experience that you can usually make a generalization the other way, that is, most of the non-replicating antigens give you brief immunity, with the notable exception of the bacterial toxoids, which I think almost stand out as an exception. I think, indeed, that is going to be one of the problems, going back to Dr Tyrrell's talk: when we come down to the oligopeptides, and the smaller the antigen the less it is involved in intimate relationship to the host cells, the more difficulty there seems to be in immunogenicity.

While I have the microphone, I wonder if I could go back to the point of Dr Schild's approach and ask whether we might have some problems if we go over to cultivation in mammalian cells in terms of hazard to personnel and preservation of virulence of the virus more effectively. I think there is perhaps not very good direct evidence, but there is almost consensus evidence that when you take things into the chick embryo they become pretty markedly attenuated. One would have to be cautious in defining the exact host cell system one wanted to work in.

Dowdle I would like to go back to Dr Assaad's point and several others on inactivated vaccine. I think we have to remember that, even with the present antigen concentration, we still may be working in an area of very small antigen dosage. In fact, the question has come up on a number of occasions as to whether we should be working with a much higher dosage to achieve maximum immune response. He chose our antigen dosage on the basis of adverse reactions rather than the best dosage required to produce the immunity. I am not sure in some ways that the inactivated vaccine has been given a fair trial. We probably have been working in a range of minimum antigenic potencies.

The other point to be made is whether we should consider producing the antigen in some other way than we are doing now, simply by harvesting viruses. Although we are splitting viruses at the moment, are there other ways to reduce the reactogenicity of the vaccine and give much larger doses? The expense would increase but at the same time you might even have the opportunity of giving the vaccine every other year or every third year if you could provide adequate immunity. After all, I think Bob Couch showed us that natural infection may provide five to ten years of protection. That is not bad considering how the virus drifts. If we could achieve anywhere near that with inactivated vaccines, we would not be doing badly.

Couch I should like to turn the attitude round a bit, if I have properly interpreted the opinions expressed. I am not sure we can say that inactivated vaccines are not particularly effective. In fact, I would like to take the view that they are effective. I think most of us would agree that they are not as desirably effective as we would like them to be. We would like to be speaking of 90% or 95% protection instead of 60% and 70% but let us not denigrate 60% and 70% when the alternative is zero.

I do not think a discussion on the problems of antigenic mass in properly prepared vaccine, and quality control, is appropriate at this point but I should like to second Dowdle's comment about dose. I don't believe we have done a great deal, otherwise, in improving and understanding inactivated vaccines.

One additional comment I would like to make is that I do not think we have any idea what is the duration of effect of inactivated vaccine. With modern vaccines and perhaps with dosages that many of us think we should be using, we may be able to approach the degree of duration of effectiveness that we have been seeing after live infection. I think that ought to be considered an open question and we should not say that inactivated vaccine leads to protection for only one year so that it is necessary to repeat vaccine every year. In fact, it may be that the lesson to be learned from Hoskins *et al.* (1979), is that we have not been properly immunizing by giving the immunization every year. We should consider this an open question for evaluation.

Finally, we have one bit of data that relates to this question. In sera from a group of individuals immunized annually over a course of years, we have, thus far, looked at responses to the B component and find interesting results among these individuals who had vaccination four years in succession. With B/Hong Kong, there were a reduced number of responses, as you might guess, in the second and third year. Then when the B/Singapore component was given, both new and old vaccinees responded very nicely with neutralizing antibody. If we are going to say that new specific neutralizing antibody is not effective, then we are saying that something very strange is happening with vaccines that is contrary to a number of our current concepts of immunity. I am certainly not willing to accept that until we have more information than we have at present.

J. W. G. Smith Is it not true, Dr Kilbourne, that in the case of killed polio vaccine a durable immunity can result in the absence of stimulation with infection as appears to happen in Sweden? In other words, the possibility does exist that with a viral antigen you could get a durable immunity.

Kilbourne Of course, in that situation, as I understand it, repeated inoculation is necessary, and also the magnitude of challenge and the opportunity for challenge is certainly less in that kind of an ecological situation, which can be both good and bad. You do not have the reinforcement from boosting from natural infection but it also means your protection statistics look pretty good.

Schild I would just like to comment on the situation with recipients of inactivated poliovaccine. Studies on viruses in Sweden show that the antibody levels are maintained excellently for some 20 years and in the apparent absence of continued stimulation by circulating polioviruses.

I entirely agree with Dowdle about the need for more information on antigenic potency of influenza vaccines. There is good evidence from the UK and I think, in the United States, that when graded-dose studies of inactivated vaccines have been done, starting from the conventional dose of 10 to 15 μgm and going up to ten times this dose, you do not reach a plateau. The larger amount of antigen you give, the better the level of antibody. Another point is that we do tend to neglect studies for antibody to the "second best" antigen. Some of the existing vaccines do not stimulate anti-neuraminidase antibody very efficiently and this is an area with scope for technical improvement in vaccine design. There are also methods of presenting purified glycoprotein antigens not with adjuvants but using new ways of aggregating and complexing them into multivalent structures; these have recently been reported from Sweden. I think there is much to be learned about optimum methods of presentation of glycoprotein antigens.

Chu I should think the analogy between polio and influenza is not really close because the vaccine for polio presumably prevents the spread of virus by the blood stream to the central nervous system. A little antibody is adequate to prevent disease, whereas with influenza you have a surface infection and really you can produce a very high antibody by neutralization tests or haemagglutination tests with the present killed vaccine but they are not so effective. With the same antibody level for polio, you will be protected.

Kilbourne I am afraid Dr Schild has opened the door for me to say something, because he referred to the second best antigen, and it is my position, of course, that influenza virus neuraminidase is the best antigen. I think at least it should be mentioned that there is a stratagem which has been proposed by which you can get infection-permissive immunization by the use of neuraminidase which is not mediated by neutralizing antibody in the strict sense of our definition the other day. The reason I am reinforced in my feeling about this is because of the failures that we have both with the live virus and current inactivated virus approaches, and it seems to me—not wishing to be the eternal compromiser—that some combination of those approaches might be what we have to resort to eventually; in other words, if you put some kind of a floor of basic immunity down with neuraminidase antibody, then you need not be concerned about the level of attenuation or avirulence of each new live virus vaccine, or that you could, indeed, rely on natural infection as being reinforcing.

Skehel I should like to ask why the Christ's Hospital study is not an indictment of inactivated vaccines in general?

Tyrrell I do not think I can say that for absolutely certain. It seems to me likely that the phenomenon was related to the fact that the subjects were young children, relatively immature immunologically; whereas the policy at the moment is to give vaccine to people with serious disease who tend to be a lot older. I think it is at least plausible that at that stage, with the amount of experience they have had of influenza infections, they would not show this phenomenon. That is my intuition, and I would think it is very important at some time, somehow, somebody does such an experiment. I know that people have thought of it, but I was in fact talking to Dr Chanock during coffee and saying how incredibly difficult it would be because I do not think that serological studies are really of very much value. You have to do an experiment which shows protection on challenge with the virus.

Kendal So far as the Christ's Hospital study is concerned, my recollection is that in every year the wrong vaccine was used for the epidemic strain of virus. Is that not correct?

J. W. G. Smith It was certainly correct for four of the years.

Kendal So, again I think that the principle of indicting inactivated influenza vaccine is somewhat premature. There are factors which are partially under control—namely the selection of the strain—and there are factors such as Dr Tyrrell referred to this morning to changing the strategy for use of vaccine based on more aggressive attempts at epidemic protection. Again, one of the reasons that some people here may be of the view that there are instances where influenza vaccines have been ineffective, stems partially from publications in MMWR over the last few years, particularly in relation to influenza B outbreaks. One feature of all these outbreaks, however, is the fact that they tend to occur very late in the winter, really in early spring, and the administration of vaccine in many cases is probably far earlier than need be. In these cases the decline of antibody over the intervening period may well have resulted in increased susceptibility to infection.

For those who are coming to the Royal Free this afternoon, I will try to overcome some of the cynicism about inactivated influenza vaccines by presenting some data which show that at least during the last season in the United States, and at least with H3N2 influenza, there was a statistically significant reduction in both hospitalization and pneumonia assessed by mortality in nursing home residents who were vaccinated versus those who were unvaccinated. That was based on an investigation of a totally unselected population of every nursing home in a single county in one State. So we are trying to avoid the problems that we have had in the past of reporting on outbreaks that come to attention because of their severity.

Schild I think it is a little misleading to say that the wrong vaccines were used at Christ's Hospital. Although they were not identical, perhaps, with the current epidemic strains they could hardly be expected to be nearer. Up-to-date epidemiological information was used to formulate those vaccines. You are never going to get better than that. If their lack of identity with the epidemic strains was the essential problem, then we have a permanent problem with this strategy for vaccination.

Glezen I would probably look at the Christ's Hospital experience in a somewhat different light. My understanding was that this was a boarding school which I would consider a closed population. The attack rate for the children not recognized to have had previous infection or vaccination was 21%. That is very low for school children for influenza. In Houston we have observed attack rates of 40% regularly for illness severe enough to keep children from attending school. Certainly there has been some protective effect by vaccination or previous infection which has diminished the attack rate in this population to considerably below the average. It seems to me the observation is that natural infection with the previous variant protected better than the killed vaccine with the previous variant. That is about all you can say. I have trouble seeing this as an indictment of vaccination. In the first place it was not designed as a study to examine that question and to make an interpretation, I think, is carrying matters too far.

Skehel If one of the conclusions from the study is that previous vaccination leads to subsequent recalling antibodies against the first and not giving antibodies against the second vaccine in a significant number of vaccinees, then it seems to me an important thing to consider when using inactivated vaccines.

Murphy I think we really are talking about two different things here. First of all, the current inactivated vaccines in the United States are targeted for people who are over 65 years old. I think the Hoskins study demonstrates that repeated annual vaccination is probably not efficient in preventing the tracheobronchitis that children or young adults experience but this does not mean that the inactivated vaccines administered annually would be ineffective for preventing the serious pneumonic complications that occur in populations over 65. It is not necessarily fair to extrapolate from the experience in younger children to people who have compromised pulmonary function and who are experiencing a more severe disease. In this latter case, the serum antibody that is induced by annual vaccination might be more effective in preventing the pneumonia than the tracheobronchitis. Until the "Hoskins effect" is demonstrated in the people over 65 I do not think we would like to extrapolate the data from the young to the old. It might be true, but I would not extrapolate until we had the specific information.

Tyrrell Brian said it so much better than I tried to earlier but I would like to ask Dr Kendal whether it will be at all possible to continue his study and to expand current vaccines in further years and see whether protection persists or whether the Christ's Hospital model is followed?

Kendal In answer to Dr Tyrrell's question, the particular study that is done this year certainly could be done in subsequent years if there is a high enough local impact of influenza to make it geographically practical. We have another prospective study in progress with approximately 6000 nursing home residents in some 50 or 60 nursing homes who were enrolled last year with the intent to follow them over the long term (at least more than one year), and try to determine whether there are variations in mortality rates in vaccinated and unvaccinated, taking account other underlying factors.

I should add that one of the other things that we have shown is that apparently vaccine utilization appears to be similar regardless of the level of medical care of the persons resident in the nursing homes, which is one of the biases we have been concerned might have existed in the past.

J. W. G. Smith I am sorry, Dr Kendal, could you elucidate that again? I did not quite follow it.

Kendal We have always been concerned that one of the reasons why vaccine might appear to be ineffective was that there might be a selection factor exercised within the target population, i.e. those people who were at highest risk were, for various reasons, not receiving vaccine. The results of the latter survey that I have just described indicated that the administration of vaccine in this sample of 50 to 60 nursing homes has been fairly flat, regardless of whether the residents had minimal care, intermediate care, or skilled nursing care requirements. So it does not appear that that should be a factor which would bias the outcome of vaccine efficacy determinations.

I have two other points. First, I would stand by my comment about Christ's Hospital, that the wrong vaccine was used. I certainly am known in some circles to be a hawk for changing virus strains. I think we all recognize that decisions for changing, updating, influenza vaccines are affected by both scientific issues and the practical issues of what this means in terms of the vaccine manufacturers' capabilities and costs, and timetables for distribution. However, I think it is fair to say that if we had tended to be as aggressive as we were theoretically capable of being in several of the years when the Christ's Hospital study was running, a different virus could, in fact, have been in the vaccine if one is prepared to have very fast reaction times upon the detection of new strains. That is clearly a controversial and personal point of view but I am very hawkish on the fact that this is at least theoretically possible if we want to take that approach.

Secondly, I wanted to comment on something that Dr Tyrrell said this morning about the fact that influenza is perhaps a decreasing problem. Indeed he may be right that improving health care will decrease the relative mortality rates of persons who are infected, but the demographic trends are such that we would assume that during the next twenty years influenza might, in fact, be an increasing problem as the number of persons over 65 and with other underlying medical conditions increases as a proportion of the total population. It could be a very significant trend over the next ten or 20 years and considerations about the use of influenza vaccine should perhaps take this into account.

Schild I should like to be a devil's advocate. If you are really going to keep absolutely up-to-date with your vaccine composition, this will mean taking risks in that you would be putting a strain into a vaccine almost as soon as it appears at any point on the globe. In taking such risks you may do more harm than good. There may be many occasions when you make the vaccine and arrange to use it and you are absolutely wrong. It is clearly a question of compromise. I think that in general the system that is now used gets it about as right as you possibly can. There is probably little scope for improvement except, of course, by a major increase in surveillance.

Murphy I think the comment that in the Hoskins studies the wrong vaccine was used does not take into account the findings from that study which demonstrated that one dose of the Port Chalmers vaccine protected against the Victoria virus as a level that has been generally observed for inactivated vaccines. I think the data from the Hoskins study also demonstrated that each of the inactivated vaccines that were used behaved as a single dose according to the general experience with vaccines. So calling the Port Chalmers vaccine the wrong vaccine is not fair. It might perhaps have been somewhat better, but it certainly was not wrong. The data from that study should not be put in the context of incorrect vaccines being used. I think that the study had the correct vaccines and the interpretations from that study were fairly clear-cut, simple and straightforward.

Kilbourne My comment was going to be much like Dr Murphy's but I would go beyond that and say that I really think you could take the position that within the decade or so of prevalence of a given sub-type, the experiment has not really been done of sticking with the initial isolate using its antigens in reinforcing inoculations through the entire period. We know that there is substantial heterotypic immunity among strains within a sub-type and one could make the point that perhaps it might be better to have a quantitatively greater level of high affinity antibody heterotypic to the new strain than a lower level of antibody homotypic to it. In other words, you take advantage of original antigenic sin to keep boosting heterotypic antibody. The point is not just a theoretical one; some time it should really be tried.

Skehel I was under the impression that the reason for designating H1 as a sub-type was due to a vaccine failure initially. Clearly that points to the idea that you should try and keep the vaccine as up to date as possible.

Kilbourne Here we come into the old Geneva conference arguments about what is really a sub-type. On molecular biological evidence, nucleotide sequencing and so forth, there was wisdom in classifying 1947 H1N1 viruses with PR8 and swine viruses. I think it is a practical matter. The challenge in the field, the fact that there was a pandemic in 1947, shows that the 1946–7 virus had wandered a fair distance away antigenically. It is again almost a semantic argument about what is a sub-type or not; but I am talking about, for example, intra-sub-type variation within the H2N2 period and within the more recent H3 prevalence period where there has been a lot of evidence of overlapping immunity. Many studies have brought that out, particularly some of Meiklejohn's with his Air Force Academy studies where he has shown substantial heterotypic protection. Since we have never done the experiment of trying really good reinforcement of homotypic response with heterotypic stimulation as new strains come, I think that this is an experiment yet to be done.

Murphy I think that the Hoskins studies would lead an advocate of live virus vaccine to a different conclusion, i.e. that we need to give children live virus vaccines. It will be important to see whether a similar phenomenon occurred after repeated annual immunizations with a live virus. Dr Glezen's studies earlier really emphasized the importance of the influenza virus as a pathogen for children of all ages. One of the great potentials for live virus vaccines in the possibility for the range of individuals who currently receive influenza vaccines to include all ages. In this way the morbidity associated with infectious diseases can be handled a little more efficiently than we are dealing with it at present.

Kendal Just to set my comments on three pages of the record straight, my question that it was the wrong vaccine was that it was the wrong vaccine in terms of reaching the conclusion that annual re-vaccination will prove to be an ineffective control strategy and that, in fact, with different vaccines annual re-vaccination might prove to be successful. I certainly think that that includes the use of live vaccines as an alternative to inactivated vaccine.

It is also unfortunate that nobody from NIH in Japan is here. I can recount second-hand information which I hope holds up to be correct in the final analysis. As most people know, in Japan there is a mandatory annual school-child vaccination policy and, due to the concerns which have existed in Japan in some quarters about the validity of this approach, apparently two winters ago at least one prefecture decided to buck the trend and did not administer influenza vaccine to school children in their locality. During the winter's epidemic apparently the attack-rate of influenza in schools in that locality was very dramatically higher than that in the neighbouring locality, which was presumably affected by the same strain with similar epidemiologic potential. I hope that that becomes hard information and available for us all to see.

Dowdle The question I might pose for the group is that when we meet again in the next few years, as I am sure some of the group will, are we going to be in a better position at that time to use words other than homotypic and heterotypic? With the introduction now of the newer knowledge from molecular biology can we better define antigenic relationships and can we plan our strategies a little better? Can we plan our vaccines a little better based on what we know about the antigenic sites which may be involved?

Tyrrell Can I raise a point that is a little hobby horse of mine? It is, in fact, possible in various ways to look at the binding of particular antibodies to particular antigens, and I think we should use these to describe the antibody a host has made in these terms in more detail. Dowdle looks at cross-reacting and specific antibody, but this is, I think, only a partial description of what is really going on. It is not a complete analysis. Maybe some of the things which we regard as paradoxical would disappear if we realized that what we record as haemagglutination-inhibiting antibody are binding weakly or to a bit of the molecule which is not so important.

This is really a call to go to the molecular immunochemistry, if you like, of antibody/virus interactions and try to bring them along, perhaps in a rather selected area, to some of the paradoxes which we find in whether vaccines work or whether particular individuals are immune, to see if there is not something of an answer there.

Schild Some attempts have been made to evaluate the biological significance of the various antihaemagglutinin antibodies of different specificities, i.e. cross-reactive and strain-specific anti-HA. By far the largest element of the anti-haemagglutinin antibody response to inactivated vaccines in the interpandemic periods is directed against the older strains, rather than the vaccine strain, and most individuals, in our experience, who have had a conventional dose of vaccine fail to demonstrate production of strain-specific antibody to the virus in the vaccine. Work on the passive transfer of the strain-specific or cross-reactive antibodies in mice and also in cell culture work suggest that the cross-reactive antibody is much less efficient than strain-specific antibody in neutralizing virus and in protecting mice. Some work along the lines you suggest has been done, but of course we need a lot more studies to understand the whole problem.

Couch We looked at this question in volunteers with Webster's vaccines and cross-reacting antibody was very clearly associated with protection. A person need not have strain-specific antibody so long as the cross-reacting antibody was capable of neutralizing virus. If you have heterotypic antibody that is not capable of neutralizing virus, then I do not think anyone would expect that antibody to be protective.

Webster I should like to go back to some experiments that Dr Fazekas did with Dr Francis. It really comes back to the suggestion by Dowdle that providing you give enough antigen, you can overcome original antigenic sin and get specific antibody produced in addition to antibody produced in response to the original virus. These kinds of experiments have not been done in humans.

Kilbourne I made my heretical statement for the following reason. Going back to the premise, which may be debatable, that I offered a moment ago about the value of infection-permissive immunization, or partial immunity, I think that, as more and more antigenic sites are defined, and as more and more of the synthetic oligopeptides are produced, many of these are currently being thrown away if they do not fulfil the classical test of stimulating the production of neutralizing antibody in the narrow sense of antibody which scores in a neutralization test as inhibiting virus infection, *in vitro* (in pre-inoculation mixing of virus and antibody).

I think that if we were to examine antibody to some of these smaller antigens in a system in which we could look for their effect on multiple cycle replication, either in reduction of plaque size or other models of that sort, we might find that they were analogous to neuraminidase in terms of the kind of antibody they stimulate. In other words, they might stimulate antibody which would bind to the virus particle, not specifically to neutralizing sites, but could have an effect on damping virus replication cycles so that they might be of some value.

If one does think of this other stratagem of a lesser victory over the virus in terms of accepting partial immunization, then a whole new world is opened up as far as I am concerned in terms of not summarily discarding these oligopeptides simply because they are not immunogenic for neutralizing antibody antigenic.

Chu May I just mention an accidental challenge, without any intention, with a live virus? In 1971 we had a variant called Hong Kong/107/71 which did not spread worldwide but affected the Far East and quite a portion of that area. Some people in the vaccine laboratory passed it in human kidney and in monkey kidney, about seven or eight passages. They gave it to the workers in the laboratories. Altogether 11 people were given it. Five of them were double negative, i.e. they were negative against Hong Kong/68 as well as the '71 virus. Four of them got a fairly high fever—above 38°—and a mild 'flu. Those who were doubly positive with antibody against Hong Kong/68 and '71 viruses were protected. There was no clinical reaction at all and no antibody rise. There were three or four people with only cross-reacting antibody from the Hong Kong/68 virus, none against the homologous one. They gave no clinical reaction at all but there was antibody rise, so there is infection but no disease. That corroborates very well with the experience of Dr Couch that heterotypic antibody from natural infection does protect, but I do not know about heterotypic antibody from a killed vaccine. It may be different.

Tyrrell I am trying to fulfil the purpose of this meeting and link the molecular studies to the way we look at vaccination. I have learned by considering how experiments using monoclonal antibodies map the epitopes on a complete haemagglutinin, that we are making studies in an immensely complicated system when we take *whole* human serum, polyclonal serum against a *whole* virus consisting of several epitopes, and imagine individual doses of antibodies binding with different degrees of affinity to them.

Whenever you find a biological effect, if it neutralizes the virus you might find that may tell you all you need to know about the complicated mixture of antibodies and viruses, but I can think that there could be circumstances when that is not enough to known and you should look at it in more detail with the techniques which are now available.

O'Grady Could I change the subject and ask about the development of new antiviral agents for the control of influenza. It seems to me there is already enough evidence to suggest that antiviral agents are likely to be a rerun of antibacterial agents, that is to say we will have agents of a rather limited spectrum, there may well be problems with toxicity and almost certainly there will be problems with the emergence of resistant strains requiring generations of new agents.

One of the things that put manufacturers off developing antiviral agents was the failure of prescribers to take up amantadine after it was shown to be effective. How much encouragement with that background should we give to the pharmaceutical houses at this time to develop anti-influenza agents?

Tyrrell I think there were two objections to amantadine; one was that it is very difficult to make a clinical diagnosis in the sense that you cannot be sure on first seeing your patients whether they have influenza A or not; secondly, that people emphasized the importance of the prophylactic studies—which were, after all, done first.

Nowadays it is possible to recognize within one day by rapid diagnostic methods that you have an influenza patient infected with an A virus and in an epidemic situation it is probably reasonable to use a clinical diagnosis as a sufficient trigger for a drug in other similar cases. We know now that the therapeutic use of a drug does give the patient benefit. So I think the situation is a bit different from what it was.

Ribavirin was the other drug I was referring to and it can be used against influenza B as well as influenza A; incidentally, also against respiratory syncytial virus in children. So it has a wider range and as Couch and his colleagues have shown, that also works therapeutically and not just prophylactically, though it must be given by aerosol to be satisfactory. So there are widening opportunities of really influencing the course of the virus infection when a patient comes to you in whom the infection has already started.

Assaad There has been a small WHO meeting dealing with amantadine and rimantadine in August this year and I think the conclusion was that especially rimantadine was less toxic. This was with the new studies that have been carried out and it stands a good chance in treatment as well as prevention. I think the report will be out very soon.

The problem, however, is this. One of the things that came out of this report is that if you give rimantadine by itself, it can be about 60–70% effective. If you give an inactivated vaccine it is about 60–70% effective and if you give both, then you have an additive effect and there is a claim that you can be up to 90%. This is really another dimension, if you give rimantadine for prophylactic purposes to those who are at the same time vaccinated; you would protect the risk groups until the vaccine really has developed effects.

Couch Dr Assaad made one of the comments I would have made, but in answer to Professor O'Grady, I do not think we need to discuss the amantadine story; it was a mixed-up problem of bad publicity and communication and companies should not be discouraged by that experience. A major problem pharmaceutical companies had in the 1960s and 1970s was using antibacterial screening methods for finding new drugs. But these experiences should not be dampening influence on current pharmaceutical interest in antivirals.

We have not had much to work with so far, so we are not sure what the value of antivirals might be in influenza; but, at the present time, there is no question regarding the size of the market if a drug with value in all circumstances for occurrence of influenza could be identified.

I should also like to second what Tyrrell said earlier. We would all like to have a magic bullet for influenza and perhaps that will occur one of these days. However, I do not think anyone at this meeting is going to say they definitely see this in the foreseeable future. In the absence of such a probability and with the continuing kind of problem we have in the world with influenza, we ought to be willing to use any approach available for control. I think we have to put together a package of approaches to get the best public health result in the foreseeable future; a combination of vaccine and antiviral use such as Dr Assaad referred to, may be one of the first good ways to begin using a multifactorial approach.

I think there is considerable incentive for antiviral development, not the least of which is that perhaps an early and effective treatment would be the best way to prevent bacterial pneumonia deaths. There are a multitude of approaches that could be evaluated if we had the proper antivirals with which to do studies on how to best use them.

Mahy I wanted to comment on the antivirals. One thing we have learned from the molecular virology over the last five years or so is that in contrast to the surface proteins there is a great deal of conservation amongst the replicative proteins and in particular we can see very obvious targets which could be developed, one obvious one is the product of segment one, the PB2 protein which is multifunctional and acts very early on. Clearly if one could design a drug which was active against such an enzymatic target or cap-structure binding target, this would be likely to be effective against quite a wide range of viruses.

Kilbourne One of the stratagems proposed by Dr Tyrrell, and he rated it third, was the elimination of the virus from the scene. I wonder if that is actually so absurd a possibility. I would really like to direct this question to Webster and Laver as well. I would like to have their assessment of our current knowledge about the interspecific transfer of influenza virus, particularly from avian reservoirs, putting this in the context of whether indeed there will prove to be just the three haemagglutinins which are capable of replicating in man, in association with other genes. If there are limitations, if we do not plan to draw from all the 13 haemagglutinin genes as a potential, are there ways of erecting some kind of a barrier against transfer? I am thinking of a disease like brucellosis which has been effectively controlled by the control of defined animal sources. Cows, of course, are different from migratory birds—thank goodness! Bird droppings are bad enough! Could I just open this for debate? I am basically very cynical about eradication attempts for any disease, particularly influenza, but perhaps we have been too cynical and should re-think things as we have more of this new ecological information.

Webster It is an enormous question to try to answer. We have to keep in mind that there is a very large pool of influenza genetic information in the wild animal population, particularly in ducks. We monitor the Canadian wild ducks, each year and I can take you to a pond and you can dip out your own influenza virus through the months of July and August. I do not think there is any way we could hope to eradicate this reservoir or prevent it from spreading to the human population. You could approach this in several ways. We could eliminate the wild duck population and the duck hunters of the world would be very upset with you! We might stop the spread from wild ducks but we must not forget about the geese, the terns and other winter-birds. We could try to take measures to stop wild birds coming into contact with humans or with domestic species. The turkey farmers in the United States are very aware of this, and they do take steps to keep the wild ducks out. Nevertheless, I do not see that there is any approach that we could take to prevent contact between domestic birds, wild birds and humans. There is no way I can see to eradicate the influenza gene pool or to prevent it spreading to man.

The other question Kilbourne directed at me was: is there a limited number of haemagglutinins or genes that could infect humans? So far I could imagine the only restriction is that it is unlikely that the internal genes of avian species are likely to be reassorted into viruses that infect humans. Theoretically we could anticipate that all 13 haemagglutinins could eventually end up in humans.

Palese I would also like to make a comment regarding the question of a limited number of influenza virus haemagglutinins. Even if we just stick to the human haemagglutinins, there may be the potential for an unlimited number of haemagglutinins. I am very impressed about the evolution of influenza A, B and C haemagglutinins. The C virus haemagglutinin does not share sequence homologies with those of the A and B viruses, but it retains similar functions. Thus, many haemagglutinins (with different primary sequences) may be viable. Recent data also have shown that the H3 haemagglutinins of the A viruses continuously change and that this change amounts to 10% over only a 10-year period. This could mean that in a hundred years we would have 100% of the amino acids exchanged assuming that H3 viruses continue to circulate. So without even taking into account the avian haemagglutinins I feel that the human haemagglutinins may have the capability of unlimited change.

Laver Since Kilbourne's question was directed to me as well as Robert Webster perhaps I should add that one sub-type has been eliminated from the human population, and that is H2N2. I would like to know why.

The second thing is that if you want to eliminate or try to eliminate the virus, then obviously type B is the one to go for first. But the reason why H2N2 has totally disappeared may have nothing to do with the emergence of

H3N2. We do not know why it has suddenly disappeared—at least I do not anyway.

Shortridge The object of the influenza exercise at least as I see it is that we want to try to stop a pandemic. There are two fundamental problems. First we have no idea what the antigenic make-up of the next virus will be. Secondly we do not know when that virus will emerge. I think the only real information we do have is that it is probably going to come from China. This is where there should be a focus of influenza investigation. We have heard a lot about the possible transmission from animal to man and I am a little pessimistic about our ability to block or to stop the virus reaching man because of the situation in China—for whose Southern Region we have coined the term "an influenza epicentre"—is somewhat different from anywhere else in the world. There is a huge duck population containing all the known influenza virus sub-types. The reason we have a duck population is very simple, and Dr Chu will perhaps corroborate this. It is a result of farming practices that have been going on for about the last 2000 years at least, because the ducks are raised as an adjunct to rice farming. If we are going to reduce exposure to avian viruses, I think the only way we can do this is to stop rice farming which is an impossibility. Alternatively we ought to stop duck raising. Of course, the duck is very important simply because he can be raised on the flooded rice fields and after the harvest, feed on fallen grain. This is a very simplistic view of the origin of influenza but I think that it has an element of credibility in it because of the increasing evidence for the emergence of influenza from that part of the world. I have checked out government records and there appear to have been these sporadic events happening ever since the mid 1800s and we have been able to track this across to Western China as well. The problem is, of course, that we are dealing with information provided by administrators and so forth, so we are not entirely 100% sure of this information. However, it does strike me as an almost intractable problem if the duck is the source of influenza for man.

There has been a lot of discussion on vaccines and I was very interested yesterday to see, or to have had gelled for me, current approaches in vaccine technology. If some of this technology could be rapidly deployed in the region where there is evidence of an incipient pandemic that would be a very useful stop towards control.

However, this sort of problem gets difficult again because one area about which we do not have information is the actual epidemiology of influenza and, until we have really clear-cut information on the general pattern we shall not quite know what to expect should there be any unexpected behaviour. So we have a whole series of difficulties here in grappling with influenza at its apparent source.

Dowdle A comment closely related, but perhaps not quite, is that Japan had problems with Japanese encephalitis for many, many years. Transmission of the virus to man of course, required rice fields, pigs and mosquitoes. Just by sheer coincidence it became economically unfeasible to raise pigs in a family setting as they had been raising them for many hundreds of years. Once different husbandry practices became commonplace Japanese encephalitis disappeared without really much effect of the vaccine.

Shortridge This is an interesting aspect; if we do have increasing industrialization and different housing conditions, one might imagine less contact with the animals—I do take your point.

Murphy I think we learnt last night from Dr Percival's talk that the difference between a man and a duck was one amino acid. I think that this gives us great potential for either changing ducks into men, or perhaps preferably men into ducks.

Percival Could I suggest, Mr Chairman, that you try immunizing the ducks. I did not hear anything yesterday during those brief moments when I was still awake which gave conclusive evidence that the virus did come from ducks to man. Is that right?

J. W. G. Smith I think that is fair.

Chu I think that this whole problem is really in the stage of research. It is very hard to predict what will come out, at least it seems to be premature to me. We have pretty good evidence that H2N2 first started in South-west China. Assuming that H3N2 started in Hong Kong, that was just on the corner of China; the H1N1, which you are now calling the USSR, was in fact detected five months earlier and that was in North-east China, not in the South. How could you explain that?

Shortridge At the Beijing meeting in November, I did put forward the suggestion, that we have to look at the problem of emergence of pandemics over the next 100 years before we can resolve this matter. We are only dabbling within a very short period of time; this influenza virus has obviously been going through periods of changes for countless years. We are trying to do a very difficult job in a very limited time with a very variable virus.

We are dealing with a number of strands of information which circumstantially point a direction; there is the duck from which viruses can be isolated all the year round and there is no doubt that these isolations peak in summer. It is also in the summer months when the influenza pandemics appear to emerge. The duck-raising practices are different in the North. I think we are dealing with as far North as Shanghai.

Chu No, in North-east China.

Shortridge That might implicate horses.

Chu The H1N1 was first found there in May, 1977.

Lambert Leaving the animals for a minute and getting back to vaccination policies in man, could I pick up a point that Tyrrell made about the newer methods of mathematical modelling of epidemic behaviour? I think that Anderson, May and others have made quite a significant advance. It is clear, that even now with all the computing, the advance is much more easily applicable to infections like measles, rubella and pertussis than it is to this hugely difficult subject about which we are talking. However, I do not think that one should dismiss it as a future aim, to get this modelling much more precise than it has been so far. I was thinking, for example, of Dr Glezen's work. It would be of great interest to have data like that delivered to Anderson (who is in Imperial College here) and May (in Princeton) to see what they could make of it in relation to vaccine policies. If other, more detailed, pictures of epidemiology emerge in different social settings it may become more possible to devise logical vaccine policies than it has been in the past. After all, there is a huge mass of serological data available which you people round the room have provided down the years, and now there is more and more isolation data. It would be very interesting for those involved in the epidemiology of this to look at it in a way which would be able to provide the mathematical modellists with data that they could actually bring to bear.

To go back to what Tyrrell said, their contribution to the measles/rubella business, and perhaps for pertussis, has actually made a significant difference to the way we think of vaccine policies.

Tyrrell Can I just follow that up? I am glad you picked up that point. I did, in the written version, try to make it a little wider and point out that it would be valuable, if possible, to make some predictions of epidemics. That still escapes us in spite of all the serological data and monitoring which you talk about. We really cannot say whether an epidemic will happen or not, but some of the things that have come up recently are quite surprisingly simple. Dr L. Smith has published a paper in a French epidemiological journal (Smith, 1982) suggesting that by carefully monitoring the frequence of acute respiratory disease in general you can detect rises which will indicate that an influenza epidemic will come under way. It suggests that the incidence of these diseases indicates that the environment—whatever that means—is right for the influenza virus to get going. I would be ready to laugh, I think, in a way, except that he seems to have in a very empirical way, shown that it works, using the data from Colindale and the fact that at an earlier stage by equally simple methods he developed a technique for predicting crop diseases in South-east England which is based on simple examination of weather records and which is now apparently a great commercial success with the Meteorological Office because it is so economically valuable to farmers.

Some of these predictions may yet come into the field of human medicine, I hope so.

Kilbourne I just wanted to get on the record the fact that models have been looked at by Fox and Lisa Elvebach and they have proved rather interesting, but I do not know how successful they have been.

Tyrrell I think the general view would be that these were very worthwhile explorations of the subject. Elvebach's models have been taken up and applied with modern computing technology by Longini, but some of the techniques which Anderson and May are using can go even further, and we should take them further and not sit down and assume that we have done all we can with this approach.

J. W. G. Smith Of course, the Russians have used this approach quite a lot, have they not, and they claim to be able to successfully forecast the spread of epidemics between cities.

Tyrrell Their model depends, though, on having all the initial data from the beginning of the epidemic in the first city. Then what they are saying is that they can now predict how the epidemic will proceed from one city to another. But that has a number of very special features, including the structure of Russian society, which almost certainly would not apply if you did it in Europe, the Far East, or almost anywhere else.

J. W. G. Smith I remember Rvachev, the mathematician who did it, saying "We can do it in Russia, but Europe is one big city".

I wonder if we ought to think of drawing the discussion to a close now. Are there any final points anybody is burning to make?

Chu I have one practical question. Has it been demonstrated that the present vaccine will save the lives of aged people as practised in the United States? Is there any evidence that it does? Has it been demonstrated that any of the antivirals administered to 'flu patients of this high risk group will be effective in therapy?

Dowdle The first question was whether or not the vaccine has saved any lives. Is that correct?

Chu Yes.

Dowdle Of course, we have talked about this for a number of years. You cannot design an experiment where death is the end point, but I think there are some indirect bits of evidence which indicate the vaccine can save lives. Some of this evidence was described by Dr Kendal this morning. Monitoring nursing homes and institutions where there are large concentrations of people in the high-risk groups, it would appear that indeed there seems to be evidence of a sparing of mortality.

Tyrrell I think there is a misunderstanding there. Dr Chu is talking about aged people, and these are people in nursing homes for the aged. Alan

Kendal is saying that they are protected, and this is important new evidence which has not been available before.

Kendal I think it was just a communication problem there. There was a study in ambulatory aged people by Barker and Mullooly (1980, 1982) looking at data from the Kaiser Permanente Plan which also showed a reduction in mortality in aged persons, but these were ambulatory as opposed to living in institutions for the aged.

J. W. G. Smith I think we ought to draw the discussion to a close. Perhaps I could make one point that you will be interested in. We have had the data from the microphones fed into the computer here and it has come out with a very firm forecast that I think we can underline, and that is there are obviously going to be jobs for us all still in 50 year's time, unless, it says, we are taken off by influenza!

REFERENCES

Barker, W. H. and Mullooly, J. P. (1980). Impact of influenza A in a defined adult population. *Amer. J. of Epidem.* **112**, 798–811.

Barker, W. H. and Mullooly, J. P. (1982). Pneumonia and influenza deaths during epidemics. Implications for prevention. *Arch. Int. Med.* **142**, 85–89.

Hoskins, T. W., Davies, J. R., Smith, A. J., Miller, C. L. and Allchin, A. (1979). Assessment of inactivated influenza-A vaccines after three outbreaks of influenza A at Christ's Hospital. *Lancet* **i**, 33–85.

Smith, L. P. (1982). Numerical forecasting of epidemics of influenza in Great Britain and Northern Ireland. *Rev. epid. et Sante publique.* **30**, 413–422.

Index

Actinomycin-D 109
α-Amanitin 109
Amantadine 270, 273, 293, 294
Animal Influenzas 13, 55, 58
Antibody
    anti-HA 132–134, 146
    anti-IgA (secretory) 134–139, 147, 149
    anti-IgG 135–139, 147, 149, 151
    anti-NA 131, 132
    cross-reactive 73, 133
    duration 133
    transport 151
    maternal 36
Antigenic drift 9, 11, 18–22, 270, 271
Antigenic shift 8, 78, 270, 271
Aspirin 37
Avian-human reassortants 47, 214–217, 219, 227, 228
Avian influenza viruses
    genetics 46, 47, 52, 53
    host species 40
    pathogenicity 196
    reassortants 47–49, 57
    tissue tropism 47, 50, 53
Avidity 98

Breast-feeding 38

Capping RNA 102, 103, 113–115
Carboxypeptidase 198, 205–207
Cardiac failure 272
Cleavage haemagglutinin 93, 197–200, 204, 205, 207, 208
Cold-adapted mutants 219–224, 227–9, 234, 235, 243, 244

Death-rate (children) 32, 33

Deletion mutants 244–250, 252, 253, 255
Duck viruses 39, 54, 55

Endogenous pyrogen 179, 180
Epidemiology 17, 23–30, 35, 117, 118, 151, 152, 297, 298, 299
Equine virus 8, 40
Eradication of influenza 277, 278

Ferrets, pathogenicity 175–188
    distemper 1
    fever 178–180
    lower respiratory tract 180–183
    neonatal 184, 185
    upper respiratory tract 176, 177
Fusion capacity 196, 206

Genes, avian 233
    frequency, mutation 239
    reassortant 39, 234, 238
    recycling 265
    variation 264, 265
Glycosylation 69–71, 75, 77, 95
Gull virus 14, 15

Haemagglutinin 61–69
    antigenic sites 66, 67
    cross-reaction 14, 72, 73
    membrane fusion 65, 196, 197
    number 14, 296
    polypeptides 61, 64
    sequences 66
H1N1 9, 18, 20, 21, 42, 44, 45, 46, 70, 124, 129, 148
H2N2 39
H3N2 9, 18, 20, 21, 65, 66, 67, 71, 120–124
Herald-wave 22

Host cell selection 281, 282, 283
  influenza A 166, 170
  influenza B 164–169

Immunity
  cell-mediated 127, 154
  cross-reactive 125, 156, 159
  delayed hypersensitivity 129, 154
  duration 120, 121, 124, 147–149, 283
  maternal 36
  natural 124, 125, 145
  passive, newborn 36, 38, 150
  specificity, heterotypic 121–124
  specificity, homotypic 120, 121, 124
  T-cell immune cytotoxic 127–129, 154–159, 172, 173
Immunization
  active 274–276, 282–293, 300
  memory 129, 146, 155, 157, 158
  molecular 291, 292
  passive 139
Influenza A
  antigen 73, 74
  clinical 6, 270, 271
  historical 6, 7
  pandemic 7, 8, 9, 39, 271
  prediction 11, 12, 277
  WHO programme 12
Influenza B 9, 11, 73, 74, 239, 270
  MB protein 115, 263
Influenza C 34, 54, 55, 73, 74
Interferon 130, 131, 177

Latency 3, 115–118

Macrophages, alveolar 130, 189, 190
Models 35, 277, 299, 300
Monoclonal sera 48, 52, 70–72, 80–83, 86, 87, 96, 97, 164–166
Mortality
  children 32–34
  excess 6, 34
  reduced 272, 273
  relation to age 30
Mutation rate 146, 239, 296

Natural killer cells 130, 131
Neuraminidase 77–91
  antigenic drift sequence 79–83
  antigenic shift sequence 78, 79
  calcium 91, 92
  catalysis 84, 85
  immunodiffusion 86
  number 14
  pronase, action of 78, 80, 89
  trinitrobenzene sulphonic acid
    activation of 86, 87
  structure 77, 78, 84, 85
  succinic anhydride
    action of 86, 87
Neutralization 92, 93, 95, 97, 98

Pandemics 39, 40
Pathogenicity,
  ferret 175–188
  fever 179–180
  lower respiratory tract 180–184
  neonatal 184, 185, 192
  upper respiratory tract 176–178
Pneumonia, staphylococcal 193, 194, 272
PR8 70, 73, 104, 105, 176–186, 189–191, 213, 214

Rescue, of virus 249, 250, 255
Reversion rate (mutants) 226, 240, 244
Reye syndrome 36, 37, 270, 273
Rhodopsin 75
Ribavirin (aerosol) 270, 273, 294
Rimantadine 273, 294
RNA-RNA hybridization 40, 44, 53, 242
RNA segments
  membrane (M) 105, 107
  non-glycosylated 101–108
  non-structural (NS) 107, 108
  nucleoprotein (NP) 104, 105
  phosphorylation 105
  polymerases (PB1, PB2, PA) 102–104

Seal virus 40, 41, 42
  H4N5 41
  H7N7 40, 41
  human 40
  monkeys 41
  mortality 40
Shedding, of virus 217–220, 222, 223, 229, 255
Sodium salicylate 38, 179
Sudden infant deaths 34

Swine virus (H1N1) 2, 40, 42–46, 54, 55, 70
   mutants 56, 57

Temperature-sensitivity
   acquired 239–240
   natural 230
   polygenic 238
Transmission, of virus 229, 230
Turkey virus (from pigs) 42–44, 56

Vaccine
   cloned with vaccinia 253
   inactivated 274
   live, attenuated 274, 275
   peptide sequences 275
   strategy 276
Virus virulence,
   attenuated 212–244, 228, 238, 239
   enhanced 226, 230–232
   reassortant 213–216
   restricted host-range 241–244

DATE DUE

DEMCO 38-297